Hepatology

Guest Editors

P. JANE ARMSTRONG, DVM, MS, MBA
JAN ROTHUIZEN, DVM, PhD

VETERINARY CLINICS OF NORTH AMERICA: SMALL ANIMAL PRACTICE

www.vetsmall.theclinics.com

May 2009 • Volume 39 • Number 3

SAUNDERS an imprint of ELSEVIER, Inc.

W.B. SAUNDERS COMPANY
A Division of Elsevier Inc.

1600 John F. Kennedy Blvd. • Suite 1800 • Philadelphia, PA 19103-2899

http://www.vetsmall.theclinics.com

**VETERINARY CLINICS OF NORTH AMERICA: SMALL ANIMAL PRACTICE Volume 39, Number 3
May 2009 ISSN 0195-5616, ISBN-13: 978-1-4377-0562-1, ISBN-10: 1-4377-0562-6**

Editor: John Vassallo; j.vassallo@elsevier.com
Developmental Editor: Donald Mumford

Veterinary Clinics of North America: Small Animal Practice (ISSN 0195-5616) is published bimonthly (For Post Office use only: volume 39 issue 3 of 6) by Elsevier Inc., 360 Park Avenue South, New York, NY 10010-1710. Months of issue are January, March, May, July, September, and November. Business and Editorial Offices: 1600 John F. Kennedy Blvd., Suite 1800, Philadelphia, PA 19103-2899. Customer Service Office: 11830 Westline Industrial Drive, St. Louis, MO 63146. Periodicals postage paid at New York, NY and additional mailing offices. Subscription prices are $229.00 per year (domestic individuals), $366.00 per year (domestic institutions), $114.00 per year (domestic students/residents), $303.00 per year (Canadian individuals), $450.00 per year (Canadian institutions), $336.00 per year (international individuals), $450.00 per year (international institutions), and $165.00 per year (international and Canadian students/residents). To receive student/resident rate, orders must be accompanied by name of affiliated institution, date of term, and the *signature* of program/residency coordinator on institution letterhead. Orders will be billed at individual rate until proof of status is received. Foreign air speed delivery is included in all *Clinics* subscription prices. All prices are subject to change without notice. **POSTMASTER:** Send address changes to *Veterinary Clinics of North America: Small Animal Practice*, 11830 Westline Industrial Drive, St. Louis, MO 63146. Customer Service (orders, claims, online, change of address): Elsevier Periodicals Customer Service, 11830 Westline Industrial Drive, St. Louis, MO 63146. Tel: 1-800-654-2452 (U.S. and Canada). Fax: 314-523-5170. E-mail: journalscustomerservice-usa@elsevier.com (for print support); journalsonlinesupport-usa@elsevier.com (for online support).

Reprints. For copies of 100 or more of articles in this publication, please contact the Commercial Reprints Department, Elsevier Inc., 360 Park Avenue South, New York, NY 10010-1710. Tel.: 212-633-3812; Fax: 212-462-1935; E-mail: reprints@elsevier.com.

Veterinary Clinics of North America: Small Animal Practice is also published in Japanese by Inter Zoo Publishing Co., Ltd., Aoyama Crystal-Bldg 5F, 3-5-12 Kitaaoyama, Minato-ku, Tokyo 107-0061, Japan.

Veterinary Clinics of North America: Small Animal Practice is covered in *Current Contents/Agriculture, Biology and Environmental Sciences, Science Citation Index, ASCA, MEDLINE/PubMed (Index Medicus), Excerpta Medica, and BIOSIS.*

Printed in the United States of America.

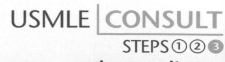

Moving?

Make sure your subscription moves with you!

To notify us of your new address, find your **Clinics Account Number** (located on your mailing label above your name), and contact customer service at:

E-mail: elspcs@elsevier.com

800-654-2452 (subscribers in the U.S. & Canada)
314-453-7041 (subscribers outside of the U.S. & Canada)

Fax number: 314-523-5170

Elsevier Periodicals Customer Service
11830 Westline Industrial Drive
St. Louis, MO 63146

*To ensure uninterrupted delivery of your subscription, please notify us at least 4 weeks in advance of move.

Contributors

GUEST EDITORS

P. JANE ARMSTRONG, DVM, MS, MBA
Diplomate, American College of Veterinary Internal Medicine (Small Animal Internal Medicine); Professor of Internal Medicine, Veterinary Clinical Sciences Department, College of Veterinary Medicine, University of Minnesota, St. Paul, Minnesota

JAN ROTHUIZEN, DVM, PhD
Diplomate, European College of Veterinary Internal Medicine; Professor of Internal Medicine, Department of Clinical Sciences of Companion Animals, Utrecht University, Utrecht, The Netherlands

AUTHORS

P. JANE ARMSTRONG, DVM, MS, MBA
Diplomate, American College of Veterinary Internal Medicine (Small Animal Internal Medicine); Professor of Internal Medicine, Veterinary Clinical Sciences Department, College of Veterinary Medicine, University of Minnesota, St. Paul, Minnesota

CHERYL BALKMAN, DVM
Diplomate, American College of Veterinary Internal Medicine; Lecturer, Department of Clinical Sciences, College of Veterinary Medicine, Clinical Programs Center, Cornell University, Ithaca, New York

ALLYSON C. BERENT, DVM
Diplomate, American College of Veterinary Internal Medicine; Adjunct Assistant Professor of Internal Medicine and Interventional Radiology, Sections of Internal Medicine and Surgery, Veterinary Hospital of the University of Pennsylvania, Philadelphia, Pennsylvania

GERALDINE BLANCHARD, DVM, PhD
Animal Nutrition Expertise SARL, Antony, France

SHARON A. CENTER, DVM
Diplomate, American College of Veterinary Internal Medicine; Professor, Department of Clinical Sciences, Cornell University, College of Veterinary Medicine, Ithaca, New York

JOHANNA COOPER, DVM
Diplomate, American College of Veterinary Internal Medicine; Small Animal Medicine Internist, Tufts VETS, Walpole, Massachusetts

JOHN M. CULLEN, VMD, PhD
Professor, Department of Population Health and Pathobiology, College of Veterinary Medicine, North Carolina State University, Raleigh, North Carolina

ROBERT P. FAVIER, DVM
Department of Clinical Sciences of Companion Animals, Faculty of Veterinary Medicine, Utrecht, The Netherlands

LORRIE GASCHEN, PhD, DVM
Diplomate, European College of Veterinary Diagnostic Imaging; Associate Professor, Section of Diagnostic Imaging, Department of Veterinary Clinical Sciences, Louisiana State University, School of Veterinary Medicine, Baton Rouge, Louisiana

GABY HOFFMANN, Dr med vet, PhD
Diplomate, American College of Veterinary Internal Medicine; Diplomate, European College of Veterinary Internal Medicine-Companion Animals; Royal Dutch Association of Veterinarians Recognized Specialist in Internal Medicine, and Section Chief of Small Animal Gastroenterology, and Senior Lecturer in Internal Medicine, Department of Clinical Sciences of Companion Animals, Utrecht University, Faculty of Veterinary Medicine, Utrecht, The Netherlands

JAN ROTHUIZEN, DVM, PhD
Diplomate, European College of Veterinary Internal Medicine; Professor of Internal Medicine, Department of Clinical Sciences of Companion Animals, Utrecht University, Utrecht, The Netherlands

KAREN M. TOBIAS, DVM, MS
Diplomate, American College of Veterinary Surgeons; Professor of Small Animal Surgery, Department of Small Animal Clinical Sciences, University of Tennessee, Knoxville, Tennessee

DAVID C. TWEDT, DVM, PhD
Diplomate, American College of Veterinary Internal Medicine; Professor of Internal Medicine, Department of Clinical Sciences, College of Veterinary Medicine and Biomedical Sciences, Colorado State University, Fort Collins, Colorado

CYNTHIA R.L. WEBSTER, DVM
Diplomate, American College of Veterinary Internal Medicine; Professor, Department of Clinical Sciences, Tufts Cummings School of Veterinary Medicine, North Grafton, Massachusetts

CHICK WEISSE, VMD
Diplomate, American College of Veterinary Surgeons; Assistant Professor of Surgery, and Director of Interventional Radiology Services, Veterinary Hospital of the University of Pennsylvania, Philadelphia, Pennsylvania

Contents

> Liver disease is a frequently encountered problem in small animal practice. The World Small Animal Veterinary Association has formed a group of experienced clinicians and pathologists to develop a standardized format for diagnostic terminology. This is hoped to lead to greater uniformity in diagnoses and better communication between clinicians and pathologists alike. The aim is to find a sound scientific basis of diagnostic and treatment protocols for hepatobiliary diseases. This article provides an overview of that monograph.

> Several clinical syndromes can develop in many different liver diseases. They are important to understanding the clinical manifestations of hepatobiliary diseases. The signs, diagnostic procedures, and specific diseases associated with these syndromes are discussed.

> Radiography and ultrasonography are the most well-established and frequently used imaging modalities for diagnosing hepatic disease in veterinary medicine. Contrast-enhanced harmonic ultrasound imaging of the liver is being established in veterinary medicine for the assessment of liver perfusion, hemodynamic alterations in the presence of portosystemic shunts (PSSs), and differentiation of benign from malignant hepatic nodules. New techniques in nuclear medicine include splenic portal scintigraphy and hepatic function tests. CT is now being used to diagnosis PSSs noninvasively. The roles of CT and MR imaging in the diagnosis of hepatic disease are currently being validated. Although less broadly available than

ultrasound, advanced imaging is becoming more accessible, not only through academic institutions, but through the increasing number of specialty practices worldwide.

A liver biopsy is required to make the diagnosis of most non-vascular liver diseases. Liver biopsy samples can be obtained with several techniques. With proper training and adequate operator experience, the liver biopsy is a safe technique. It is important to evaluate blood coagulation and to use the biopsy in the context of evaluation of the liver and associated structures with ultrasonography, laparoscopy, or other imaging methods. The histological evaluation should be done using international standards as summarized by John Cullen elsewhere in this issue.

Poor understanding of the causes of primary hepatitis, especially idiopathic chronic hepatitis, results in limited options for adequate treatment and variable results. Elucidating the causes, aside from the copper-associated form of hepatitis, is of utmost importance to find etiology-based treatments for canine (chronic) hepatitis, when possible, most likely resulting in a better prognosis.

The liver is essential for copper metabolism. Copper metabolism is highly conserved between different species. This article provides the reader with an overview of copper storage disorders in humans and animals. Diagnosis and treatment of copper-associated hepatitis are described, and breed-specific characteristics of the disease are explained. A literature review references publications about the disease in companion animals.

Portovascular anomalies are most commonly seen as congenital communications in dogs and cats. Fixation, whether surgical or interventional, should be considered in all cases for which it is possible to improve perfusion to the liver, and ultimately liver function. Medical management before fixation is always recommended. If surgery is not recommended or not possible, long-term medical management can be successful in approximately 30% of cases. New modalities, such as percutaneous transjugular coil embolization or glue embolization, facilitate treatment of more complicated conditions, such as intrahepatic portosystemic shunts and hepatic arteriovenous malformations.

Most disorders of the biliary system are associated with increased activity of parenchymal transaminases (alanine aminotransferase, aspartate aminotransferase) and cholestatic enzymes (alkaline phosphatase and gamma glutamyl transferase) with or without hyperbilirubinemia or jaundice. While parenchymal liver disease is most common in the dog, inflammatory disorders involving the small- and medium-sized bile ducts and zone 1 (periportal) hepatocytes predominate in the cat. Historically, the incidence of disorders restricted to the gallbladder is low in both species; however, with routine diagnostic use of abdominal ultrasonography, the incidence of gallbladder mucoceles and cholelithiasis has increased. Extrahepatic bile duct obstruction is a well-recognized syndrome because of its association with pancreatitis and obvious jaundice. Less common disorders of the biliary system include a cadre of diverse conditions, including necroinflammatory processes, cholelithiasis, malformations, neoplasia, and an emerging syndrome of gallblader dysmotility.

Hepatic lipidosis (fatty liver syndrome) is the most common form of liver disease in cats. Especially in obese cats, it occurs subsequent to a period of anorexia because of an underlying disease or stressors such as a change in food or lifestyle. Jaundice, increased liver enzymes, and hyperechogenicity of the liver in a cat with recent, rapid weight loss are typical findings. Diagnosis is confirmed by fine needle aspiration cytology and/or liver biopsy. Absent irreversible underlying disease, the prognosis for complete recovery is good provided that nutritional support is instituted early.

Hepatobiliary tumors are uncommon in dogs and cats. They generally occur in older animals with nonspecific clinical signs, usually relating to the gastrointestinal tract. Liver enzyme concentrations are commonly elevated. Early detection for massive-type lesions may allow for surgical resection and prolonged survival especially for hepatocellular carcinomas. Chemotherapy, in general, is not effective for primary liver tumors.

> Nonresectable and metastatic liver tumors are difficult challenges in veterinary patients. As such, these animals traditionally have been treated conservatively and symptomatically. The relatively limited efficacy of routine (intravenous) chemotherapy for macroscopic disease and the cost and potential deleterious side effects associated with radiation therapy have led investigators to evaluate increasingly novel therapeutic modalities. Interventional radiology techniques offer the potential for improved tumor response rates, prolonged survival times, and enhanced quality of life in patients with minimal systemic toxicity risks.

> Many medicinal, nutraceutical, and botanic extracts have been used as cytoprotective agents in liver disease. This article explains the mechanisms of action, pertinent pharmacokinetics, side effects, and clinical indications for the use of S-adenosylmethionine, N-acetylcysteine, ursodeoxycholic acid, silymarin, and vitamin E. The literature pertaining to in vitro studies, laboratory animal models, and human and veterinary clinical trials is reviewed with regards to the efficacy and use of these cytoprotective agents in hepatobiliary disease.

RELATED INTEREST
Veterinary Clinics of North America: Exotic Animal Practice May 2005 (Vol. 8, No. 2)
Gastroenterology
Tracey K. Ritzman, DVM, Dipl. ABVP—Avian, *Guest Editor*

THE CLINICS ARE NOW AVAILABLE ONLINE!
Access your subscription at:
www.theclinics.com

Preface

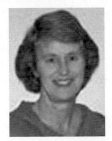 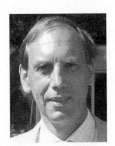

P. Jane Armstrong, DVM, MS, MBA   Jan Rothuizen, DVM, PhD
Guest Editors

Two previous issues of the *Veterinary Clinics of North America: Small Animal Practice* were devoted to liver disease in companion animals. The 1985 issue, guest edited by Dave Twedt, included comprehensive descriptions of a variety of clinical syndromes. The 1995 issue, guest edited by Donna Dimski, reflected progress in imaging techniques and our understanding of the pathophysiology of some liver disorders. In the intervening 14 years, great progress has been made in standardizing terminology relating to liver pathology and setting the stage for prospective treatment studies. This interval has also seen the identification of the genetic basis for some hepathopathies, notably copper storage disorders in the Bedlington terrier and Labrador retriever breeds. Advanced imaging has further advanced our diagnostic capabilities. In this issue, we aim to highlight new and emerging themes in hepatology. We seek to underpin the entire issue with standardized terminology developed by the World Small Animal Veterinary Association Liver Standardization group. We hope that the next 10 years will see the publication of prospective controlled treatment trials, allowing therapeutic decisions to be based on the principles of grade 1 evidence-based medicine.

The talented contributors to this issue were selected to present the most current work occurring on both sides of the Atlantic. We are indebted to them for agreeing to share their expertise even when their professional "plates" were already very full. We also thank John Vassallo at Elsevier for his encouragement and patience in the development and publication of this issue. We hope that the information presented here will prove valuable to internists, general practitioners, and students seeking a deeper understanding of topical areas in companion animal hepatology. We look forward to a time when the talents of veterinary students, graduate students, and residents join those already in the field and contribute to future advances and discoveries in companion animal hepatology.

P. Jane Armstrong, DVM, MS, MBA
Veterinary Clinical Sciences Department
College of Veterinary Medicine
University of Minnesota
1352 Boyd Avenue
St. Paul, MN 55108, USA

Vet Clin Small Anim 39 (2009) xi–xii
doi:10.1016/j.cvsm.2009.03.002
vetsmall.theclinics.com

Jan Rothuizen, DVM, PhD
Department of Clinical Sciences of Companion Animals
Utrecht University
Yalelaan 108, PO Box 80.154
3508 TD Utrecht, The Netherlands

E-mail addresses:
armst002@umn.edu (P.J. Armstrong)
j.rothuizen@uu.nl (J. Rothuizen)

Erratum
Making Sense of Blood Gas Results

Shane W. Bateman, DVM, DVSc

In the May 2008 issue (volume 38, number 3), there were two errors. On page 547, in the second column of **Table 3**, last row, it should read "Primary non-respiratory acidosis" and not "Primary non-respiratory alkalosis." The corrected table is printed below.

Table 3
Primary (with compensation) and mixed acid-base disturbance patterns

	Primary Non-Respiratory Alkalosis ± Compensation	Primary Respiratory Alkalosis ± Compensation	Not Possible	Mixed Alkalosis	If pH > 7.4 Use This Row ⇐
CO_2 ⇑		⇓	⇑	⇓	
HCO_3 ⇑		⇓	⇓	⇑	
	Primary respiratory acidosis ± compensation	Primary non-respiratory acidosis ± compensation	Mixed acidosis	Not possible	If pH < 7.4 use this row ⇐

Abbreviations: CO_2, partial pressure of carbon dioxide; HCO_3, bicarbonate

On page 554, the first full word on the last line should be "hyperkalemia" and not "hypokalemia."

Department of Veterinary Clinical Sciences, The Ohio State University, 601 Vernon L. Tharp Street, Columbus, OH 43210-1089, USA

Vet Clin Small Anim 39 (2009) xiii
doi:10.1016/j.cvsm.2009.03.001
0195-5616/09/$ – see front matter

Summary of the World Small Animal Veterinary Association Standardization Committee Guide to Classification of Liver Disease in Dogs and Cats

John M. Cullen, VMD, PhD

KEYWORDS
- Pathology • Histopathology • Liver • Classification • Dog
- Cat

Liver disease is a frequently encountered problem in small animal practice. The diagnostic terminology to describe liver diseases used by pathologists from various countries and even different training programs is often inconsistent, leading to confusion for clinicians interpreting pathology reports and those who would like to compare the pathology results from separate studies. Because of these issues, the World Small Animal Veterinary Association (WSAVA) has formed a group of experienced clinicians and pathologists to develop a standardized format for diagnostic terminology that, it is hoped, leads to greater uniformity in diagnoses and better communication between clinicians and pathologists alike. Standardized criteria and nomenclature are also mandatory for setting up multicenter clinical trials. Based on the developed system, several international studies are now getting started. The aim is to find a sound scientific basis of diagnostic and treatment protocols for hepatobiliary diseases. An overview of that monograph[1] follows.

MORPHOLOGIC CLASSIFICATION OF CIRCULATORY DISORDERS OF THE LIVER

There are several congenital disorders of the vascular supply to the liver recognized in dogs and cats. The liver responds to insufficient portal blood flow in a relatively

Department of Population Health and Pathobiology, College of Veterinary Medicine, North Carolina State University, 4700 Hillsborough Street, Raleigh, NC 27606, USA
E-mail address: john_cullen@ncsu.edu

Vet Clin Small Anim 39 (2009) 395–418
doi:10.1016/j.cvsm.2009.02.003
0195-5616/09/$ – see front matter © 2009 Elsevier Inc. All rights reserved.
vetsmall.theclinics.com

stereotypic fashion regardless of the impediment to normal perfusion. Consequently, there is considerable overlap in the histologic appearance of these disorders. Typical features include absent or diminished portal vein profiles in the portal tracts; an increase in arteriolar profiles in the portal tracts and periportal sinusoidal dilation may also occur, presumably attributable to the local increased blood pressure that accompanies the arteriolar blood flow into the sinusoids (**Fig. 1**). Bile duct proliferation may be evident as well. Hepatocytic atrophy is also common. Nonuniform distribution of portal flow most likely leads to irregular residual lobular architecture and the presence of abundant lipogranulomas formed from areas of hepatocyte loss, although other explanations are possible.

Abnormal venous anastomoses are often difficult to identify post mortem without benefit of antemortem imaging studies. Clinical data, such as the presence or absence of shunt vessels and the determination of portal vein pressure, are essential to achieve a final diagnosis.

Congenital Portosystemic Shunts

Congenital portosystemic shunts occur in the dog and cat. Congenital portosystemic shunts are single (almost always) large-caliber connections between the portal vein and systemic veins. A congenital shunt can be intrahepatic or extrahepatic in location. Intrahepatic congenital shunts, often attributable to a patent ductus venosus, occur most often in large-breed dogs. Extrahepatic congenital shunts, which occur in small-breed dogs more often than the intrahepatic shunts, may connect the portal vein to any of several veins, including the splenic, azygous, or renal vein, or to the caudal vena cava.

The typical histologic appearance is characterized by loss or diminution of portal veins; arteriolar proliferation; hepatocytic atrophy, often with abnormal lobule formation; and the presence of lipogranulomas. Dogs with congenital portosystemic shunts do not develop portal hypertension, because any increased portal pressure would lead to increased flow into the systemic venous system, restoring normal blood pressure.

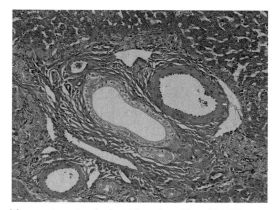

Fig.1. Portal tract with a portosystemic shunt in a dog. The alterations are similar in a variety of disorders leading to portal vein hypoperfusion of the liver. These changes include an absent or dramatically reduced portal vein profile, prominent hepatic artery branches, arteriolar proliferation, and atrophy of hepatocytes.

Disorders Associated with Portal Hypertension

Portal vein obstruction

Flow through the portal vein can be obstructed through thrombosis or invasive neoplasms or through compression from local inflammatory processes, such as pancreatitis or peritonitis. Infection with schistosomal parasites can also produce disturbed portal vein blood flow. Because the disorder is typically acquired rather than congenital, the liver is characterized histologically by diminution of the portal vein profiles depending on the proportion of the flow that is interrupted, but without prominent arteriolar changes.

Primary hypoplasia of the portal vein (microvascular dysplasia and noncirrhotic portal hypertension)

There has been considerable confusion surrounding this disorder because of the various terms used to describe it, including *microvascular dysplasia* and *noncirrhotic portal hypertension*. The preferred term proposed by the WSAVA Liver Study Group is *portal vein hypoplasia*. Portal vein hypoplasia is a congenital vascular anomaly that occurs in dogs, and occasionally in cats, in which the intrahepatic vein and, in some circumstances, the extrahepatic portal vein are abnormally small or absent. The abnormally small or absent extrahepatic vein or intrahepatic portal vein results in diminished hepatic perfusion. There is potential for portal hypertension, along with ascites and the formation of acquired shunt vessels because of the restricted intrahepatic portal blood flow. These alterations can be present early in the course of the disease or may develop over time or not at all. Affected animals have small livers and the typical histologic pattern of portal vein hypoperfusion. It is important to remember that this condition differs from portosystemic shunts, because there is no abnormal connection between the portal vein and systemic venous system.

There are histologic variants of this disorder that are characterized by increased, possibly abnormal, connective tissue within the portal tracts that may bridge between portal tracts in some cases. This variant has previously been called noncirrhotic portal hypertension or, when the portal tract connective tissue is particularly abundant, hepatoportal sclerosis.

Intrahepatic arteriovenous fistulas

Intrahepatic arteriovenous fistulas, acquired or congenital, occur in the dog and cat. These shunts arise from a direct communication between a branch of the hepatic artery and branches of the portal vein. They may occur anywhere within the liver and can be single or multiple. A distended throbbing fistula can often be appreciated at surgery. Affected areas of the liver contain a convoluted hepatic artery branch and an aneurysmal portal vein branch with abnormal thickened walls. The liver adjacent to the fistula has the typical appearance of portal hypoperfusion. Shunting of blood may lead to portal hypertension or reversal of the direction of portal blood flow, subsequent development of acquired portocaval shunts, and ascites. Most of these lesions are diagnosed before biopsy.

Incidental Vascular Disorders

Peliosis hepatis

Peliosis hepatis is defined as a random distribution of dilated vascular spaces in the hepatic parenchyma. Grossly, these areas appear as variably sized dark blue foci within the liver that vary from pinpoint to several centimeters in size. It occurs in old cats, and occasionally in dogs, in which it can be mistaken for a vascular tumor, such as hemangioma or hemangiosarcoma.

MORPHOLOGIC CLASSIFICATION OF BILIARY DISORDERS

Acquired and congenital biliary diseases can be divided into four categories:

1. Biliary cystic diseases
2. Cholestasis and cholate stasis
3. Inflammation (cholangitis and cholangiohepatitis)
4. Diseases of the gallbladder

Solitary Biliary Cysts

These lesions are uncommon in cats and dogs. They are single round cysts lined with a flattened single layer of biliary epithelium. They may be acquired or a congenital disorder.

Congenital Biliary Cystic Disease

Congenital biliary cystic diseases are a complex and often confusing collection of conditions that affect dogs and especially cats. They can all be attributed to an abnormality of the development of the primordial biliary ductular system arising from the ductal plate. Congenital cystic disease is characterized by dilation of portions of the biliary tree and associated fibrosis. Lesions may affect only the large extrahepatic bile ducts in a pattern resembling Caroli's disease in human beings or may affect only the small-caliber ducts, with formation of fibrotic portal tracts and abnormal, often dilated, irregular profiles of biliary epithelial-lined ducts that can lead to extensive lesions with bridging fibrosis and associated abnormal bile ducts, diagnosed as congenital hepatic fibrosis (**Fig. 2**). A third pattern is characterized by multiple unilocular or multilocular biliary cysts that range from a few millimeters to several centimeters in diameter and contain clear fluid (**Fig. 3**). In animals affected with this form of so-called "Von Myenburg complexes," discrete fibrous areas with small, often irregular, bile duct profiles are also frequently found. These lesions are often confused with benign tumors of the bile duct epithelium. Dilated renal tubules can also occur in some circumstances as well. The pattern of lesions and inheritance in domestic animals is not as clearly separated in domestic animals as it is in human beings. Persian cats are more frequently affected than other feline breeds.

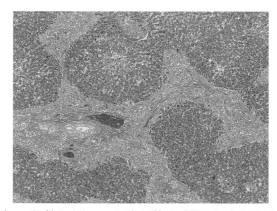

Fig. 2. Congenital hepatic fibrosis in a cat. The affected liver is characterized by thick bands of connective tissue that bridge between portal tracts and contain proliferated small bile ducts.

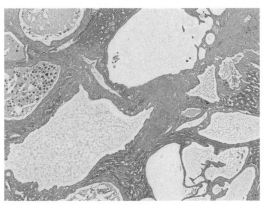

Fig. 3. Biliary cystic disease in a cat. Multiple biliary cysts, lined by a single layer of cuboidal to flattened biliary epithelium, are present within the hepatic parenchyma. Occasional hepatocytes are entrapped between the cysts.

Cholestasis

Cholestasis is an accumulation of substances normally secreted in the bile (eg, bilirubin, bile acids) in the blood. Cholestasis can be categorized as follows:

Intrahepatic cholestasis (attributable to decreased or blocked bile flow in the canaliculi) occurs in association with a wide spectrum of conditions affecting hepatocytes (drug toxicity, lipidosis, necrosis, hepatitis, and others) or, in some circumstances, dramatically increased bile production associated with hemolysis.

Extrahepatic cholestasis (attributable to blockage of extrahepatic bile ducts) results from luminal obstruction by bile calculi (gall stones), inspissated bile (often associated with gallbladder mucoceles in dogs), or extraluminal compression attributable to neoplasia or inflammation (particularly of the pancreas or duodenum).

Histologically, the most prominent feature of intrahepatic cholestasis is the presence of bile, seen as fine linear deposits between hepatocytes. These deposits are called canalicular bile plugs, and they are most abundant in the centrilobular region. Bile may also be found within Kupffer cells. Retention of bile salts is damaging to cell membranes, and swollen and pigmented hepatocytes (termed *feathery degeneration*) may also be found in the periportal region. Extrahepatic cholestasis is typically characterized by edema and neutrophils in portal areas and ductal bile plugs. Over time, concentric rings of fibroblasts or myofibroblasts expand, forming an "onion skin" appearance around interlobular bile ducts, proliferation of bile ducts, and, eventually, bridging portal-portal fibrosis (**Fig. 4**).

INFLAMMATION
Cholangitis

Cholangitis, inflammation of the bile ducts, can be differentiated in (1) neutrophilic cholangitis, (2) lymphocytic cholangitis, (3) destructive cholangitis, and (4) chronic cholangitis associated with liver fluke infestation.

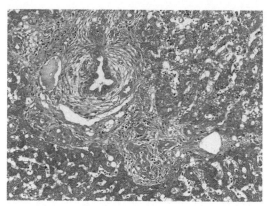

Fig. 4. Chronic biliary obstruction in a dog. Affected bile ducts typically have concentric spindle-shaped cells that may be myofibroblasts. Biliary hyperplasia of small ducts is also present. Moderate numbers of mononuclear inflammatory cells and pigmented macrophages are usually present.

Neutrophilic cholangitis

Neutrophilic cholangitis is more common in cats than in dogs. The pathogenesis is thought to involve ascending bacterial infections, but this is not always demonstrated. Affected bile ducts have neutrophils in their lumen, between the biliary epithelial cells, or in close association with the bile ducts (**Fig. 5**). When the inflammation extends beyond the limiting plate and spills into the hepatic parenchyma, the diagnosis becomes cholangiohepatitis. This can be the result of bile duct rupture and release of the contents of the bile duct, leading to necrosis and abscesses. This term should no longer be used for mild accumulations of inflammatory cells within the portal tracts.

Lymphocytic cholangitis

This condition occurs in cats. It is characterized by dense aggregates of lymphocytes that form a cuff around bile ducts but usually do not penetrate the lumen of affected ducts or invade the biliary epithelium (**Fig. 6**). Biliary hyperplasia is usually also present but can be difficult to appreciate when the inflammation is intense. The primary

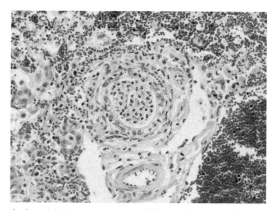

Fig. 5. Neutrophilic cholangitis in a cat. Neutrophils are found within the lumen and invade the biliary epithelium.

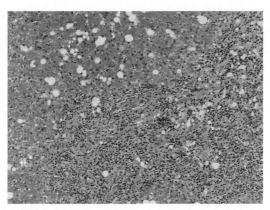

Fig. 6. Lymphocytic cholangitis in a cat. Moderate to intense infiltrates of mature lymphocytes centered on bile ducts and associated biliary hyperplasia are characteristic of lymphocytic cholangitis in cats.

differential diagnosis is hepatic lymphoma. The presence of biliary hyperplasia supports a diagnosis of lymphocytic cholangitis and lymphoid aggregates in such areas as the periphery of the central vein, suggesting lymphoma. Use of special techniques, such as the polymerase chain reaction for antigen receptor rearrangements assay, to assess the presence or absence of monoclonal lymphocyte populations (characteristic of lymphoma) may be needed in difficult cases.

Destructive cholangitis
Destructive cholangitis is uncommon and is the result of biliary epithelial necrosis in smaller branches of the biliary tree. Histologically, portal tracts from affected animals lack a normal-caliber bile duct and contain aggregates of pigmented macrophages and small numbers of inflammatory cells, predominantly neutrophils or eosinophils (**Fig. 7**). Portal fibrosis can also occur. Destructive cholangitis is most likely attributable to an idiosyncratic reaction to some drugs (ie, trimethoprim sulfa). It is not known if ducts can completely recover.

Chronic cholangitis
In chronic cholangitis, the inflammatory cells include lymphocytes and plasma cells, often in association with neutrophils. There are varying amounts of bile duct hyperplasia and fibrosis. Portal-portal bridging fibrosis is present in severe cases. This condition results from persistent inflammation, such as unresolved bacterial infections or, particularly in cats, liver fluke infestation, in which dramatic ductular distention and fibrosis can occur.

Chronic cholangitis associated with liver fluke infestation
Chronic cholangitis associated with liver fluke infestation is regularly observed in cats, and less frequently in dogs, in endemic areas. Infections are caused by members of the family Opisthorchiidae. The lesion is microscopically characterized by dilated larger bile ducts with papillary projections and marked periductal and portal fibrosis (**Fig. 8**). A slight to moderate inflammation may be seen within the ducts (neutrophils and macrophages) and in the portal areas (neutrophils, lymphocytes, and plasma cells). Eosinophils may be present. The number of liver flukes and eggs within the dilated bile ducts varies markedly, and it is often difficult to find liver flukes or eggs.

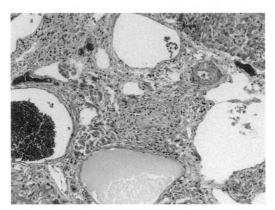

Fig. 7. Destructive cholangitis in a dog. The affected liver is characterized by loss of the normal bile duct profile in the portal tract. In the center of the field, there is a remnant outline of the bile duct with peripheral accumulation of mononuclear inflammatory cells.

GALLBLADDER LESIONS
Cholelithiasis

Cholelithiasis is not common in any domestic species, although bile calculi can occur in dogs and cats. Inspissated bile may cause bile duct obstructions. A histologic pattern typical of extrahepatic obstruction can result.

Cystic Mucosal Hyperplasia

This condition is relatively common in older dogs. The mucosa is thickened, sometimes dramatically, and contains variably sized mucus-containing cysts lined by hyperplastic columnar epithelium.

Gallbladder Mucocele

This is a condition characterized by the presence of a distended gallbladder filled with firm tenacious mucoid material, which may lead to gallbladder rupture (**Fig. 9**). The

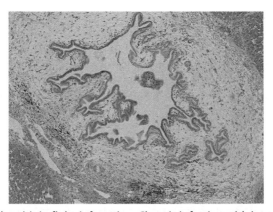

Fig. 8. Chronic cholangitis in fluke infestation. Chronic infection with intrabiliary flukes typically produces prominent ductular distention and an associated dramatic peripheral deposition of connective tissue and mononuclear inflammatory infiltrate. It is uncommon to find flukes in tissue sections, however.

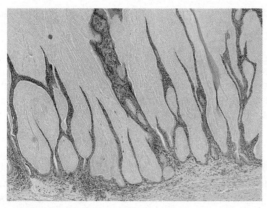

Fig. 9. Gallbladder mucocele in a dog. The affected gallbladder is characterized by distention attributable to an excess of tenacious mucus that fills the lumen of the organ. The gallbladder mucosa is often mildly proliferative with fine fronds of mucosa projecting into the lumen.

mucosa is variably hyperplastic. The viscous mucus may extend into the cystic or common bile duct, causing obstruction.

Gallbladder Infarcts

Gallbladder infarction is characterized histologically by transmural coagulation necrosis of the wall of the gallbladder, with minimal inflammation. The primary lesion seems to be thrombosis of arteries in the wall of the gallbladder without evidence of concurrent cholecystitis. Affected animals may have severe bile peritonitis as a result of rupture of the infarcted gallbladder.

Cholecystitis

Cholecystitis is an inflammation of the gallbladder. It can be acute or chronic and may be associated with inflammation in other areas of the biliary tree. Neutrophilic cholecystitis is frequently seen in cats, and rarely in dogs, and is, in general, associated with bacterial infection. The lesion is characterized by the presence of neutrophils in the lumen, epithelium, or wall of the gallbladder. Neutrophilic cholecystitis can be present as a solitary lesion or in combination with neutrophilic cholangitis.

Lymphoplasmacytic and follicular cholecystitis are characterized by the presence of a lymphoplasmacytic infiltrate or the presence of lymphoid follicles in the mucosa of the gallbladder. The gallbladder lining, like other mucosal surfaces, can normally contain a small number of lymphocytes and occasional lymphoid follicles.

MORPHOLOGIC CLASSIFICATION OF PARENCHYMAL DISORDERS OF THE CANINE AND FELINE LIVER
Introduction to Parenchymal Diseases

Parenchymal disorders of the liver in dogs and cats can be grouped into seven categories: (1) reversible injury (cell swelling, excess glycogen accumulation, and lipidosis); (2) amyloidosis; (3) hepatocellular death, apoptosis, and necrosis; (4) acute and chronic hepatitis; (5) hepatic abscesses and granulomas; (6) hepatic metabolic storage disorders; and (7) miscellaneous conditions.

Lesions involving the hepatocytes are the hallmarks of most of these disorders; however, inflammation, necrosis, fibrosis, and bile duct proliferation are not restricted to parenchymal disorders and may be prominent in primary biliary or circulatory disorders.

Reversible Injury

Hepatocellular swelling

The earliest manifestation of injury is termed *cloudy swelling* and is attributed to loss of cell membrane functionality, leading to an influx of water into the cytoplasm. This change is difficult to appreciate histologically because of its subtlety in most circumstances.

Vacuolar change

Cytoplasmic accumulation of various substances leading to vacuole formation in hepatocytes can occur for a variety of reasons. The finding of vacuolar hepatopathy is consequently a vague and often uninformative diagnosis. In young animals, particularly those with abnormal growth, storage disorders should be considered. In older animals, the vacuoles are almost always lipid or glycogen containing. Identification of the contents can aid in sorting out the pathogenesis; however, in many circumstances, the diagnosis of hepatocellular vacuoles in an animal with altered liver-related biochemistry does not provide much assistance in determining the pathogenesis of the problem. Some disorders associated with vacuole formation are discussed here.

Steroid-induced hepatopathy

This condition occurs in dogs and is characterized by excessive accumulation of cytoplasmic glycogen. Typically, hepatocytes are swollen with clear cytoplasm attributable to glycogen accumulation and contain fine irregular strands of eosinophilic cytoplasm and a central nucleus (**Fig. 10**). The distribution can be diffuse or zonal or may involve individual cells. Periodic acid–Schiff staining with or without diastase may help to identify glycogen accumulation in mild cases, although frozen sections are usually needed to preserve glycogen content. Other hepatic changes associated with glycogen accumulation are marginated neutrophils in sinusoids and occasional foci of extramedullary hematopoiesis. This condition is caused by an excess of endogenous or exogenous corticosteroids. Possible additional causes include an excess of other types of steroid hormones and, occasionally, drugs, such as D-penicillamine.

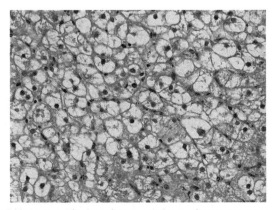

Fig.10. Corticosteroid hepatopathy in a dog. Excessive endogenous or exogenous corticosteroids can produce distended hepatocytes with irregular clear vacuoles and diaphanous strands of cytoplasm. The vacuoles contain glycogen that is removed during fixation and processing.

Hepatocellular steatosis (lipidosis and fatty change)

Hepatocellular steatosis is a nonspecific accumulation of lipid-filled vacuoles in the cytoplasm of hepatocytes, is a reversible form of cellular change, and can be a physiologic change in some circumstances.

Hepatic steatosis has two phenotypic forms. In macrovesicular hepatocellular steatosis, the accumulation of lipids forms vacuoles that are larger than the size of the nucleus and tend to displace the hepatocellular nucleus (**Fig. 11**). These lipid vacuoles most commonly form as a result of dietary excess or starvation or in some forms of feline hepatic lipidosis. A particular form of lipidosis, identified as microvesicular lipidosis (vacuoles smaller than the size of the nucleus), is associated with injury to mitochondria and more severe liver dysfunction than macrovesicular lipidosis (**Fig. 12**). This form occurs in juvenile hypoglycemia of small-breed puppies and in uncontrolled diabetes mellitus, and it may occur after exposure to some toxins. Mixed microvesicular and microvesicular lipidosis is common in the syndrome of feline hepatic lipidosis.

Hepatocellular steatosis should be described by distribution (zonal or diffuse), severity, and size of the cytoplasmic vacuoles (microvesicular, macrovesicular, or mixed).

In routine formalin-fixed paraffin-embedded tissues, lipid vacuoles are empty vacuoles because of the loss of fat in processing. Frozen sections of unfixed or fixed tissue can be stained for fat using special stains, such as oil red O, Sudan IV, or osmium tetroxide, and are helpful in recognizing microvesicular lipidosis and in differentiating fat from other substances that may accumulate in vacuoles.

Amyloidosis

Amyloid in the liver is almost always secondary or reactive (serum amyloid associated) and develops over the course of a chronic inflammatory disorder. Hepatic amyloidosis is commonly associated with inflammatory conditions in other organ systems; however, in breeds with a predisposition to amyloid deposition (Chinese shar-pei dogs and Abyssinian, Siamese, and other oriental cats), inflammation in other organs may be slight or negligible. Amyloid appears as eosinophilic material in the space of Disse and sometimes in the walls of vessels and in portal areas (**Fig. 13**). Deposition may be diffuse, zonal, or multifocal, and there is frequently atrophy of the adjacent hepatocytes and dilation of the sinusoids because of disruption of the blood hepatocyte interface. Special stains (Congo red or Stokes) may be needed to identify or

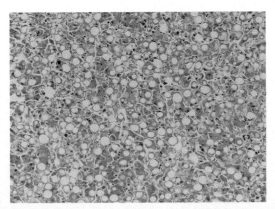

Fig. 11. Macrovesicular steatosis in a dog. Lipid vacuoles are distinct, round, and clear. Typically, these vacuoles displace the nucleus to the edge of the cell.

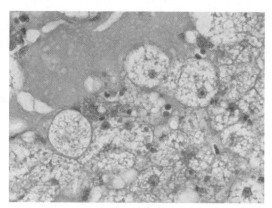

Fig. 12. Microvesicular steatosis in a cat. Microvesicular lipid vacuoles are smaller than the nucleus but retain a clear round outline, and the nucleus remains central in affected cells.

confirm the presence of amyloid. Spontaneous or biopsy-induced liver rupture with hemorrhage and hemoabdomen may occur in amyloid-infiltrated livers.

HEPATOCYTE DEATH (APOPTOSIS AND NECROSIS)

Hepatocytes may be killed by a broad variety of insults, including hypoxia, toxins, infectious agents, immunologic events, and severe metabolic disturbances. Cell death has been considered to occur through apoptosis or necrosis; however, recent evidence suggests overlap between the processes, because moderate exposure to some toxins causes apoptosis, whereas greater exposure may result in necrosis. Apoptosis is an active process of programmed cell death that results in shrinkage of the cell without loss of integrity of the cell membrane and subsequent fragmentation. Necrosis involves cytoplasmic swelling and abnormal cell membrane permeability and may result in coagulative necrosis or liquefactive necrosis. Coagulative necrosis is the result of sudden and catastrophic denaturation of the cytosolic protein and appears as swollen hepatocytes with acidophilic cytoplasm; preservation of the basic outline of the coagulated cell; and pyknosis, karyorrhexis, or karyolysis.

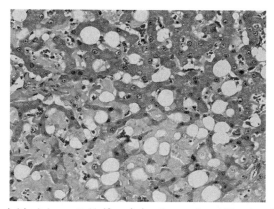

Fig. 13. Hepatic amyloidosis in a cat. Uniformly hyaline eosinophilic material within the sinusoids distends the sinusoids and leads to atrophy of the hepatocytes that remain.

Liquefactive necrosis appears as loss of hepatocytes and is the result of osmotic swelling and disintegration of hepatocytes, with subsequent collapse of the residual reticulin network or replacement by erythrocytes and, eventually, the presence of ceroid-laden macrophages. Necrosis may be followed by proliferation of Kupffer cells and infiltration of phagocytic cells, with subsequent resorption and lysis of the necrotic cells. Necrosis should be characterized by the pattern of injury, including focal, multifocal, confluent, bridging, massive, or piecemeal, because the pattern of necrosis can provide insight into the pathogenesis of the lesion.

Response of the Liver to Hepatocellular Injury

After destruction of hepatic parenchyma, regeneration of parenchyma, fibrosis, and ductular proliferation (bile duct hyperplasia) may occur. When hepatocyte destruction is limited and the reticulin network remains intact, regeneration with almost complete restitution of the liver structure can occur. Severe parenchymal destruction with extensive loss of hepatocytes is often followed by ductular proliferation, termed the *ductular reaction*, which may involve hepatic progenitor cells. With persistent parenchymal damage, fibrosis and postnecrotic scarring may occur, which may result in regenerative parenchymal nodules. In areas of collapse or fibrosis, intrahepatic portovenous vascular shunts may form.

Controversy still exists about the nomenclature of hepatic necrosis and acute inflammation. A morphologic diagnosis should emphasize the primary or most important process (necrosis versus inflammation), with appropriate modifiers indicating chronicity, severity, distribution, presence of inflammatory cells, and evidence of the cause, if known.

Acute Hepatitis

Acute hepatitis is characterized morphologically by a combination of inflammation, hepatocellular apoptosis, necrosis, and, in some instances, regeneration (**Fig. 14**). The proportion and detailed nature of these components vary widely according to the cause, the host response, and the passage of time, and it is necessary to include in the diagnosis the type, pattern, and extent of the necrosis and inflammation, in addition to the possible cause. The lesions are usually sufficiently diffuse within the liver to be diagnosed with confidence on small biopsy samples; however, although there may be histologic clues for a specific cause, it may be difficult to distinguish a cause for

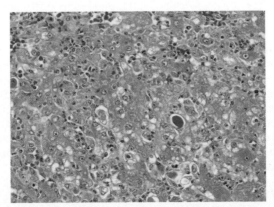

Fig. 14. Acute hepatitis in a dog. There is a diffuse distribution of neutrophils and mononuclear inflammatory cells, with scattered hepatocellular apoptosis evident.

hepatitis by morphologic means alone. The distinction between acute and chronic hepatitis can sometimes be difficult to distinguish because of overlapping features.

SPECIFIC INFECTIOUS CAUSES OF ACUTE HEPATOCELLULAR NECROSIS AND INFLAMMATION
Viral Diseases

Herpes virus
Canine and feline herpes virus infections in neonates often involve the liver in addition to other organs. Injury is characterized by multifocal randomly dispersed areas of acute hepatocellular and biliary necrosis, typically without inflammation. Inclusion bodies are intranuclear and eosinophilic but are difficult to find. The main differential diagnosis is acute bacterial septicemia.

Adenovirus
Infectious canine hepatitis attributable to canine adenovirus 1 causes a multisystemic disease involving the liver, kidney, brain, and other organs because of the ability of the virus to kill endothelial cells. Unlike most random multifocal patterns seen with viral infection, severe centrilobular to bridging necrosis with or without inflammation is typical. The centrilobular accentuation is attributed to the combined injury to hepatocytes and sinusoidal endothelial cells. Amphophilic to basophilic intranuclear inclusion bodies are usually easily found in hepatocytes and may also occur in endothelial cells and bile duct epithelium.

Corona virus
Feline infectious peritonitis involvement in the liver is characterized by multifocal random areas of necrosis, often extending in the portal and perivenular connective tissue, with a moderate to marked infiltration of macrophages and, at the periphery, plasma cells. Fibrosis may be present. A layer of fibrin with neutrophils and macrophages may be found on the liver capsule, with infiltration of the subcapsular parenchyma by plasma cells and some lymphocytes.

Bacterial Diseases

Septicemic bacterial diseases may lead to multifocal random and confluent necrosis with macrophage proliferation or infiltration with neutrophils and, in later stages, lymphocytes and plasma cells or may cause nonspecific reactive hepatitis. Enteric bacteria, such as *Escherichia coli* and *Salmonella* spp, are relatively common, as are *Streptococcus* spp, *Pasteurella* spp, and *Brucella* spp, and many other organisms are possible.

Clostridium piliformis (Tyzzer's disease) occurs in dogs and cats and is characterized by randomly dispersed areas of confluent necrosis restricted to the parenchyma with or without an inflammatory reaction. There are long slender bacilli within viable hepatocytes at the margin of the necrotic foci. These can sometimes be seen in hematoxylin-eosin preparations but are best seen with Giemsa or silver (Warthin-Starry) stains.

Leptospirosis occurs in dogs, and various serovars produce an acute multisystemic disease. Hepatocellular necrosis is usually unremarkable or minimal. The main and characteristic lesion is dissociation and separation of liver cell plates (particularly evident in postmortem material), with the presence of many hepatocytes with mitotic figures or binucleation.

Protozoal Diseases

Toxoplasma gondii causes multisystemic disease involving the liver, lung, brain, and other organs in the cat and dog. In the liver, there is confluent to panlobular necrosis, often with neutrophils, macrophages, and other inflammatory cells. Areas of necrosis and the adjacent parenchyma often contain free tachyzoites or cysts containing bradyzoites.

Toxic liver injury

Many hepatotoxins affect dogs and cats, and the list of individual toxins is too extensive to cover in this article. Manifestations of liver toxicity, one or more of which may occur with each toxin, include no morphologic abnormalities, hepatocellular swelling, lipidosis, necrosis (usually in a specific pattern), inflammation, and eventual fibrosis if exposure is long term. Most acute drug toxicity produces lesions in the centrilobular region. This is attributable to the increased abundance of the cytochrome p450 enzymes in this area. Metabolism of parent drugs by the cytochrome p450 system can produce injurious metabolites in certain circumstances and can lead to regional or massive hepatocytic necrosis depending on the dose of the toxicant (**Fig. 15**).

Some hepatotoxins are found in the environment, such as aflatoxin B1; others are therapeutic agents that are given in toxic doses or have rare and usually unpredictable toxicity. Some toxins are termed *predictable*. This group affects most animals in a dose-related fashion, such as acetaminophen. Another class of toxins, idiosyncratic toxins, affects a tiny percentage of patients, however, and the effect can be unrelated to dose, as can be seen with various therapeutic drugs. Thus, drug toxicity should be considered in most cases of acute hepatic injury. Chronic intoxication can lead to fibrosis or cirrhosis, particularly in dogs.

Chronic hepatitis

Chronic inflammation of the liver is rare in cats but is a common problem in dogs. In most cases, the pathogenesis of this process remains unclear. It is likely that chronic hepatitis has many possible causes that may include infectious, autoimmune, drug-induced, and copper-associated causes. Copper-associated hepatitis, the most well-characterized form of chronic hepatitis, is discussed in more detail elsewhere in this article. Chronic hepatitis is characterized by hepatocellular apoptosis or necrosis, a variable mononuclear or mixed inflammatory infiltrate, regeneration, and fibrosis (**Fig. 16**). The proportion and distribution of these components vary widely. It is desirable for the pathologist to provide a subjective evaluation of the activity and stage of the disease to facilitate comparison among cases. The activity of the

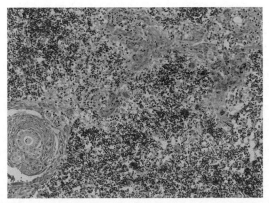

Fig. 15. Acute toxic injury in a cat. Acute hepatocytic necrosis and hemorrhage with a centrilobular and midzonal lobular distribution from a cat with diazepam-related toxicity.

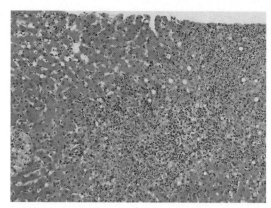

Fig. 16. Chronic hepatitis in a dog. There is pyogranulomatous inflammation, characterized by aggregates of macrophages and a diffuse infiltration of neutrophils within the lesion, in this section of tissue.

disease is determined by the amount of inflammation and extent of hepatocellular apoptosis and necrosis. The stage of the disease, and the prognosis, may be determined by the extent and pattern of fibrosis and the possible presence of architectural distortion. Fibrosis may be portoportal, portocentral, or centrocentral bridging, or it may dissect the lobule. Fibrosis may occur associated with interface hepatitis (inflammation extending from the portal tract and through the limiting plate) after parenchymal collapse with condensation of the residual reticulin network or by means of activation of hepatic stellate cells or related myofibroblasts, which synthesize collagen in the perisinusoidal space or in the portal tracts and around the central veins, respectively. Hepatocellular regeneration and regenerative nodules of hepatic parenchyma are often seen, in addition to proliferation of ductular structures at the periphery of the parenchyma and within fibrous septa. The amount and pattern of fibrosis, particularly in early and mild disease, can be best appreciated with appropriate stains, such as Sirius red or Masson's trichrome.

Copper-associated chronic hepatitis
In the Bedlington terrier, a genetic mutation in the COMM-D (formerly Murr 1) gene produces a defective protein involved in copper transport and leads to excessive accumulation of copper in hepatocytes, resulting in injury or necrosis. Copper accumulation leading to inflammation and necrosis seems to be familial in the West Highland white terrier, Skye terrier, Doberman pinscher, Labrador retriever, and Dalmatian. Typically, copper first accumulates in the centrolobular regions and, with progressive accumulation, results in hepatocyte necrosis, inflammation with copper-laden macrophages, and eventual chronic hepatitis and cirrhosis (**Fig. 17**).

Healthy dogs with normal livers may have copper levels up to 500 µg/g dry weight, and diseased dogs may have copper levels more than 2000 ppm dry weight. Hepatic copper levels in breeds with primary copper storage disease vary among individual animals and among breeds. In many circumstances, it is not clear if copper elevations are primary or secondary. Copper-induced chronic hepatitis and cirrhosis can occur in cats.

CIRRHOSIS

Cirrhosis is the end stage of chronic hepatitis and is a diffuse process of the liver characterized by fibrous septa, shunting of afferent and efferent vessels, and conversion of

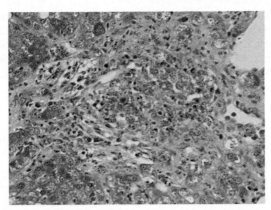

Fig. 17. Copper-related chronic hepatitis in a dog. In this liver, the aggregates of macrophages contain granular pigment, typical of copper, with an abundance of mononuclear inflammatory cells within the lesion. Surrounding hepatocytes also contain fine granular pigment as a result of copper retention.

normal liver architecture into abnormally structured parenchymal nodules (**Fig. 18**). As in chronic hepatitis, it is essential to include in the diagnosis the extent of the fibrosis, the activity of the disease, and the possible cause.

Cirrhosis is a relatively common condition in dogs and is often associated with the presence of multiple portosystemic collaterals. Some animals may have compensated cirrhotic disease and show no or minor clinical signs, whereas other animals may show decompensation of liver function and liver failure. Cirrhosis is only rarely seen in cats.

Lobular Dissecting Hepatitis

Lobular dissecting hepatitis is a particular form of cirrhosis with a rapid clinical course that is seen in young or young adult dogs as isolated cases or in groups of dogs from the same litter or kennel. The liver usually has a normal size with a smooth capsular

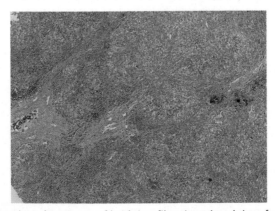

Fig. 18. Cirrhotic liver in a dog. Areas of bridging fibrosis and nodules of regenerative hepatocytes, characteristics of cirrhosis, are evident, along with aggregates of pigmented macrophages and a moderate mononuclear inflammatory infiltrate along the fibrous septa.

surface or some small nodules of regeneration. Microscopically, bands of fibroblasts and thin strands of extracellular matrix are seen between individual and small groups of hepatocytes, which cause dissection of the original lobular architecture (**Fig. 19**). Connective tissue stains (especially for reticulin) are helpful in demonstrating the pattern of connective tissue alterations. Inflammation and hepatocellular apoptosis or necrosis are usually slight to moderate.

Nonspecific Reactive Hepatitis

Nonspecific reactive hepatitis is an inflammatory response of the liver to a variety of extrahepatic disease processes, especially febrile illnesses and inflammation some-where in the splanchnic bed, or it may be the residuum of previous inflammatory intra-hepatic disease. The lesion is characterized by an inflammatory infiltrate in portal areas and in the parenchyma, without evident hepatocellular necrosis. In acute extra-hepatic diseases, there is a slight to moderate infiltrate in the parenchyma or the portal areas composed mainly of neutrophils. The infiltrate varies in intensity among portal areas, and some normal portal areas may be found (**Fig. 20**). There is slight to marked leukocytosis, Kupffer cell proliferation in the sinusoids, and some neutrophils in the connective tissue around the hepatic veins. In chronic extrahepatic diseases or in the case of residual intrahepatic disease, the inflammation is usually mononuclear,

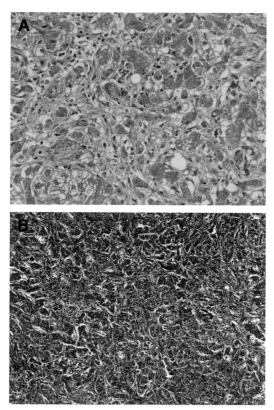

Fig. 19. Lobular dissecting hepatitis in a dog. (*A*) Normal hepatic parenchyma is disrupted by fine strands of collagen that separate hepatocytes and disrupt the normal architecture. (*B*) Trichrome stain aids the detection of the red collagen bundles that divide the hepatocytes.

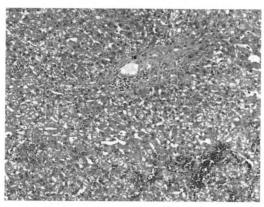

Fig. 20. Nonspecific reactive hepatitis in a dog. There is a light infiltration of lymphocytes and plasma cells in the portal tract connective tissue without evidence of hepatocellular necrosis.

with plasma cells, lymphocytes, and pigmented macrophages in the portal areas and around the hepatic veins, in addition to some plasma cells and lymphocytes with or without single or small aggregates of pigment-laden macrophages in the parenchyma.

Eosinophilic Hepatitis

Eosinophilic hepatitis is most likely a form of nonspecific reactive hepatitis. Eosinophils appear mostly as scattered elements in portal and perivenous infiltrates and, less frequently, within the sinusoids. Marked eosinophilic inflammation in the liver is a rare condition in dogs and cats and may be associated with parasitic infections (eg, migrating nematode larvae, schistosomiasis, liver fluke infestation) usually at and near the site of the parasitic lesion; a more diffuse lesion is sometimes seen in drug-induced liver lesions.

Hepatic Abscesses and Granulomas

Hepatic abscesses usually are the result of bacterial infections with subsequent neutrophil accumulation and lysis. Hepatic abscesses in dogs and cats are particularly seen in newborn animals as a result of umbilical infection by bacteria. In adult animals, hepatic abscesses may be the result of infections with *Yersinia* spp, *Nocardia asteroides*, and *Actinomyces* spp (**Fig. 21**). Hepatic abscesses may occur in association with central necrosis in hepatocellular neoplasms.

Hepatic granulomas may occur in a wide variety of diseases, but most are part of a generalized disease process. They consist of aggregates of epithelioid macrophages or multinucleated giant cells with or without lymphocytes and plasma cells. Infectious causes for hepatic granulomas in dogs include mycobacteria (eg, *Mycobacterium avium intracellulare*, *Mycobacterium tuberculosis*), *Bartonella* spp, systemic mycoses (eg, *Blastomyces dermatitidis*, *Cryptococcus neoformans*, *Histoplasma capsulatum*, *Coccidioides immitis*), *Leishmania* spp, and other parasitic infections.

Hepatic Storage Disorders

Hepatic metabolic storage disorders are usually inherited but can be acquired in certain circumstances. The histologic appearance of hepatic storage disorders can be quite varied but is most often characterized by pigment or vacuole accumulation within the hepatic cytoplasm. The types of contents range from clear to granular or

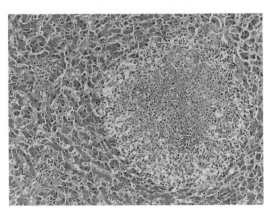

Fig. 21. Hepatic abscesses in a cat infected with *Yersinia*.

hyaline, and pigment may be evident in other circumstances. In addition to hepato-cytes, Kupffer cells and macrophages may be affected. Some storage disorders may be limited to the liver, but others affect other organs as well. Metabolic storage disorders are usually evident early in life, and the index of suspicion should be higher in young animals that do not have normal growth patterns than in adult dogs. Identi-fication of the abnormal stored material can be facilitated by ultrastructural examina-tion and the use of special stains and frozen liver samples. A metabolic screening test is most likely to clarify the metabolic disorder, however.

HEPATIC NEOPLASIA AND HYPERPLASIA
Nodular Hyperplasia

Nodular hyperplasia of hepatocytes is a common proliferative lesion in dogs older than 8 years of age. Nearly all dogs are affected by 14 years of age. Nodular hyperplasia is of no clinical significance but should be distinguished from metastatic masses. Cats have a low incidence of nodular hyperplasia.

Nodular hyperplasia of the liver is characterized by multiple distinct spherical to oval masses that are randomly distributed throughout the liver. The liver is usually normal otherwise. They can be difficult to distinguish from hepatocellular adenomas by gross pathologic morphology alone.

Histologically, nodular hyperplasia is characterized by an expansile nodule of hepa-tocytes that retains normal lobular architecture and may compress adjacent normal tissue. Hepatocytes within the nodules are often vacuolated.

Regenerative Nodules

Nodules of regenerative hyperplasia are distinct from nodular hyperplasia for several reasons. They are much more common in dogs than cats. They are believed to orig-inate from the outgrowth of surviving hepatocytes in a chronically injured liver. As a result of the outgrowth, regenerative nodules lack normal lobular architecture and there is typically only a single portal tract within the regenerative nodules. Regenera-tive nodules can be difficult to distinguish from hepatocellular adenomas on the basis of histology alone, although there are a few distinguishing features. Regenerative nodules are composed of hepatic plates that are no more than two cells thick, and adenomas may have thicker hepatic plates. Hepatocellular adenomas are more likely to be solitary lesions and usually do not typically arise in a background of hepatic injury and fibrosis.

Hepatocellular Adenoma

Hepatocellular adenomas are benign neoplasms of hepatocytes. They have most likely been under-diagnosed for many years by veterinary pathologists, because older diagnostic terminology in dogs and cats tended to include only nodular hyperplasia, regenerative nodules, and hepatocellular carcinomas. The neoplasms usually are single, unencapsulated, variably sized, red or brown masses that compress adjacent parenchyma. They lack normal nodular architecture and are composed of well-differentiated hepatocytes, which form uniform plates that may be two to three cells thick. The adenomatous hepatocytes tend to abut normal adjacent hepatocytes at right angles. Cystic areas containing hemorrhage or serum and foci of extramedullary hematopoiesis can be present.

Hepatocellular Carcinoma

Hepatocellular carcinomas are malignant neoplasms composed of hepatocytes. They are uncommon in dogs and cats. These neoplasms are often solitary, frequently involve an entire lobe, and are well demarcated, although diffuse involvement of large portions of the liver may occur. They usually arise in a liver that is otherwise normal. Metastasis occurs within the liver (intrahepatic metastasis) and to the hepatic lymph nodes most often, but distant metastasis can occur.

Histologically, hepatocellular carcinomas can be composed of trabecular, pseudoglandular, and solid patterns. Mixtures of these patterns can be found within individual tumors. In the trabecular pattern, hepatocytes form irregular trabeculae three or more cells thick and with distended vascular spaces between the trabeculae. Pseudoglandular patterns are formed by malignant hepatocytes that are arranged into complete or incomplete acinar structures. The solid pattern lacks acini or trabeculae and is characterized by sheets of neoplastic hepatocytes; this pattern often contains the least well-differentiated hepatocytes. Cells forming the neoplasm range from well-differentiated hepatocytes to atypical or bizarre forms (**Fig. 22**). Mitoses are common, and multinucleate cells can occur. In the absence of metastasis, which is obviously indicative of malignancy, the separation of a well-differentiated carcinoma from an adenoma can be difficult, although invasion by malignant hepatocytes at the margin of the adjacent compressed normal hepatocytes and hepatocellular pleomorphism and atypia are useful indicators of malignancy. Metastasis is uncommon in the author's experience.

Cholangiocellular Adenoma (Biliary Adenoma)

Biliary adenomas are nonencapsulated, irregular, pale white to pale gray, multilocular masses. Adenomas of the biliary ducts are rare in dogs and cats. They are usually small and asymptomatic, discovered as an incidental finding at necropsy.

Histologically, they are characterized by circular acini lined with well-differentiated biliary epithelial cells. Cysts may be mildly dilated. Biliary adenomas should be differentiated from solitary biliary cysts, multilocular cysts, or von Meyenberg complexes.

Cholangiocellular Carcinoma (Biliary Carcinoma)

Cholangiocellular carcinomas are malignant neoplasms of biliary epithelium that usually arise from the intrahepatic ducts, but extrahepatic bile ducts can be affected. They are found in dogs and cats.

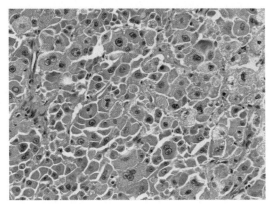

Fig. 22. Hepatocellular carcinoma in a dog. Neoplastic hepatocytes form a broad sheet of pleomorphic and multinucleate hepatocytes.

Tumors are typically white and firm, often with an umbilicated and lobulated appearance. The borders of the lesions are generally well delineated from the adjacent hepatic parenchyma, although the border is frequently irregular because of local invasion. Areas of necrosis can be found in the central regions. The tumors are composed of cells that can be quite pleomorphic but usually retain a resemblance to biliary epithelium. Characteristically, well-differentiated carcinomas are organized into a tubular or acinar arrangement (**Fig. 23**). In less well-differentiated neoplasms, some acinar arrangements can be detected among solid masses of neoplastic cells. Mucin is frequently evident in the lumen of well-differentiated areas of the tumors. The epithelial components of the neoplasms are usually separated by abundant fibrous connective tissue, termed a *scirrhous response*. Metastasis to extrahepatic sites is common.

Mixed Hepatocellular and Cholangiocellular Carcinomas

Occasionally, carcinomas with a mixture of hepatocellular and biliary characteristics can arise.

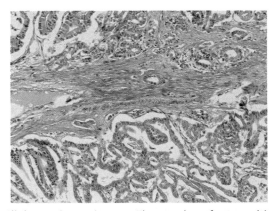

Fig. 23. Cholangiocellular carcinoma in a cat. The neoplasm forms multiple papillary projections lined by moderately pleomorphic biliary epithelial cells. Bands of fibrous tissue separate the neoplastic cells.

Carcinoids
Carcinoids are uncommon tumors of the liver. They are believed to arise from neuro-endocrine cells that lie within the intra- or extrahepatic biliary epithelium ductular tree, gallbladder, or, possibly, hepatic progenitor cells. Often, they form a single mass, but multiple nodules can occur, probably secondary to intrahepatic metastasis. They tend to have an aggressive course, and extrahepatic metastasis can occur. Cells tend to be small, elongated, or spindle shaped and form ribbons or rosettes, and the tumors are highly vascular (**Fig. 24**). Immunohistochemical detection of neuroendocrine markers, such as chromogranin A or neuron-specific enolase, may be used to confirm the diagnosis in some cases, but there are no definitive markers.

Miscellaneous primary mesenchymal neoplasms of the liver
Primary neoplasms can arise from any of the normal cellular constituents of the liver. Primary hepatic hemangiosarcoma is well recognized in dogs, although it is a relatively uncommon site of origin for this neoplasm compared with the skin and spleen. Other primary tumor types can involve mesenchymal neoplasms derived from the liver's connective tissue, including fibrosarcoma, leiomyosarcoma, and osteosarcoma (probably secondary to another mesenchymal tumor initially). Myelolipomas are well-demarcated benign tumors of cats and wild felids characterized by a mix of adipose tissue and myeloid elements.

Metastatic neoplasms
The liver is one of the two more common sites for metastatic spread of malignant neoplasms, a distinction shared with the lung. Given the higher frequency of metas-tasis compared with primary neoplasia, a complete necropsy and medical or surgical history are necessary to distinguish metastatic neoplasms from primary neoplasia of the hepatobiliary tissue.

Hematopoietic neoplasms, particularly lymphoma, frequently involve the liver as part of the generalized disease process. Neoplastic lymphocytes are characteristically distributed around the vessels of the portal tract and, to a lesser extent, the central and sublobular veins. The gamut of other myeloid neoplasms can also involve the liver.

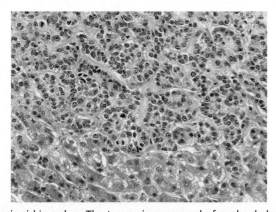

Fig. 24. Hepatic carcinoid in a dog. The tumor is composed of oval pale basophilic cells with oval to carrot-shaped nuclei that form ribbon-like arrays or rosettes, as in this case. Mitotic figures are common.

FURTHER READINGS

BOOKS

Crawford JM, Haschek WM, Rousseaux CG. In: Fundamentals of toxicologic pathology; 1998. p. 127–51.

Crawford JM. The liver and biliary tract. In: Robbins pathologic basis of disease. 7th Edition. Philadelphia: Elsevier Saunders; 2005. p. 877–938.

Rothuizen J, Bunch S, Charles J, et al. Standards for clinical and histological diagnosis of canine and feline liver diseases (WSAVA). Philadelphia: Elsevier Saunders; 2006.

Stalker MJ, Hayes MA. Liver and biliary system. In: Maxie GM, editor. Jubb, Kennedy, and Palmer's pathology of domestic animals. 5th edition, vol. 2. Philadelphia: Elsevier; 2007. p. 297–388.

BILIARY

Aguirre AL, Center SA, Randolph JF, et al. Gallbladder diseases in Shetland sheepdogs: 38 cases (1995–2005). J Am Vet Med Assoc 2007;231:79–88.

Gagne JM, Weiss DJ, Armstrong PJ. Histopathologic evaluation of feline inflammatory liver disease. Vet Pathol 1996;33:521–6.

Greiter-Wilke A, Scanziani E, Soldati S, et al. Association of *Helicobacter* with cholangiohepatitis in cats. J Vet Intern Med 2006;20:822–7.

Holt DE, Mehler S, Mayhew PD, et al. Canine gallbladder infarction: 12 cases (1993–2003). Vet Pathol 2004;41:416–8.

Weiss DJ, Gagne JM, Armstrong PJ. Characterization of portal lymphocytic infiltrates in feline liver. Vet Clin Pathol 1995;24:91–5.

Yoshioka K, Enaga S, Taniguchi K, et al. Morphologic characterization of ductular reactions in canine liver disease. J Comp Pathol 2004;130:92–8.

PARENCHYMAL

Hoffman G, van den Ingh TS, Bode P, et al. Copper-associated chronic hepatitis in Labrador retrievers. J Vet Intern Med 2006;20:856–61.

Kalaizakis E, Roubies N, Panousis N, et al. Clinicopathologic evaluation of hepatic lipidosis in periparturient dairy cattle. J Vet Intern Med 2007;21:835–45.

Mandigers PJJ, van den Ingh TS, Bode P, et al. Improvement in liver pathology after 4 months of D-penicillamine in 5 Doberman pinschers with subclinical hepatitis. J Vet Intern Med 2005;19:40–3.

Sepesy LM, Center SA, Randolph JF, et al. Vacuolar hepatopathy in dogs: 336 cases (1993–2005). J Am Vet Med Assoc 2006;229:246–52.

Shih JL, Keating JH, Freeman LM, et al. Chronic hepatitis in Labrador retrievers: clinical presentation and prognostic factors. J Vet Intern Med 2007;21:33–9.

Spee B, Arends B, van den Ingh TS, et al. Copper metabolism and oxidative stress in chronic inflammatory and cholestatic liver diseases in dogs. J Vet Intern Med 2006;20:1085–92.

REFERENCE

1. Cullen JM. Liver, biliary system and exocrine pancreas. In: McGavin MD, Zachary JF, editors. Pathologic basis of veterinary disease. Philadelphia: Elsevier Saunders; 2007. p. 393–461.

Important Clinical Syndromes Associated with Liver Disease

Jan Rothuizen, DVM, PhD

KEYWORDS

• Icterus • Cholestasis • Bilirubin • Bile acids
• Hepatic encephalopathy • Portal hypertension
• Portosystemic shunting • Ascites • Coagulopathy
• Liver disease

Several clinical syndromes can develop in many different liver diseases. They are important to understand the clinical manifestations of hepatobiliary diseases. The signs, diagnostic procedures, and specific diseases associated with these syndromes are discussed.

ICTERUS AND CHOLESTASIS
Bile Production and Flow

Cholestasis is a reduced bile flow. Normally, the flow in the biliary tree results from bile production in the proximal part and concentration of bile in the distal part. Only the flow of bile in the common bile duct is influenced by active transport due to peristalsis (gall bladder contractions and closure or relaxation of the sphincter of Oddi).[1,2] More than 50% of the bile is immediately released into the duodenum,[3] the rest being stored and concentrated in the gallbladder. The major trigger for gallbladder contraction is the hormone cholecystokinine,[4–7] which is secreted by the duodenal mucosa under the influence of fat or protein (amino acids). The gallbladder does not contract suddenly, like the urinary bladder, but gradually over 1 to 2 hours. Furthermore, the gallbladder is emptied incompletely and variably following a meal (5%–65%).[3] Bile is concentrated about tenfold in the gallbladder and in the larger bile ducts by active absorption of Na^+, HCO_3^-, and water.[8–11]

Some 50% of bile production depends on active excretion of bile salts by the hepatocytes into the canaliculi. Bile acids are produced by the liver from cholesterol, which is a major route of cholesterol excretion. The 2 acids formed are cholic acid and chenodeoxycholic acid (the so-called primary bile acids). Bile acids are made hydrophilic before excretion into bile by conjugation with glycine and taurine. A small fraction of

Department of Clinical Sciences of Companion Animals, University Utrecht, Yalelaan 108, P.O. Box 80.154, 3508 TD Utrecht, The Netherlands
E-mail address: j.rothuizen@uu.nl

Vet Clin Small Anim 39 (2009) 419–437
doi:10.1016/j.cvsm.2009.02.007
0195-5616/09/$ – see front matter © 2009 Elsevier Inc. All rights reserved.

the membrane (about 15%) of hepatocytes surrounds the smallest bile ducts (canaliculi) and contains active transporters. Active bile acid excretion creates a huge concentration gradient between the cells and the canaliculi with a factor of 2,000. The osmotic gradient induced causes excretion of water into the canaliculi, which is a major driving force of the bile flow.

When bile reaches the intestinal tract, conjugated bile acids are partly transformed by enteral bacteria in 2 ways. The secondary bile acids, deoxycholate and lithocholate, are produced by hydroxylation from cholic acid and chenodeoxycholic acid, respectively. Lithocholic acid is poorly absorbed, but it is hepatotoxic and may induce severe cholestasis. The small reabsorbed fraction is sulfated (tertiary sulfolithocholic acid) in the liver; in this form it is not reabsorbable in the next enteric cycle. Conjugated bile acids are actively reabsorbed in the ileum. The second bacterial transformation of bile acids is deconjugation. Unconjugated bile acids are absorbed in the entire intestinal tract by passive diffusion. All reabsorbed bile acids are transported to the liver by the portal blood flow, efficiently (90% in each passage) cleared by the liver, and if necessary reconjugated and then re-excreted into the canaliculi. Only a small fraction of the bile acid pool is lost in this enterohepatic circulation which cycles 10 to 15 times per day. The lost fraction is replenished by de novo synthesis in the liver.

Some bile production occurs by secretion by hepatocytes of Na^+ into the canaliculi, passively followed by water. The remaining 30% of the bile is produced by the epithelium of the intrahepatic bile ducts by excretion of water in combination with bicarbonate and chloride.

Cholestasis

Cholestasis is a reduced bile flow in the biliary tract. The cause of cholestasis may be inside (intrahepatic) or outside the liver in the common bile duct (extrahepatic). Intrahepatic cholestasis occurs in most clinical cases.[12,13] Due to the large reserve capacity of the hepatobiliary system, clinical signs of cholestasis (eg, icterus) only develop when the entire liver is affected diffusely. Obstruction of the bile flow by focal lesions is easily compensated for by the remaining liver. Intrahepatic cholestasis occurs predominantly at the level of hepatocytes and canaliculi or in bile ductuli in zone 1 of the liver lobules (the periportal zone). Extrahepatic cholestasis occurs by obstruction of the common bile duct. Again, due to the reserve of the liver, clinical signs occur only when there is nearly complete blockage of the passage.

Intrahepatic cholestasis

Intrahepatic cholestasis may occur due to leakage of the tight junctions that separate bile canaliculi from blood sinusoids. This situation occurs in endotoxemia and sepsis, and in cases of adverse reaction to drugs. Leptospira produce enzymes that destroy the tight junctions, leading to severe intrahepatic cholestasis in leptospirosis without severe reduction of other liver functions. Another reason for intrahepatic cholestasis is swelling of hepatocytes, which occlude the canaliculi and bile ductules (feline liver lipidosis). Necrosis of liver cells may occur in almost all liver diseases and gives a direct connection between canaliculi and the sinusoidal/perisinusoidal lymph and blood flow. Because active excretion of bile components with water causes pressure in the biliary system, bile leaks easily back into the low pressure blood and lymphatic system. In many liver diseases there are portal or periportal processes that block the bile flow out of the liver lobules. Examples are infiltration of inflammatory cells (hepatitis), tumor cells (malignant lymphoma and other forms), and deposition of collagen (chronic hepatitis, other fibrotic diseases, cirrhosis). Diffuse swelling of hepatocytes (lipidosis), diffusely spread space-occupying lesions (tumor metastases), and disruption of the normal acinar architecture (cirrhosis) affect the bile flow at different levels in the liver lobules. The most severe form of intrahepatic cholestasis is seen in dogs with destructive cholangitis, whereby many or all peripheral intrahepatic branches of the biliary tree become necrotic (eg, due to idiosyncratic reaction to sulfonamides/trimethoprim-sulfamethoxazole).[14] Such dogs may have a completely disrupted bile flow, which may be detectable by an empty gall bladder at ultrasonography, and severe icterus. In all cases of cholestasis (also extrahepatic) the hepatocytes may become overloaded with substances that cannot be adequately excreted. Due to diffusion through the sinusoidal membrane, they may enter the perisinusoidal space of Disse. With the hepatic lymph flow, all such compounds will then enter the blood circulation.

Extrahepatic cholestasis, extrahepatic bile duct obstruction

Extrahepatic causes of cholestasis are rare. In dogs and cats, clinical cases of extrahepatic cholestasis have common bile duct obstruction. In most cases, tumors of the pancreas or the duodenum underlie the obstruction. Gallstones may also block the common bile duct at the level of Vater's papilla. Hyperplasia of the biliary epithelium due to long-term high doses of progestins may also occlude the extrahepatic bile ducts. Cholangiocarcinomas may spread through the biliary tree and cause severe extrahepatic (and intrahepatic) cholestasis. Nematodes ascending into the biliary system have been reported to cause common bile duct obstruction, but this is a rare event, if it occurs at all in vivo. The common bile duct or lobular ducts may become obstructed if (part of) the liver is dislocated in a diaphragmatic herniation. In such cases cholestasis and icterus may occur intermittently. Cholangitis may cause diffuse intra- and extrahepatic cholestasis, which is rare in dogs, but the most common cause in cats. Chronic EHBDO causes dilatation of the extrahepatic bile ducts, which become wide and tortuous. These changes are easily detectable with ultrasonography. The gallbladder is not always distended, and in chronic cases it may even be abnormally small, containing highly concentrated mucinous bile from which the pigment has been resorbed (white bile).[12] Therefore, due to the physiologic variability of gallbladder filling, the size of the gallbladder is not an indicator of EHBDO. Morphine derivatives induce complete closure of the sphincter of Oddi,[15] so that a full gallbladder during surgery may be normal. Complete EHBDO causes absence of bile components in the feces, so that the normal color (due to the black-brown degradation products of bilirubin) may change. Bile acid-driven fat resorption is then also disturbed, resulting in soft grey feces with a high fat content (acholic feces). This finding, always in association with severe icterus, is diagnostic for EHBDO.[16] Hepatobiliary scintigraphy may be used to quantify the degree of cholestasis.[15,17]

Histology of cholestasis

Cholestasis may be visible in the canaliculi, the hepatocytes. and in the macrophages and Kupffer cells. In the canaliculi, cellular debris and bile may produce bile thrombi, visible as brown casts in the canaliculi. However, these casts are easily washed out of the liver tissue on the slide during staining procedures. Cellular debris and bile plugs containing bile pigment (bilirubin) are phagocytosed by Kupffer cells and are seen as intracellular brown-yellow material. Accumulation of bile pigment in hepatocytes may also be visible as brown-yellow pigmentation. In animals with EHBDO high levels of toxic bile acids cause hepatocellular degeneration and necrosis in the periportal zone with a secondary inflammatory reaction of polymorphonuclear cells. In acute cases periportal edema also occurs. In cases with chronic (several weeks) EHBDO, the edema disappears and concentric periportal fibrosis develops, which may give a unionlike aspect. In chronic cases bile ducts proliferate and become tortuous, which is visible as multiple bile ducts instead of just one in the portal areas. In severe chronic cholestasis of any origin the biliary excretion of copper may be decreased, leading to increased concentration in the liver. With histochemical staining slight accumulation of copper may be detectable in the periportal zone (primary copper storage diseases give more severe accumulation in the centrilobular area).

Biochemistry of cholestasis

Biochemically, cholestasis leads to increased concentration of all bile constituents, such as cholesterol, bile acids, and bilirubin, and also of enzymes that are highly active in biliary epithelial cells or the specialized biliary part of the membrane of hepatocytes: It is not possible to differentiate between extra- and intrahepatic cholestasis with biochemistry.

Bilirubin Metabolism and Icterus

Bilirubin is the pigment that gives bile its yellow-brown color. It is the normal end-product of the catabolism of heme. Heme resides in red cell hemoglobin and in many enzyme systems, which are preferentially localized in the liver (cytochromes, catalase, and peroxidase). Although the pool size of hemoproteins in the liver is small compared with the hemoglobin pool, the production of bilirubin from hepatic heme accounts for 30% of the total production, because the hepatic heme turnover rate is much higher (2 hours to 4 days versus 98 days for hemoglobin). Bilirubin is cleared from the plasma by the liver, and has to be conjugated by the hepatocytes preceding biliary excretion. The unconjugated form is stringently hydrophobic and bound to albumin in the circulation. On conjugation, bilirubin is excreted into bile and the conjugate is not reabsorbed from the intestines. Rarely, in cases of bacterial overgrowth, bilirubin is deconjugated by bacterial enzymes and the unconjugated pigment is reabsorbed in the small intestines into an enterohepatic cycle. Bacterial degradation of bilirubin in the colon produces stercobilins, black and brown pigments that give feces its normal color.

Healthy animals have only unconjugated bilirubin in their circulation. Cholestasis causes accumulation of conjugated bilirubin in plasma, which is not only re-excreted by the liver but may also be excreted by the kidneys in the urine. Bilirubin in feline urine is abnormal and indicates liver disease. However, the kidney in dogs, particularly males, has all the enzymes to produce bilirubin out of heme and to conjugate it, so that it can be excreted into urine. Therefore, the urine of healthy male dogs may contain detectable concentrations of bilirubin.

Urobilinogen is a colorless product, a small fraction of which is absorbed into the portal blood. Most of it is cleared by the liver, but a minor part reaches the systemic circulation and can be excreted by the kidneys. In cases of EHBDO much less bilirubin reaches the intestinal tract so that the amount of urobilinogen in the urine is even lower than normally. Measurement of urobilinogen in urine has been used to differentiate between different forms of icterus and cholestasis. However, due to many physiologic variations and technical errors, this parameter has no clinical value.

Bilirubin is cleared from the blood, conjugated, and excreted into bile by the liver. The clearance is not an efficient process[18,19] in contrast to the hepatic clearance of bile acids. Whereas bile acids are nearly completely cleared during the first passage, bilirubin requires many passages to become cleared completely (**Fig. 1**). As a consequence, bilirubin is equally distributed over the entire circulation, but bile acids are highly concentrated in the portal blood and have a low concentration in the systemic circulation. This explains the differences in the reaction pattern of bilirubin and bile

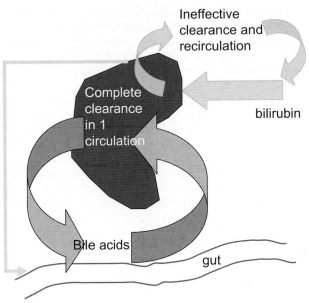

Fig. 1. The differences between bilirubin and bile acid metabolism. Both metabolites are produced in the liver. Bile acids are reabsorbed and undergo an enterohepatic circulation, which is maintained by an efficient clearance of bile acids from the portal vein. Bilirubin is not absorbed from the small intestines and its hepatic clearance from the blood has low efficiency. Consequently, there is a high gradient between the portal and systemic concentrations of bile acids, but not of bilirubin. Furthermore, systemic bile acids are increased due to portosystemic shunting and cholestasis; bilirubin is only increased due to cholestasis (or increased production in case of severe hemolysis).

acids in different liver diseases. In diseases with cholestasis, all bile components including bilirubin and bile acids gain entry to the systemic circulation with the hepatic lymph. This process is not related to hepatic clearance or portal perfusion of the liver. Conversely, in diseases characterized by portosystemic shunting (congenital portosystemic shunts, portal hypertension, acquired collateral circulation, and so forth), the high portal bile acid concentration reaches the systemic circulation giving a high plasma bile acid concentration. However, the bilirubin concentration is not influenced by abnormal liver perfusion. Animals with congenital portosystemic shunts will never have icterus.

The main processes by which plasma bilirubin may increase are increased production and cholestasis. The bilirubin concentration in health is low (<3.5 μmol/L). An increased level becomes clinically visible only as icterus (yellow discoloration of sclerae, mucous membranes and skin) when the concentration exceeds 15 μmol/L. Due to the huge liver reserve capacity, most patients remain in the subclinical region and do not become icteric, despite the fact that nearly all nonvascular liver diseases lead to some degree of cholestasis. Some 10% of all liver patients have clinical jaundice.

Given the 2 main reasons for hyperbilirubinemia, increased production and cholestasis, measurement of unconjugated and conjugated bilirubin has been used as an expression of these 2 processes. However, with sensitive techniques, it has been shown that hemolytic (increased production) and hepatobiliary diseases (cholestasis) are not different with respect to the fraction of unconjugated bilirubin, which always varies between 15% and 40%. In liver diseases, there is considerable hemolysis (eg, due to portal hypertension causing reduced splanchnic blood flow with prolonged trapping and degradation of red blood cells in the spleen, and altered erythrocyte membrane fluidity caused by high plasma bile acid concentrations). Furthermore, animals with liver disease may have increased bilirubin production from hepatocyte hemoproteins. Hepatic and hemolytic diseases also have comparable reductions of the bile flow as an expression of cholestasis.[20] Cholestasis in hemolytic disease is caused by liver cell necrosis in the centrolobular region of the liver lobules due to hypoxia with a secondary inflammatory reaction. Such liver damage occurs only in sudden, severe types of hemolysis. With mild anemia, the liver is not damaged and the reserve capacity of the liver prevents such patients from becoming icteric. As hepatic and hemolytic jaundice always consist of a mixed type of hyperbilirubinemia, the measurement of unconjugated and conjugated bilirubin is clinically useless. Furthermore, if only severe hemolysis leads to jaundice, such animals should have pale mucous membranes (and hematocrit <20%). Moderately pale or normally colored mucous membranes in the presence of icterus immediately indicate the presence of a primary disease of the liver or biliary tract.[20,21]

A final remark with respect to bilirubin concerns its binding to albumin. Conjugated bilirubin in plasma binds covalently (irreversibly) to protein albumin. This bilirubin can only escape the circulation when albumin becomes catabolized; its half-life is about 2 weeks. Therefore, after complete recovery from the underlying cholestatic disease, icterus may remain for several weeks and does not necessarily reflect the actual situation, which may be important when evaluating the effect of therapy.[22]

In summary: (1) jaundice is the result of cholestasis; the underlying cause (hemolysis or hepatobiliary disease) is visible by clinical examination of the mucous membranes; (2) cholestasis occurs in most hepatobiliary diseases but in most cases there is no icterus; (3) animals with congenital portosystemic shunts or portal vein hypoplasia do not have icterus; (4) increased (basal or postprandial) bile acid concentrations are not specific for cholestasis or portosystemic shunting; (5) acholic feces is diagnostic for EHBDO, but is not present in all cases; (6) icterus due to intrahepatic cholestasis indicates a disease that affects the entire liver diffusely.

PORTAL HYPERTENSION, ASCITES AND ACQUIRED PORTOSYSTEMIC COLLATERAL CIRCULATION
Portal Hypertension

Portal hypertension is an abnormally high pressure in the portal circulation. The normal blood pressure in the portal vein is low, 0 to 5 mmHg. Portal hypertension can be caused by an increased delivery of blood to the portal system, or by an increased resistance to the passage of portal blood. An increased delivery of blood occurs animals with arteriovenous shunts in the splanchnic circulation, usually in the liver, causing the direct connection of the arterial blood pressure with the portal system.[23] This is a rare condition, usually visible with ultrasonography as a pulsating bunch of vessels within 1 liver lobe. Usually, however, portal hypertension is caused by an increased resistance to the portal blood stream. The cause can be prehepatic (in the portal vein itself), intrahepatic, or posthepatic (hepatic veins, caudal vena cava, heart). Posthepatic causes have little influence on the liver functions, but increased hydrostatic portal blood pressure may cause ascites.

Most cases of clinically relevant portal hypertension have a cause inside the liver.[23] As applies for most liver dysfunctions, clinical problems develop only when the entire liver is affected. Liver diseases causing portal hypertension give rise to different liver dysfunctions, such as reduced protein and albumin production. However, even in severe liver dysfunction, the capacity of the liver to produce proteins is only moderately affected due to the large plasticity of the liver. Therefore, albumin levels usually do not fall below 18 to 20 g/L, which is more than the concentration that, by itself, may cause edema and ascites (<15 g/L). However, the combination of portal hypertension and moderate hypoalbuminemia often produces ascites in such animals. The hindrance to the portal circulation develops by way of compression of the portal veins in the portal and periportal area of the liver lobules. Because the cause lies at the site of entry of blood into the liver lobules, the liver itself is not congested. Due to loss of functional tissue, most of these diseases are associated with an abnormally small liver. The most frequent cause of portal vein compression is deposition of collagen (fibrosis)[23,24] and infiltration of inflammatory cells (chronic hepatitis). In advanced cases, cirrhosis, defined as disruption of the normal lobular architecture of the liver by fibrous tissue, occurs. Then, resistance to the portal blood flow occurs at different levels of the lobule and is most severe. The other most frequent cause of portal hypertension is portal vein hypoplasia,[25–27] a congenital disease in which the peripheral portal vein branches have not been formed or are incomplete, making the portal system a dead end. Portal vein hypoplasia (formerly called microvascular dysplasia) is associated with variable degrees of liver fibrosis, which may increase the resistance to normal liver perfusion.

The main prehepatic cause of portal hypertension is portal vein thrombosis. Portal vein thrombosis is a rare condition, which may result from an abnormal portal vein intima (eg, hemangiosarcoma), from hypercoagulability due to decreased antithrombin III activity (usually caused by severe proteinuria). Other predisposing conditions are Cushing's disease, pancreatitis, and liver cirrhosis.

Posthepatic causes of portal hypertension may be localized in the inferior vena cava and the heart. Obstruction of the hepatic veins either intra- or extrahepatic (Budd-Chiari syndrome and veno-occlusive disease, respectively) occur in other species, but not in cats or dogs. Heart failure is the most common posthepatic cause of portal hypertension. Thrombosis of the inferior vena cava is rare, and is often caused by an adrenal tumor giving local thrombophlebitis. Such a thrombus grows out in the direction of the blood stream and may occlude the lumen over a long distance. In posthepatic causes of portal hypertension the liver is congested and enlarged. Liver functions, however, remain adequate and biochemical examination usually reveals no or only slight liver cell damage and dysfunction.

If disorders affecting the afferent portal system cause reduced perfusion of the liver, there is secondary hypoplasia of the portal veins and increased growth of tortuous hepatic arteries (arterialization) in the portal areas.[23] These distinct histologic features occur with portal vein thrombosis, congenital portosystemic shunts, portal vein hypoplasia, and arteriovenous fistulas. With the exception of congenital shunts, all of these diseases cause increased resistance for the portal blood flow through the liver, and therefore portal hypertension.

In posthepatic causes of portal hypertension, the central vein branches may be distended and the liver cells in zone 3 degenerated. In chronic cases, fibrous tissue develops around the terminal veins and hepatocyte hyperplasia may occur in zone 1 (periportally).

In portal hypertension there is reduced portal blood flow to the liver.[28–30] With intrahepatic causes, if the hindrance of the portal flow is at the sinusoidal or postsinusoidal level of the acini, the inflowing arterial blood may cause a reversion of the portal blood flow from the liver back into the portal vein; the normal hepatopetal (into the liver) flow then becomes hepatofugal (back out of the liver). The stasis or reversion of the portal flow may be visualized with Doppler ultrasonography. Reversed portal flow is only possible if there are acquired portosystemic collateral vessels, and thus is there is chronic severe portal hypertension (see later discussion). Such abnormal flow patterns may occur in the case of portal vein hypoplasia (microvascular dysplasia), arteriovenous fistula, and advanced cirrhosis.

The clinically recognizable effects of portal hypertension may be ascites and the occurrence of hepatic encephalopathy (HE) due to acquired portosystemic shunting.

Ascites

Accumulation of free abdominal fluid may result from severe portal hypertension, or from the combination of moderately increased portal blood pressure and hypoalbuminemia. Because of the high reserve capacity of the liver, hypoalbuminemia occurs only when liver function is chronically and severely impaired. Examples are chronic hepatitis/cirrhosis, congenital portosystemic shunts, and severe forms of portal vein hypoplasia.[23,26–28,31] However, even in the most severe cases, the synthesis of albumin is only moderately reduced, typically resulting in plasma albumin concentrations of 18 to 22 g/L. Reduced oncotic pressure may be the only cause of edema/ascites when albumin concentrations are $\leq$15 g/L. Therefore portal hypertension must be present in liver diseases in order to cause ascites.

In posthepatic causes of portal hypertension (eg, heart failure), the liver functions are not or only slightly impaired; protein production remains adequate. In such cases, the hydrostatic blood pressure is the only factor causing ascites, which occurs only if the blood pressure is high. This situation occurs only in cases of near-complete obstruction of the inferior vena cava or severe cardiac failure.

Prehepatic portal hypertension (portal vein thrombosis), if located in the stem of the portal vein, may cause near-complete obstruction. The severely increased hydrostatic blood pressure may then cause ascites. This situation does not occur if only a branch of the portal vein is occluded.

In dogs with severe cholestasis, associated with high systemic plasma levels of bile acids, a specific mechanism of ascites formation may occur. In man, rats, cats, and dogs, different bile acids have been shown to inhibit the activity of 11β-hydroxysteroid dehydrogenase (OHSD). the function of OHSD is to prevent cortisol from binding to the aldosterone receptor. Cortisol is present in about tenfold excess to aldosterone, and has the same affinity for the aldosterone receptor. On binding, cortisol activates the intracellular aldosterone pathways and then acts as aldosterone. To keep the aldosterone receptor free to bind its specific ligand, the membranes of cells that express the aldosterone receptor also express OHSD. OHSD converts cortisol into cortisone, which does not bind to the receptor.[32–38] Inhibition of the enzyme by bile acids may cause unexpected hyperaldosteronism, exerted by cortisol. The author has seen this only in cases with severe cholestasis, such as in dogs with destructive cholangitis. Such cases may develop ascites, hydrothorax, or edema as a result, which is refractory to most diuretics but responds well to spironolactone, an aldosterone receptor antagonist.

The cause of ascites formation is reflected in the type of ascitic fluid.[28,39] With pre- and posthepatic causes there is a high portal blood pressure and congestion of the splanchnic vascular bed. The abdominal free fluid then contains lymph, plasma, and erythrocytes. The fluid is more or less turbid and pink-colored. If the cause is intrahepatic, there is only moderate portal hypertension and hypoalbuminemia. In these cases there is increased hepatic and splanchnic lymph production, which exceeds the capacity of the lymphatic system, causing a clear, nonhemorrhagic, colorless transudate (or yellowish in cases of icterus).

The diagnosis of the underlying cause of ascites starts by examining a few milliliters of ascitic fluid. If cardiac failure can be excluded with physical examination, pink-colored fluid indicates either portal vein or thoracic vena cava obstruction. Clear colorless transudate indicates an intrahepatic disease requiring liver biopsy for final diagnosis. Clear colorless transudate may also occur in nonhepatic diseases associated with severe albumin loss (nephrotic syndrome and protein-losing enteropathy); in these conditions the plasma albumin concentration is ≤ 15 g/L. Pink-colored fluid may be seen with some abdominal tumors, although this is rare.

The ascitic fluid may contain a large amount of albumin due to diffusion of this low molecular weight protein out of the circulation. Complete removal of the abdominal fluid in animals with portal hypertension is useless (the cause remains and the ascites recurs quickly) and undesirable. Some of the body's albumin stores is removed with the fluid, leading to accelerated ascites formation. During this process, hypovolemia occurs, which stimulates compensatory aldosterone production (Na^+ retention, K^+ excretion). The loss of K^+ may cause a marked worsening of the clinical or subclinical HE. The ascites can be treated more effectively by a low-sodium diet and potassium-sparing diuretics.

Portosystemic Collaterals

There are small, nonfunctional blood vessels in the omentum and mesentery, which expand and become functional as a result of a high portal pressure. Acquired portosystemic shunting develops only in the case of a high pressure gradient between the portal vein and the vena cava, and is seen only if the cause is pre- or intrahepatic. High pressure in the caval and the portal vein induces no portosystemic shunting. Functional portosystemic shunting develops gradually over time; it usually takes 6 to 8 weeks before measurable dysfunction occurs. The degree of shunting may vary from slight to 100%, depending on the cause and the stage of the process. Acquired portosystemic collaterals are always multiple and they are typically localized in the mesorectum, in the omentum just caudal to the left kidney, and along the gastric cardia and in the esophageal wall. Intraluminal bleeding into the esophagus from these tortuous vessels is a feared complication of portal hypertension in humans, but it does not occur in dogs or cats, due to the submucosal location in man, in contrast to the subserosal collaterals in dogs and cats.

The collateral circulation may cause HE. In addition, toxins from the gastrointestinal tract are inadequately cleared by the liver, causing excitation of the vomiting center and nausea, inappetence, and vomiting.

The presence of portosystemic shunting resulting from formed collaterals can be determined with an ammonia tolerance test; the postprandial bile acid test is not specific to distinguish portosystemic shunting from cholestasis, which are both present in such cases.[39,40]

HEPATIC ENCEPHALOPATHY
Forms of Hepatic Encephalopathy and Diseases Involved

HE is a dysfunction of the brain secondary to liver dysfunction.[41] HE is a frequent liver-associated syndrome in dogs and is less frequent in cats. Like portal hypertension and cholestasis, HE is not a disease but a manifestation of clinical symptoms that may develop in different liver diseases.

There are 2 different forms of HE: a rare acute type and a common chronic type. The acute form of HE, caused by fulminant hepatic failure, results in a fatal failure of all liver functions. Such animals will die within a few days and the encephalopathy is severe.

Therefore, they are comatose, and total liver failure causes severe icterus and coagulopathy due to disseminated intravascular coagulation (DIC). All liver enzymes in plasma will be raised dramatically. This form cannot be treated but is easily diagnosed.

The chronic form of HE is more common by far.[41,42] In dogs and cats (and humans), the underlying lesion is portosystemic collateral circulation, which may be due to acquired multiple collaterals due to portal hypertension or a single congenital portosystemic shunt. This form of HE is often called portosystemic encephalopathy (PSE). The reserve capacity of the liver prevents the development of HE even in severe parenchymal liver diseases (with the exception of fulminant failure) that are not accompanied by portosystemic shunting. Therefore, PSE occurs only if significantly reduced parenchymal liver function occurs in combination with portosystemic shunting. Either one of the components will not lead to HE.

The combination of shunting and impaired liver function occurs in all pre- and intrahepatic diseases causing portal hypertension, and also in animals with congenital portosystemic shunt. In the latter condition, the liver has been deprived of growth factors from birth and is therefore abnormally small with a too small, hypofunctional parenchymal mass.

The strict association of chronic HE with portosystemic shunting has 2 exceptions. In cats, chronic HE may occur in liver steatosis (lipidosis) due to prolonged fasting. Because cats cannot synthesize arginine in their liver, depletion of this essential amino acid occurs during fasting. Arginine is an important intermediate in the urea cycle. Therefore anorexia in cats may cause the combination of liver lipidosis and impaired ammonia detoxification. HE is a frequent phenomenon in such cats. In contrast to all other forms of HE, this form should not be treated by dietary protein reduction, but instead by forced feeding of amino acid (protein)-rich nutrients. In all species there may be rare congenital errors of metabolism in which one of the enzymes involved in ammonia metabolism fails. These animals may have severe hyperammonemia and HE in the absence of portosystemic shunting and or liver pathology. In contrast to all other forms of HE, these cases are characterized by high plasma ammonia and low bile acid concentrations.

Symptoms

The clinical symptoms of HE are variable. The neurologic signs in the first stage are aspecific and are often only recognized retrospectively, when more specific signs have developed. The subtle first signs are apathy, listlessness, and decreased mental alertness. In more advanced cases, signs include ataxia, circling, head pressing against obstacles, salivation, stupor, and coma. Epilepsy is uncommon but may occur occasionally in association with and subordinate to other signs of HE. Epilepsia alone in the absence of other signs of HE is never caused by HE. the episodic nature of HE is characteristic, with fluctuations between grade 1 and the more advanced stages in the same animal. Usually 1 or a few days of severe signs of HE alternate with more or less normal periods lasting 1 or several weeks. In addition to the neurologic signs of HE, nonneurologic signs related to the underlying disease may be seen. These signs are associated with the underlying chronic liver diseases and may include polyuria, vomiting, diarrhea, weight loss, decreased endurance, and, in case of congenital portosystemic shunt, retarded or insufficient growth and dysuria due to ammonium biurate crystalluria.

The signs of HE are classified according to the schedule in **Table 1**.

Pathogenesis

HE is a biochemical disorder of the metabolism of the brain as result of hepatic dysfunction. Because the integrity of the brain is not involved unless in advanced stages, the

Table 1	
Classification of hepatic encephalopathy signs	
Stage	**Signs**
Stage 1	Apathy, decreased mental alertness, staring glance, unawareness of surroundings
Stage 2	Ataxia, circling, head pressing against obstacles, blindness, salivation
Stage 3	Stupor, severe salivation, completely inactive but can be aroused
Stage 4	Coma, total irresponsiveness
Nonneurologic signs associated with liver diseases causing HE	
All stages	Nonneurologic signs associated with the underlying disease: polyuria/polydipsia, vomiting, dysuria due to ammonium biurate crystals, and so forth
General	Periodic occurrence is typical

neurologic signs are completely reversible if the underlying liver disease can be treated. Essentially, HE is a neurotransmitter dysfunction involving several transmitter systems in the brain. The most important neurotransmitter systems involved are the glutamate, dopamine/noradrenaline, and gamma-aminobutyric acid and benzodiazepine (GABA/BZ) pathways. Only the most important features directly relevant for understanding the clinical findings and treatment of HE are discussed here.

Glutamate neurotransmission and ammonia metabolism

Glutamate is one of the most important excitatory neurotransmitters. It is regulated by the hepatic metabolism of ammonia and deranged in cases of hyperammonemia.[41–43] Ammonia is mainly produced in the intestinal tract, in the colonic lumen by bacterial degradation of nitrogenous compounds (proteins, amines, urea) and by the intermediary metabolism in the small and large intestinal mucosa, which liberates ammonia from glutamine. Much of the intestinal ammonia is resorbed and enters the portal vein. The healthy liver is extremely efficient and has a huge reserve capacity for removing ammonia from the blood. Ammonia is nearly completely removed from the portal blood during one passage through the liver. Therefore, even severe liver dysfunction does not critically affect the liver's capacity to detoxify ammonia, which explains why HE occurs only if the ammonia-rich portal blood bypasses the liver due to (congenital or acquired) portosystemic shunting. One-way for the liver to handle ammonia is conversion into urea by the urea cycle of hepatocytes. Urea formation is concentrated in periportal zone 1 of the liver lobules and occurs exclusively in the liver. Urea is released into the blood and most of it is excreted permanently by the kidneys in the urine. Some urea enters the saliva and recirculates in an enterohepatic cycle. Normally, only a small amount of ammonia escapes this pathway and plasma ammonia concentrations in peripheral blood in healthy animals are low (<45 μmol/L). In most tissues of the body (eg, muscle, brain, and liver) ammonia is further metabolized by enzymatic incorporation into glutamate and glutamine. The end product, glutamine, enters the circulation and becomes metabolized in the intestinal mucosa and the kidneys to liberate ammonia again. Intestinal ammonia enters the cycle again; the kidneys can excrete ammonia produced in the tubular cells into the urine. The definite fate of ammonia in the kidneys depends on the pH of the urine. Normally most of the ammonia is permanently lost in the urine. However, if the kidneys produce alkaline urine, ammonia is reabsorbed and released into the renal veins. The liver itself is one of the most important tissues for glutamine formation, which is concentrated around the central veins. The dual mechanism for ammonia metabolism in the liver is important in pH regulation; in acidosis zone 1 urea synthesis decreases to spare bicarbonate and ammonia detoxification is taken over by zone 3 hepatocytes, which produce glutamine.

In the case of portosystemic shunting, ammonia-containing blood bypasses the liver and systemic concentrations increase. High plasma ammonia levels become toxic to neurons if the defense of the protecting astrocytes becomes overwhelmed. Neuronal cells are separated from the blood by a layer of astrocytes, and substances from the circulation have to pass the astrocytes before they can reach the neurons. Blood ammonia enters the astrocytes, and these cells incorporate it into glutamine by a 2-step reaction catalyzed by glutamine synthetase. Under normal conditions, glutamine diffuses into the adjacent neurons where it is converted into glutamate by glutaminase, and glutamate in the neurons is partly converted into GABA (**Fig. 2**). These 2 compounds are important neurotransmitters. Excitatory glutamate and inhibitory GABA form a finely tuned equilibrium determining the excitability of postsynaptic neurons. In hyperammonemia, the capacity of astrocytic glutamine synthetase becomes exhausted and free ammonia diffuses into neurons. High neuronal ammonia concentrations inhibit glutaminase activity leading to accumulation of glutamine and depletion of the neurotransmitter glutamate. The disturbed glutamate-glutamine ammonia shuttle between astrocytes and neurons is one of the most important factors in the pathogenesis of HE.

To understand the clinical implications of hyperammonemia, it is important to know that only the molecular, nonionized form (NH_3) passes cell membranes, whereas NH_4^+ does not. Intracellularly, both forms have equal metabolic effects. In extra- and intracellular fluid, there is an equilibrium between NH_4^+ and $NH_3 + H^+$ ($pK_a = 9.15$). The ionic form of ammonia is thus pH dependent, with more NH_3 in the case of alkalosis. Alkalosis aggravates the neurotoxic effect of hyperammonemia. Alkalosis is compensated by the formation of alkaline urine from which the nonionized ammonia is readily

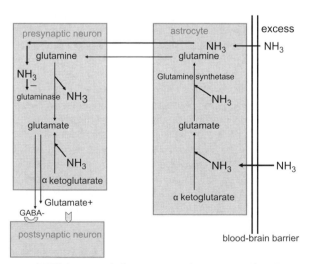

Fig. 2. A major cause of HE is increased plasma ammonia concentration. Excess ammonia is not detoxified by the astrocytes, and reaches the neurons in the brain. High neuronal ammonia inhibits glutaminase, so that the production of the neurotransmitter, glutamate, is decreased and the equilibrium between glutamate and GABA is disturbed causing neural dysfunction.

reabsorbed. This process may change the kidney from an ammonia-excreting organ into an ammonia-generating organ. The most severe form of alkalosis is associated with hypokalemia (**Fig. 3**). Low plasma potassium is replenished by exchange of intracellular potassium against sodium and hydrogen; the hydrogen shift induces extracellular alkalosis and intracellular acidosis. In the case of hypokalemic alkalosis, ammonia penetrates the cells easily but becomes ionized intracellularly and is trapped in the cell. Cells (also neurons) then act as one-way scavengers of this toxic compound.

Conditions of alkalosis and hypokalemia may well occur in chronic liver diseases. Hypokalemia may be caused by diarrhea, insufficient intake due to anorexia or vomiting, and loss due to salivation (a sign of HE). Portal hypertension causing ascites results in hypovolemia, which activates the renine angiotensine aldosterone system and causes renal loss of potassium. Therefore, one should never remove much ascitic fluid from a liver patient; the induced hypokalemic alkalosis may aggravate even subclinical HE to a severe degree within a few hours. Animals with ascites should only be treated with potassium-sparing diuretics (spironolactone).

Catabolic conditions are common in advanced liver disease and may contribute to the onset of HE. Increased breakdown of peripheral proteins liberates glutamine, which has to be metabolized in zone 3 hepatocytes, in the renal tubules, or in the intestinal mucosa, always leading to ammonia formation. The neurotoxic action of ammonia is further enhanced by methane- and ethanethiol formed by the intestinal flora from methionine. Oral administration of methionine should therefore be prevented in HE-related liver disease.

The GABA/BZ receptor complex

Neurotransmission by way of the GABA/BZ receptor system is one of the most important inhibitory systems in the brain. In HE, the GABA tone is abnormally high inducing suppression of normal brain functions.[44,45] The pathophysiology of this mechanism is complex and not fully understood. BZ-related ligands may be formed in the intestinal tract or locally in the brain. The GABA/BZ receptor complex binds many different drugs that are related to GABA, BZ, or barbiturates. Reversal of hepatic coma by injection of benzodiazepine antagonists such as flumazenil has been reported in humans and experimental animals, but there are no long-acting antagonists available for practical use. The increased GABA/BZ tone in animals with HE causes an enhanced effect

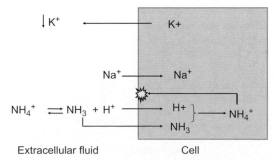

Fig. 3. Hypokalemic alkalosis. Hypokalemia causes a shift of K^+ from the cells to plasma, in exchange with H^+. The resulting extracellular alkalosis and intracellular acidosis cause free entrance of ammonia into the cells, whereby the ammonia is transformed into the ionized form (NH_4^+) which cannot escape, making (neural and other) cells a one-way trap for ammonia.

of sedative and anesthetic drugs. Such drugs should be avoided or at least used with much caution in such animals.

Catecholaminergic neurotransmission

Dopamine and norepinephrine also play a role in the pathogenesis of HE, related to the role of the liver in the metabolism of amino acids. Normally, the liver removes the aromatic amino acids (AAA; tryptophan, tyrosine, and phenylalanine) efficiently from the portal circulation, resulting in low systemic concentrations. The brain needs low concentrations of AAA, which are the precursors of dopamine and norepinephrine. In this catecholamine pathway, the capacity of the enzyme, tyrosine 3-hydroxylase, is rate limiting. The high systemic concentrations of AAA that are associated with portosystemic shunting are being processed by way of alternative metabolic routes, giving rise to alternative products such as octopamine and tyramine. These compounds bind to the catecholamine receptors, but have only weak intrinsic activity. Such false neurotransmitters block the normal catecholamine neurotransmission, which contributes to the pathogenesis of HE (**Fig. 4**). The branched-chain amino acids (BCAA), valine, leucine, and isoleucine, are passively involved in this process. Together with the AAA they form the neutral amino acids that use the same carrier system to enter the brain through the blood-brain barrier. Plasma BCAA levels are reduced in catabolic chronic liver disease because they are used as an alternative energy source in muscles and other tissues. The low BCAA/AAA ratio in plasma gives AAA even easier access to the brain because they experience less competition for the common carrier.

Blockage of central catecholamine receptors may partially explain the polyuria[46,47] that occurs in many dogs with chronic liver disease. Catecholamines inhibit the release of ACTH from the intermediate lobe of the pituitary. In health, the anterior rather than the intermediate pituitary lobe is involved in the pituitary-adrenocortical feedback system. However, in animals with HE the intermediate lobe may change from a silent organ to a secreting organ leading to hyperadrenocorticism. Hyperadrenocorticism is a complicating factor in HE by the induction of catabolism. Like all manifestations of HE, it disappears with the successful treatment of the underlying cause.

Diagnosis of hepatic encephalopathy

Ammonia measurement in plasma is the only practical way to diagnose HE.[41–43,48,49] Due to the incorporation of ammonia into glutamine in many tissues, the arterial

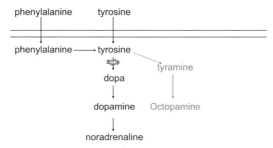

Fig. 4. Dopaminergic blockade. Dopaminergic dysfunction is one factor underlying HE. Excess aromatic amino acids (eg, tyrosine), which are not cleared from the portal blood by the liver, enter the brain. The low capacity for conversion of tyrosine into catecholamines (dopamine, norepinephrine) is overwhelmed, causing production of alternative transmitters, which block the receptor and prevent normal neurotransmission.

concentration may be much higher than that in venous blood. Therefore moderate increments of plasma ammonia may be missed in venous samples. In case of doubt an ammonia tolerance test (ATT, using venous samples) always gives a clear result. This test is sensitive and specific to detect all forms of portosystemic shunting, and is not abnormal in liver diseases without shunting (except fulminant liver failure).

The ATT can best be performed by administering 2 mL/kg of a 5% NH_4Cl solution deep (10–20 cm) rectally by way of a soft catheter.[40] Sampling should be done before and at 20 and 40 min after administration. With this protocol the test gives a semi-quantitative estimate of the degree of shunting. The ATT should not be done in animals in which the basal ammonia value is already high (>150 μmol/L). In other cases, the additional ammonia load is safe and does not increase the signs of HE. In animals without portosystemic shunting, the basal values are within normal limits and they show no increase of ammonia with this test. In cases with high basal values, the ATT is pointless because this already proves HE and portosytemic shunting.

Ammonia should be measured in freshly sampled blood collected in an EDTA coated tube. Samples may be stored in melting ice for 30 minutes. These restrictions are necessary because ammonia is spontaneously liberated from nitrogenic sources such as amino groups in proteins and urea, if kept at room temperature. Ammonia measurement is easy and reliable with sophisticated desktop equipment.[49]

In about half of the dogs with HE, ammonium biurate crystals may be detectable in the urine sediment. If present, this is an indication for conditions causing HE. The dysfunctioning liver not only fails to process ammonia but also converts uric acid into allantoin. Ammonia and uric acid flocculate easily in acidic urine to form crystals and sometimes larger calculi in the renal pelvis or urine bladder. Such animals sometimes present with major symptoms of hematuria or dysuria. The urinary crystals are not diagnostic because they also occur in dogs with congenital defects of uric acid metabolism.

Treatment of hepatic encephalopathy

HE is a complex of symptoms that may occur in a variety of liver diseases. Therefore, it is of importance to diagnose and, if possible, treat the underlying disease. HE disappears immediately on recovery of the causal disease. It is important to give symptomatic support for HE and gain time for treatment of the underlying disease, prepare a patient for surgery, or for life-long support in cases in which liver functions are permanently insufficient.

HE can be treated by feeding a low-level high-quality protein diet.[41–43] The commercial hepatic support diets are more effective than kidney diets. Low protein of high quality reduces intestinal ammonia and aromatic amino acid production. The animal's caloric requirement should always be fulfilled to prevent catabolism. The degree of protein restriction depends on the given indication. In cases of chronic active hepatitis and cirrhosis, the hepatitis can be cured but the fibrosis and often the portosystemic collaterals remain. Such animals need life-long protein restriction at a level just enough to prevent HE, in order not to compromise hepatic protein synthesis, which could induce ascites formation. Cats require about twice as much protein as dogs, but, taking this into account, the recommendations for dogs can be followed.

Oral administration of disaccharides such as lactulose (1–3 ml/kg/day divided into 2 to 3 doses) may be helpful. Lactulose is not absorbed in the small intestines and is degraded into volatile free fatty acids by colonic bacteria.[43] The resulting acidification gives a shift to nonabsorbable ionized ammonia, increased colon motility, and an altered and less ammoniagenic flora. The ammonia formation from glutamine metabolism in the intestinal mucosa may also be reduced by lactulose. In animals with advanced HE, forced intravenous diuresis may be helpful to excrete as much ammonia as possible (100 ml/kg/day). Here too, lactulose and correction of catabolism are essential.

In all cases, conditions that aggravate HE, such as hypovolemia, hypokalemia, and alkalosis, should be corrected and drugs like benzodiazepines, barbiturates, and methionine should be avoided. Glucocorticoid medication, which induces catabolism, should be avoided if possible.

BLOOD COAGULOPATHY IN LIVER DISEASE

Normal blood coagulation occurs by way of the intrinsic and extrinsic pathways; the activity can be measured by the activated partial thromboplastin (cephalin) time and the prothrombin time, respectively. Both pathways unite in the formation of thrombin from prothrombin. All of the clotting factors except the Von Willebrand subtype of factor VIII are synthesized in the liver. The activation of factors II, VII, IX, and X depends on the availability of vitamin K. The equilibrium between activation and inactivation of the coagulation cascade also depends on the activity of several clotting inhibiting proteins, primarily antithrombin III, a low molecular weight protein synthesized in the liver. In addition, the clearance of activated clotting factors and of antithrombin depends on the reticuloendothelial system, which is largely localized in the liver. Some of the clotting factors such as fibrinogen behave as acute phase reactants, and are produced in excess by the hepatocytes in cases of inflammatory or neoplastic disease. The liver may also affect the primary hemostasis by splanchnic pooling of blood and hence prolonged capturing of thrombocytes at their site of degradation, the spleen. This may induce abnormally low thrombocyte counts.

This brief outline of hepatic involvement in hemostasis indicates that the liver may affect blood coagulation in many ways.[50–53] In practice, however, most of them never give rise to clinical manifestations of coagulopathy. Biochemically, the extrinsic and intrinsic clotting times may be slightly prolonged due to insufficient protein synthesis. In chronic complete EBDO, inadequate fat resorption may lead to lack of vitamin K, with the relevant clotting factors not being activated. This does not lead to clinical coagulopathy, but biochemically the prothrombin time may be prolonged.[54,55] Administration of vitamin K normalizes blood clotting in such cases, but is pointless in other liver diseases.

A frequent mechanism behind coagulopathy in hepatobiliary diseases is DIC. This is especially the case if there is diffuse liver cell necrosis, as in several forms of hepatitis, lymphosarcoma, or metastatic tumors. Depending on the activity of the process (the amount of thromboplastin released from necrotic cells per unit of time), coagulopathy may then be subclinical or clinically apparent. Biochemically, low fibrinogen and thrombocyte levels and the presence of fibrin degradation products indicate DIC. For this reason, it is essential to measure blood coagulation, especially plasma fibrinogen, before taking a liver biopsy. Fibrinogen levels less than 50% of the lower reference value are a contraindication for taking a liver biopsy. Once the disease causing the hepatocellular necrosis is being treated, DIC disappears spontaneously. In dogs with chronic hepatitis and DIC, the coagulation usually normalizes within 1 to 2 weeks after starting prednisone medication.

REFERENCES

1. Shafik A. Cholecysto-sphincter inhibitory reflex: identification of a reflex and its role in bile flow in a canine model. J Invest Surg 1998;11:199–205.

2. Abiru H, Sarna SK, Condon RE. Contractile mechanisms of gallbladder filling and emptying in dogs. Gastroenterology 1994;106(6):1652–61.
3. Rothuizen J, de Vries-Chalmers H, van Papendrecht R, et al. Post prandial and cholecystokinin-induced emptying of the gall bladder in dogs. Vet Rec 1990; 126:505–7.
4. Pozo MJ, Salido GM, Madrid JA. Action of cholecystokinin on the dog sphincter of Oddi: influence of anti-cholinergic agents. Arch Int Physiol Biochim 1990;98: 353–60.
5. Westfall SG, Deshpande YG, Kaminski DL. Role of glucagon and insulin in canine bile flow stimulated by endogenous cholecystokinin release. Am J Surg 1989;157: 130–6.
6. Kaminski DL, Deshpande YG, Beinfeld MC. Role of glucagon in cholecystokinin-stimulated bile flow in dogs. Am J Physiol 1988;254:G864–9.
7. Westfall S, Andrus C, Schlarman D, et al. The effect of cholecystokinin-receptor antagonists on cholecystokinin-stimulated bile flow in dogs. Surgery 1991;109: 294–300.
8. Mochinaga N, Sarna SK, Condon RE, et al. Gastroduodenal regulation of common duct bile flow in the dog. Gastroenterology 1988;94:755–61.
9. Center SA. Serum bile acids in companion animal medicine. Vet Clin North Am Small Anim Pract 1993;23(3):625–57.
10. Mahmood I. Interspecies scaling of biliary excreted drugs: a comparison of several methods. J Pharm Sci 2005;94:883–92.
11. Matsumura J, Neri K, Rege RV. Hypercholeresis with cholate infusion in dogs with pigment gallstones. Dig Dis Sci 1996;41:272–81.
12. Ingh TS, Cullen JM, Twedt DC, et al. Morphological classification of biliary disorders of the canine and feline liver. In: WSAVA Liver Standardization Group, editor. WSAVA standards for clinical and histological diagnosis of canine and feline liver diseases. Edinburgh (UK): Churchill Livingstone; 2006. p. 61–76.
13. Tierney S, Nakeeb A, Wong O, et al. Progesterone alters biliary flow dynamics. Ann Surg 1999;229:205–9.
14. van den Ingh TS, Rothuizen J, van Zinnicq Bergman HMS. Destructive cholangiolitis in seven dogs. Vet Q 1988;10:240–5.
15. Rothuizen J, van den Brom WE. Quantitative hepatobiliary scintigraphy as a measure of bile flow in dogs with cholestatic disease. Am J Vet Res 1990;51: 253–6.
16. van den Ingh TS, Rothuizen J, van den Brom WE. Extrahepatic cholestasis in the dog and the differentiation of extrahepatic and intrahepatic cholestasis. Vet Q 1986;150:150–7.
17. Boothe HW, Boothe DM, Komkov A, et al. Use of hepatobiliary scintigraphy in the diagnosis of extrahepatic biliary obstruction in dogs and cats: 25 cases (1982–1989). J Am Vet Med Assoc 1992;201:134–41.
18. Usui R, Ise H, Kitayama O, et al. Bilirubin conjugation and biliary bilirubin excretion after intravenous bilirubin injection in dogs. Tohoku J Exp Med 1991;165:67–77.
19. Rothuizen J, van den Brom WE, Fevery J. The origins and kinetics of bilirubin in healthy dogs, in comparison with man. J Hepatol 1992;15:25–34.
20. Rothuizen J, van den Brom WE, Fevery J. The origins and kinetics of bilirubin in dogs with hepatobiliary and haemolytic diseases. J Hepatol 1992;15:17–24.
21. Rothuizen J, van den Brom WE. Bilirubin metabolism in canine hepatobiliary and haemolytic disease. Vet Q 1987;9:235–40.
22. Rothuizen J, van den Ingh T. Covalently protein-bound bilirubin conjugates in cholestatic disease of dogs. Am J Vet Res 1988;49:702–4.

23. Cullen JM, van den Ingh T, Bunch SE, et al. Morphological classification of circulatory disorders of the canine and feline liver. In: WSAVA Liver Standardization Group, editor. WSAVA standards for clinical and histological diagnosis of canine and feline liver diseases. Edinburgh (UK): Churchill Livingstone; 2006. p. 41–59.
24. Spee B, Penning LC, van den Ingh TS, et al. Regenerative and fibrotic pathways in canine hepatic portosystemic shunt and portal vein hypoplasia, new models for clinical hepatocyte growth factor treatment. Comp Hepatol 2005;4:7–13.
25. Zandvliet MM, Szatmari V, van den Ingh T, et al. Acquired portosystemic shunting in 2 cats secondary to congenital hepatic fibrosis. J Vet Intern Med 2005;19:765–7.
26. Van den Ingh TS, Rothuizen J. Portal hypertension associated with primary hypoplasia of the hepatic portal vein in dogs. Vet Rec 1995;137:424–7.
27. Schermerhorn T, Center SA, Dykes NL, et al. Characterization of hepatoportal microvascular dysplasia in a kindred of cairn terriers. J Vet Intern Med 1996; 10:219–30.
28. Hess PR, Bunch SE. Management of portal hypertension and its consequences. Vet Clin North Am Small Anim Pract 1995;25:461–83.
29. Szatmari V, Rothuizen J, van den Ingh TS, et al. Ultrasonographic findings in dogs with hyperammonemia: 90 cases (2000–2002). J Am Vet Med Assoc 2004;224: 717–27.
30. Szatmari V, Rothuizen J, Voorhout G. Standard planes for ultrasonographic examination of the portal system in dogs. J Am Vet Med Assoc 2004;224:713–6, 698–9.
31. Szatmari V, Rothuizen J. Ultrasonographic identification and characterization of congenital portosystemic shunts and portal hypertensive disorders in dogs and cats. In: WSAVA Liver Standardization Group, editor. WSAVA standards for clinical and histological diagnosis of canine and feline liver diseases. Edinburgh (UK): Churchill Livingstone; 2006. p. 15–40.
32. Schipper L, Spee B, Rothuizen J, et al. Characterisation of 11 beta-hydroxysteroid dehydrogenases in feline kidney and liver. Biochim Biophys Acta 2004; 1688:68–77.
33. Frey FJ. Impaired 11 beta-hydroxysteroid dehydrogenase contributes to renal sodium avidity in cirrhosis: hypothesis or fact? Hepatology 2006;44:795–801.
34. Morris DJ, Souness GW, Latif SA, et al. Effect of chenodeoxycholic acid on 11beta-hydroxysteroid dehydrogenase in various target tissues. Metabolism 2004;53:811–6.
35. Stauffer AT, Rochat MK, Dick B, et al. Chenodeoxycholic acid and deoxycholic acid inhibit 11 beta-hydroxysteroid dehydrogenase type 2 and cause cortisol-induced transcriptional activation of the mineralocorticoid receptor. J Biol Chem 2002;277:26286–92.
36. Quattropani C, Vogt B, Odermatt A, et al. Reduced activity of 11beta-hydroxysteroid dehydrogenase in patients with cholestasis. J Clin Invest 2001;108: 1299–305.
37. Ackermann D, Vogt B, Escher G, et al. Inhibition of 11beta-hydroxysteroid dehydrogenase by bile acids in rats with cirrhosis. Hepatology 1999;30:623–9.
38. Gomez-Sanchez EP, Gomez-Sanchez CE. Central hypertensinogenic effects of glycyrrhizic acid and carbenoxolone. Am J Physiol 1992;263:E1125–30.
39. Gerritzen-Bruing MJ, van den Ingh TS, Rothuizen J. Diagnostic value of fasting plasma ammonia and bile acid concentrations in identification of portosystemic shunting in dogs. J Vet Intern Med 2006;20:13–9.
40. Rothuizen J, van den Ingh TS. Rectal ammonia tolerance test in the evaluation of portal circulation in dogs with liver disease. Res Vet Sci 1982;33:22–5.

41. Maddison JE. Hepatic encephalopathy. Current concepts of the pathogenesis. J Vet Intern Med 1992;6:341–53.
42. Butterworth RF. Hepatic encephalopathy. In: Arias IM, editor. Liver: biology and pathobiology. 3rd edition. New York: Raven Press; 1994. p. 1193–208.
43. Conn HO, Bircher J. Hepatic encephalopathy: management with lactulose and related carbohydrates. East Lansing (MI): Medi-Ed Press; 1988.
44. Jones EA, Schafer DF, Ferenci P, et al. The GABA hypothesis of the pathogenesis of hepatic encephalopathy: current status. Yale J Biol Med 1984;57:301–16.
45. Ferenci P, Riederer P, Jellinger K, et al. Changes in cerebral receptors for gamma aminobutyric acid in patients with hepatic encephalopathy. Liver 1988;8:225–30.
46. Meyer HP, Chamuleau RA, Legemate DA, et al. Effects of a branched-chain amino acid-enriched diet on chronic hepatic encephalopathy in dogs. Metab Brain Dis 1999;14:103–15.
47. Rothuizen J, Biewenga WJ, Mol JA. Chronic glucocorticoid excess and impaired osmoregulation of vasopressin release in dogs with hepatic encephalopathy. Domest Anim Endocrinol 1995;12:13–24.
48. Rothuizen J, van den Ingh TS. Arterial and venous ammonia concentrations in the diagnosis of canine hepato-encephalopathy. Res Vet Sci 1982;33:17–21.
49. Sterczer A, Meyer HP, Boswijk HC, et al. Evaluation of ammonia measurements in dogs with two analysers for use in veterinary practice. Vet Rec 1999;144:523–6.
50. Bigge LA, Brown DJ, Penninck DG. Correlation between coagulation profile findings and bleeding complications after ultrasound-guided biopsies: 434 cases (1993–1996). J Am Anim Hosp Assoc 2001;37:228–33.
51. Léveillé R, Partington BP, Biller DS, et al. Complications after ultrasound-guided biopsy of abdominal structures in dogs and cats: 246 cases (1984–1991). J Am Vet Med Assoc 1993;203:413–5.
52. Badylak S, Dodds WJ, Van Vleet JF. Plasma coagulation factor abnormalities in dogs with naturally occurring hepatic disease. Am J Vet Res 1983;44:2336–40.
53. Badylak S, Van Vleet JF. Alterations of prothrombin time and activated partial thromboplastin time in dogs with hepatic disease. Am J Vet Res 1981;42:2053–6.
54. Plourde V, Gascon-Barré M, Willems B, et al. Severe cholestasis leads to vitamin D depletion without perturbing its C-25 hydroxylation in the dog. Hepatology 1988; 8(6):1577–85.
55. Mount ME, Kim BU, Kass PH. Use of a test for proteins induced by vitamin K absence or antagonism in diagnosis or anticoagulant poisoning in dogs. J Am Vet Med Assoc 2003;222:194–8.

Update on Hepatobiliary Imaging

Lorrie Gaschen, PhD, DVM

KEYWORDS

- Biliary obstruction • Portal scintigraphy
- Computed tomographic angiography
- Portosystemic shunt
- Contrast-enhanced harmonic ultrasound
- Tissue sampling

Ultrasound is the most common modality used to screen animals with suspected liver disease, including vascular anomalies. Contrast-enhanced harmonic ultrasound (CEHU) is a noninvasive and highly accurate method of differentiating benign from malignant hepatic nodules in dogs. Ultrasound-guided tissue sampling has also become a mainstay of hepatic diagnostics. The use of nuclear medicine in the diagnosis of hepatic diseases in dogs and cats has become well established, and alternative imaging modalities, such as CT and MRI, are being validated for their diagnostic roles. These advanced technologies are more widely available than ever before through academic institutions and the rapid growth of specialty clinics offering these diagnostic services.

Radiography is widely available and recommended in dogs and cats suspected of having hepatic disease, but it is an insensitive method.[1] Radiographic contrast studies, such as intravenous cholangiocystography and percutaneous transhepatic cholangiocystography, for the diagnosis of biliary obstruction are described[1,2] but have not come into common use and have mostly been replaced by ultrasonography. Ultrasound is complementary to the abdominal radiograph and provides a more detailed examination of the inner structure of the liver and surrounding organs. This update on hepatobiliary imaging does not include a description of survey and contrast radiographic examinations of the liver or the basic principles of hepatic sonography. The reader is referred to the many complete and excellent sources available on these topics.[1–5]

The World Small Animal Veterinary Association's Liver Standardization Group recently categorized canine and feline hepatic disease into four main groups: parenchymal disease, neoplastic disease, biliary disorders, and vascular disorders.[6] An update on the sonographic, CT and MR Imaging, and nuclear medicine imaging examinations necessary to make diagnoses in each category is provided in this article.

Section of Diagnostic Imaging, Department of Veterinary Clinical Sciences, Louisiana State University, School of Veterinary Medicine, Skip Bertman Drive, Baton Rouge, LA 70803, USA
E-mail address: lgaschen@vetmed.lsu.edu

Vet Clin Small Anim 39 (2009) 439–467
doi:10.1016/j.cvsm.2009.02.005
0195-5616/09/$ – see front matter © 2009 Elsevier Inc. All rights reserved.

vetsmall.theclinics.com

PARENCHYMAL DISEASE

Nonneoplastic canine and feline parenchymal diseases include steroid-induced hepatopathy, hepatic lipidosis, amyloidosis, acute and chronic hepatitis, cirrhosis, necrosis (eg, toxic insult, ischemia, immune mediated), abscessation, granulomas, and metabolic storage diseases.

Sonography

Hepatic parenchymal abnormalities are characterized as being diffuse, focal, or multifocal. Ultrasound is sensitive at detecting focal and multifocal disease but can be poor at detecting diffuse changes. Therefore, a definitive diagnosis should be based on a minimum combination of ultrasound features, blood test results, and tissue sampling results.

An enlarged liver is a subjective finding and may be generalized or focal. Causes include steroid hepatopathy, lipidosis, amyloidosis, diabetes, hepatitis, congestion, neoplasia (eg, lymphoma, histiocytic sarcoma, mast cell tumor), and hepatocellular carcinoma (HCC).[4] In cats, large amounts of falciform fat may be present and can be mistaken for an enlarged liver sonographically (**Fig. 1**). The ventral capsule of the liver can be observed in almost all instances and allows the liver to be visually separated from the falciform fat next to it. In obese cats, the liver may even become hyperechoic to the falciform fat.[7]

Focal or lobar enlargement can be caused by primary or metastatic disease or by cysts, hematomas, abscesses, granulomas, lobar torsion, or thrombosis. In dogs that have portosystemic shunts (PSSs), cirrhosis, or fibrosis, the liver is typically small and the stomach appears closer to the diaphragm than usual.

Diffuse parenchymal disease

Diffuse parenchymal disease generally affects all lobes and may appear normal, isoechoic, or hyperechoic. A large group of hepatic diseases exists that can lead to infiltration of the liver without disruption of the architecture, making disease difficult to detect.[8] These diseases include cholangiohepatitis, diffuse prenodular (early) metastatic carcinoma or sarcoma, round-cell neoplasia (eg, lymphoma, mast cell disease, histiocytic sarcoma), patchy or diffuse fatty infiltration, vacuolar hepatopathy, storage diseases (eg, amyloidosis, copper), toxic hepatopathy, and early degenerative changes associated with micronodular hyperplasia and fibrosis (**Fig. 2**). **Table 1**

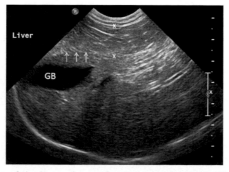

Fig. 1. Ultrasound image of the liver of a cat shows large amounts of falciform fat that can be mistaken for being part of the liver and misdiagnosed as hepatomegaly. Note the hyperechoic interface (*arrows*) marking the separation between the fat and the liver. The liver is of normal size.

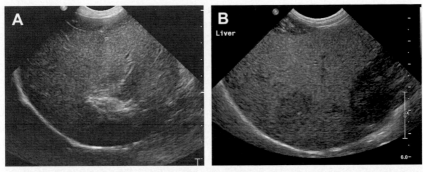

Fig. 2. (*A*) Ultrasound image of a diffusely enlarged canine liver with a mildly hyperechoic but homogeneous echotexture. The histologic diagnosis was amyloidosis. (*B*) Ultrasound image of a dog that was being treated with oral prednisone. The liver is enlarged and diffusely hyperechoic with rounded borders.

summarizes the ultrasound findings in different causes of diffuse liver disease. Mast cell disease affecting the liver may appear sonographically normal or diffusely hyperechoic.[9] The overall accuracy of ultrasound as the sole criterion for discriminating among the categories of diffuse liver disease is less than 40% in dogs and less than 60% in cats.[8] Adding biochemical or hematologic information in the assessment of

Table 1
Sonographic findings that can be seen with diffuse hepatic parenchymal diseases

Disease	Ultrasound Findings				
	Normal	Enlarged	Hyperechoic	Hypoechoic	Mixed Echogenicity
Acute hepatitis	√	√	—	√	—
Chronic hepatitis	—	—	√	—	—
Lipidosis	√	√	√	—	—
Steroid hepatopathy	√	√	√	—	√
Other vacuolar disease	—	√	√	—	—
Amyloidosis	√	√	—	√	√
Copper storage disease	√	—	—	—	—
Toxic insult	√	—	√	—	—
Micronodular hyperplasia	√	—	—	—	—
Fibrosis and cirrhosis	√	—	√	—	√
Metastatic carcinoma	√	√	—	—	√
Small round-cell neoplasia					
Lymphoma	√	√	√	√	√
Mast cell	√	√	√		
Histiocytic sarcoma	√	√	√		
Drug administration					
Phenobarbital	√	√	√		
Superficial necrolytic dermatitis	—	√	—	—	√
Congestion	—	√	—	√	—

the ultrasound findings in diffuse liver disease does not seem to improve accuracy.[8] Therefore, it is generally not possible to make a final diagnosis based on the combination of sonographic findings and biochemical and hematologic data in dogs and cats that have diffuse liver disease. Tissue sampling, preferably for histologic examination, is recommended for a definitive diagnosis in most instances, even if the liver appears sonographically normal.

Vacuolar changes in the liver associated with lipidosis and steroid hepatopathy usually cause hepatomegaly in conjunction with diffuse hyperechogenicity and rounded borders. Another feature that may occur is hyperattenuation of the ultrasound beam. This is seen as a gradual decrease in echogenicity in the far field of the image, which can be so severe that the liver in that region is not visible (**Fig. 3**).

Inflammatory disease can be associated with diffuse hypoechogenicity. If acute hepatitis or cholangiohepatitis is present, the liver may appear to have high contrast—a hypoechoic parenchyma with pronounced hyperechogenicity of the portal vein walls or periportal tissue (**Fig. 4**). Chronic inflammation of the liver usually results in hyperechoic or mixed echogenicities. When fibrosis or cirrhosis is present, the liver may be smaller and hyperechoic. If nodular hyperplasia develops, such as with vacuolar hepatopathy, the liver may appear more heterogeneous and nodular, such as in neoplastic disease. Other differential diagnoses for this pattern include amyloidosis in cats and dogs and hepatocutaneous syndrome in dogs (**Fig. 5**).[10]

Quantitative determination of hepatic echogenicity has been found to be feasible through histogram analysis and may be useful for early detection of diffuse parenchymal disease and for serially evaluating disease progression.[11] In this technique, numeric values from echogenicity data are derived that are related to the mechanical properties of the tissue being evaluated.[12] These numeric values enhance the accuracy for differentiating between tissues with a normal and abnormal ultrasonographic appearance. The analysis is generally done with the on-board computer software of the ultrasound unit or with separate image analysis software. In people, quantitative ultrasonographic methods help to diagnose diffuse abnormalities of the liver and kidney.[13] In cats, quantitative ultrasound video signal analysis has been used to correlate an increase in obesity-related hepatic lipid content to an increase in attenuation and backscatter of the ultrasound signal.[7] This method of image analysis may prove useful for the evaluation of diffuse hepatic parenchymal disease.

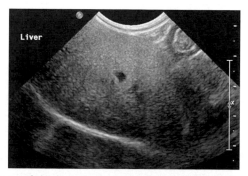

Fig. 3. Ultrasound image of the liver in a cat. The liver is markedly hyperechoic in the near field, with decreasing echogenicity in the far field. This is attributable to the beam attenuation commonly seen in cats that have hepatic lipidosis.

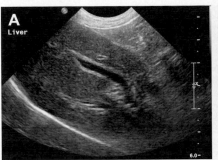
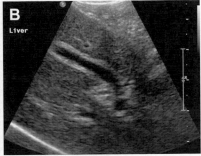

Fig. 4. (A) Ultrasound image in a dog with cholangiohepatitis diagnosed on liver tissue core biopsy samples. The liver is diffusely hypoechoic, and the portal veins seem to stand out more prominently than normal hyperechoic walls. (B) Magnification of the liver shows that the walls appear to be thickened. There are no signs of anechoic tubular structures within or adjacent to the hyperechoic walls; therefore, the intrahepatic bile ducts are likely not dilated in the periphery.

Focal parenchymal disease

Focal or multifocal changes in the liver parenchyma are easier to identify sonographically than diffuse changes.[14] Hypoechoic, hyperechoic, and anechoic lesions are easy to identify because they contrast better with the surrounding parenchyma. For this reason, cystic lesions are the easiest to detect, even when extremely small.

Anechoic cavitary structures in the liver can be attributable to necrosis, neoplasms, or cysts. Cystic structures generally have sharply defined borders, can be round or irregular in shape, and may even contain hyperechoic septa. Acoustic enhancement is typically identified in the far field, distal to the cyst. Causes include congenital cysts, posttraumatic cavitations, biliary pseudocysts, or parasitism. Unfortunately, biliary cystadenomas and cystadenocarcinomas may appear similar.[15]

Hepatic abscessation occurs rarely in small animals and may appear similar to a primary tumor, granuloma, or hematoma because of its highly variable sonographic features (**Fig. 6**).[3,16] It is usually the result of bacterial infections that reach the liver by means of the portal vein or umbilical vein, ascending by means of the bile system or by direct penetration of the liver. It may also occur secondarily to necrosis of hepatic neoplasms and can look similar to parasitic cystic structures. Sonographically, hepatic abscesses may be round to irregular in shape with a hypoechoic central region

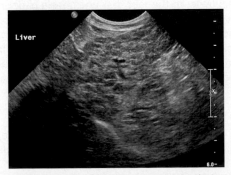

Fig. 5. Ultrasound image of the liver in a dog with chronic skin lesions. The liver has a honeycomb-like echotexture, which is commonly seen in hepatocutaneous syndrome.

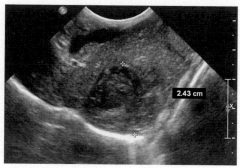

Fig. 6. Hepatic abscess in a cat. A focal heterogeneous space-occupying lesion with an ill-defined central hypoechoic zone is present. Fine-needle aspiration for cytology was diagnostic for an abscess.

or of mixed echogenicity. Reverberation artifacts may be detected because of gas accumulations within the necrotic tissue. Anechoic centers with distal acoustic enhancement also occur. Additional findings, such as regional lymphadenopathy, may be present in hepatic neoplasia and abscessation. Focal peritonitis may be seen with abscessation and may include free peritoneal fluid and focal hyperechoic mesentery.

Granulomatous causes of focal hepatic disease in dogs and cats include mycobacterial infections (*Mycobacterium tuberculosis*, *Blastomyces dermatiditis*, *Cryptococcus neoformans*, *Histoplasma capsulatum*, and *Coccidioides immitis*), migrating larvae, and schistosomiasis.[17] Foreign material is another cause of granuloma formation in the liver. Sonographically, granulomas in dogs and cats may appear as multifocal hyperechoic and well-marginated parenchymal lesions.[3]

Liver lobe torsion occurs in the dog rarely but should be included in the differential diagnosis for acute abdomen or abdominal effusion. The torsion leads to congestion and necrosis of the affected lobe or lobes.[18–22] Typically, the affected lobe appears hypoechoic, and color Doppler shows reduced or no blood flow within the lobe. Thromboembolism would have a similar appearance but is rare in the liver.

CT

There are few reports of the use of CT to assess canine or feline hepatic parenchymal diseases. This is likely attributable to the adequacy of ultrasonography and tissue sampling as diagnostic tests, to the fact that anesthesia is not required, and to CT's higher cost and lack of widespread accessibility. Hepatic volumetry has recently been described in dogs using CT.[23] Liver volume estimations may be helpful in dogs for assessing changes in liver size after shunt attenuation. In human beings, liver volume is used as a prognostic indicator in patients who have liver failure. More work is required in this field to determine its usefulness in veterinary medicine.

NEOPLASTIC DISEASE

Neoplastic disorders in dogs and cats are categorized as hepatocellular (nodular hyperplasia, adenoma, and HCC), cholangiocellular (biliary adenoma, biliary carcinoma, and mixed), hepatic carcinoids, primary vascular and mesenchymal (hemangiosarcoma and myelolipoma), hematopoietic (lymphoma and histiocytic sarcoma), and metastatic.[24]

Sonography

Neoplastic disease of the liver may manifest as diffuse, multifocal, or focal disease sonographically. Diffuse disease is usually attributable to round-cell neoplasia. Lymphoma, histiocytic sarcoma, and mast cell tumor are the most common neoplasms that may lead to diffuse changes and remain sonographically undetectable.[9,25] Diffuse hypoechogenicity or hyperechogenicity and mixed patterns may also occur.[26] Carcinomas tend to be diffusely spread throughout the liver and often lead to a mixed pattern.

Benign hyperplastic nodules are an extremely common finding in dogs, especially in older animals.[3] They are generally not more than 1 cm in diameter. Malignant nodules have a highly varied appearance and size. They may appear as hypoechoic or hyperechoic nodules, target lesions, or heterogeneous ill-defined nodules. **Table 2** summarizes the causes of nodules and compares their differences in echogenicity. Hypoechoic nodules can be attributable to nodular hyperplasia, metastases, lymphoma, histiocytic sarcoma, primary neoplasia, necrosis, hematomas, or abscesses. For this reason, tissue sampling is critical for a definitive diagnosis and the presence of hepatic nodules is not synonymous with malignancy. Hypoechoic lesions with a hyperechoic center are referred to as target lesions and have been associated with metastatic and benign processes (**Fig. 7**).[27,28] Hemangiosarcoma, HCC, carcinoma, insulinomas, bile duct carcinoma, lymphoma, and histiocytic sarcoma are malignant diseases that may cause target lesions. Benign causes of target lesions include nodular hyperplasia, pyogranulomatous hepatitis, chronic active hepatitis, and cirrhosis.[27] Hepatic target lesions have a positive predictive value for malignancy of 74%,[27] which emphasizes the fact that histologic type cannot be predicted by the presence of target lesions.

Biliary cystadenomas and cystadenocarcinomas may appear as loculated cavitary lesions. Hepatic and biliary cysts are benign diseases that may resemble their malignant counterparts.[15]

Contrast-enhanced Harmonic Ultrasound

CEHU is a new diagnostic option that allows assessment of the perfusion patterns of organs in a noninvasive manner. It requires the use of contrast ultrasound probes and on-board software designed to receive and analyze the contrast signals. The underlying principle behind these contrast agents is based on the detection of nonlinearly

Table 2
Nodular hepatic infiltration: causes and sonographic appearance

Disease	Hyperechoic	Hypoechoic	Anechoic	Isoechoic	Mixed	Mineralization	Target Lesions
Hematoma	Early	Late	Possible	—	Late	Possible	—
Cysts	—	—	√	—	√	—	—
Granuloma	√	—	—	—	—	Possible	—
Regenerative nodules	√	Most common	—	√	√	—	Possible
Abscess	√	√	√	—	√	Possible	—
Neoplasia	√	√	—	√	√	Possible	√
Myelolipoma	√	—	—	—	—	—	—

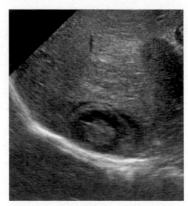

Fig. 7. Ultrasound image shows a target lesion in the liver. Fine-needle aspiration was performed, and the final diagnosis was lymphoma.

scattered signals, which are harmonic frequencies generated when the ultrasound beam interacts with the contrast media. The newest agents range from 2 to 6 μm in diameter and contain air or other gases that enhance the ultrasound signal.[29] Second-generation phospholipid shell microbubbles containing perflutren gas, such as in Definity (Lantheus Medical Imaging, Billerica, Massachussetts), elicit harmonic frequencies at much lower acoustic powers than are necessary to generate tissue harmonics. Thus, the harmonic signal of the microbubbles within the capillary bed and vessels can be separated from the tissue signals. This produces an angiogram and parenchymal perfusion effect.[30] The contrast agents are injected into a peripheral vein in small volumes, and because of their size, they act as blood pool agents ideal for assessing organ perfusion.

Studies describing the characteristics of CEHU of the liver, spleen, and kidney in normal dogs are available.[31–34] Detection and characterization of liver nodules in dogs with CEHU have been the most commonly reported uses of the technique, however. One study investigated hepatic perfusion dynamics of CEHU in normal dogs and in dogs with naturally occurring HCC and metastatic hepatic hemangiosarcoma.[35] Another study describes the ability of CEHU for detecting hepatic metastasis not identified on gray-scale ultrasound imaging in dogs that have hemangiosarcoma.[36]

Contrast-enhanced ultrasound in the liver is divided into two phases: early and late (or sinusoidal phase). The early phase is equivalent to the blood pool phase and is composed of an arterial phase (wash-in) and a portal venous phase (wash-out). In the early phase, the presence, number, distribution, and morphology of lesional vessels can be evaluated.[37] The late phase corresponds to intracellular contrast media uptake in the liver.[38,39] The main difference between benign and malignant lesions is that during the portal and late phases, all benign lesions, except cysts and thrombosed hemangiomas, exhibit isoenhancement or slight hyperenhancement as compared with surrounding liver tissue (**Fig. 8**). Malignant liver lesions exhibit hypoenhancement or do not perfuse at all, because the perfusion of malignant tumors is provided exclusively by arterial vessels and there is no portal venous supply.[40] The sensitivity, specificity, positive predictive value, negative predictive value, and accuracy of CEHU for diagnosing benign versus malignant liver nodules have been shown to be 100%, 94.1%, 93.8%, 100%, and 96.9%, respectively. No complications or morbidity has been reported in veterinary medicine using this agent. CEHU seems

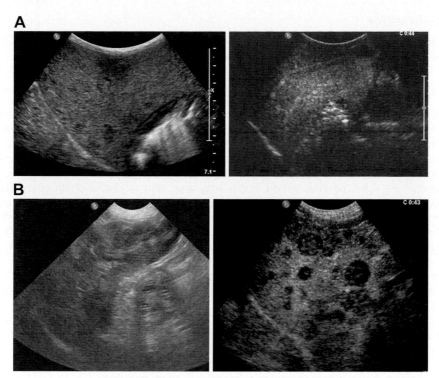

Fig. 8. (A) Non–contrast-enhanced ultrasound image of a canine liver with multifocal hypo-echoic nodules (left). The image on the right was taken 43 seconds after injection of contrast (portal phase) and shows diffuse enhancement of the liver parenchyma. The nodules are not visible and have become isoechoic with the enhanced liver parenchyma. The histologic diagnosis was nodular hyperplasia. (B) Non–contrast-enhanced ultrasound image of a canine liver with multifocal hypoechoic nodules (left). The image on the right was taken 44 seconds after injection of contrast (portal phase). The nodules are not enhanced during the portal phase and appear hypoechoic. The histologic diagnosis was HCC.

to be accurate at discriminating between naturally occurring benign and malignant nodules in the liver of dogs, but its use is currently limited to academic institutions.

CT and MRI

In humans, differentiation between benign and malignant hepatic lesions is often made with CT or MRI, and the diagnosis is determined principally from vascular information obtained as a result of contrast enhancement in the arterial and portal venous phases.[41] One study in dogs with splenic hemangiosarcoma assessed the use of CT compared with sonography for diagnosing hepatic metastases and found no significant difference between the two modalities.[42] In a pilot study examining the specificity of MRI before and after gadolinium contrast administration for benign versus malignant hepatic lesions in dogs, MRI accurately differentiated between benign versus malignant disease in 33 of 35 lesions for a sensitivity and specificity of 100% and 90%, respectively.[43] Both modalities show potential for diagnosing hepatic neoplasia, but more work in the field is required to validate them in dogs and cats.

BILIARY DISEASE

Biliary disease is divided into four main categories: biliary cystic disease, cholestasis, cholangitis, and diseases of the gallbladder (eg, mucoceles, cholecystitis).[15,44]

Sonography

Dogs and cats that have icterus may have cholestasis because of intrahepatic or extrahepatic disease. Extrahepatic cholestasis can be caused by intraluminal obstruction (eg, choleliths, mucinous cystic hyperplasia, sludge) or luminal constriction (eg, neoplasia, inflammation) of the extrahepatic biliary tree or large intrahepatic ducts.[1,44] Intramural biliary obstruction may occur secondary to biliary adenocarcinomas.[1] Enlarged perihilar lymph nodes may also lead to ductal obstruction. The duodenum should be examined for obstruction at the major duodenal papilla, wherein inflammatory and malignant diseases may be another source of obstruction (**Fig. 9**). Dilation of the ducts depends on the degree and duration of the obstruction. The common bile duct can be up to 3 mm in diameter in normal dogs and up to 4 mm in cats.[45,46] Longer standing obstructions (3–7 days) of the common bile duct may lead to dilation of the extrahepatic and intrahepatic ducts.[1,47] These are evident as anechoic tubular structures at the porta hepatis (extrahepatic ducts) or throughout the parenchyma (intrahepatic ducts). Color Doppler ultrasound should be used to assess any anechoic tubular structure in the liver to differentiate biliary from vascular structures. Relief of the obstruction does not lead to an immediate reduction in the diameter of the dilated biliary ducts. The gallbladder may remain a normal size or be enlarged with extrahepatic bile duct obstructions. The presence of a normal-sized gallbladder should not eliminate the possibility of an obstruction.

Neutrophilic cholangitis or cholangiohepatitis is more common in cats than in dogs.[44] It is usually attributable to an ascending infection from the intestinal tract. Lymphocytic cholangiohepatitis is also common in cats. The two diseases cannot be distinguished sonographically in cats and require different treatment protocols. Therefore, it is important to perform tissue sampling to differentiate between the two diseases. Sonographic features of cholangiohepatitis in cats include a diffusely

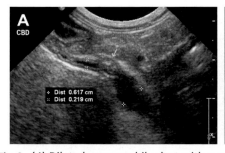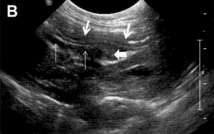

Fig. 9. (*A*) Dilated common bile duct with a small hyperechoic filing defect (*arrow*) close to the entrance of the duodenal papilla. Mild shadowing of this lesion could occasionally be seen during the examination (not shown). Note that the common bile duct is dilated proximal to the obstruction. A cholelith was confirmed during surgery (*B*) Dilated common bile duct proximal to the duodenal papilla in an icteric cat. The papilla (*short wide arrow*) is enlarged and moderately echogenic. The lumen of the bile duct (*thin arrows*) appears narrowed at the thickened and enlarged papilla. Thick arrows show the duodenal wall adjacent to the dilated bile duct. A choledochoduodenostomy was performed, and the papilla was resected. Histologic examination diagnosed a chronic inflammatory polypoid infiltration.

hypoechoic liver parenchyma with prominent-appearing portal vascular structures.[48] Included may be thickening of the gallbladder wall and bile duct wall and increased amounts of sludge in the gallbladder. Intra- and extrahepatic dilation of the biliary tree, in addition to pancreatitis, may also be present. Similar findings to neutrophilic and lymphocytic cholangiohepatitis may occur in liver fluke infestation (family Opisthorchiidae in endemic regions). Because these diseases appear similarly and even may appear normal sonographically, tissue sampling is critical for a diagnosis.[44]

Generalized gallbladder wall thickening can occur with cholecystitis, cholangiohepatitis, hepatitis, free peritoneal fluid, and hypoproteinemia.[3] The wall may appear to have a "double" layer in these instances. Neoplastic disease of the gallbladder wall causing focal thickening is less common than benign cystic hyperplasia of the mucous glands, which appear as broad-based or pedunculated hyperechoic structures. Choleliths can occur, more commonly in dogs, and appear as hyperechoic structures of variable size, number, and shape that produce acoustic shadowing. They are not always associated with clinical signs and can be incidental findings, especially in older dogs. Mineralized and nonmineralized material may also be found in the bile ducts. Sludge balls are accumulations of thick or inspissated bile that can be found in the gallbladder lumen or within the bile duct, wherein they can potentially cause obstruction (**Fig. 10**). They appear as rounded or irregularly shaped structures of moderate echogenicity and can be found to move freely within the gallbladder.

Gallbladder mucoceles occur in dogs and are an important cause of icterus and obstructive disease. They are caused by cystic mucinous hyperplasia leading to increased mucin production that distends the gallbladder and can eventually cause wall necrosis and rupture. Sonographically, they have a varied appearance. The classic finding is that of a "kiwi fruit" pattern of hyperechoic striations radiating from a central point (**Fig. 11**). Variations include irregular or striated nongravitationally dependent content or content with a stellate pattern.[49] They can also lead to

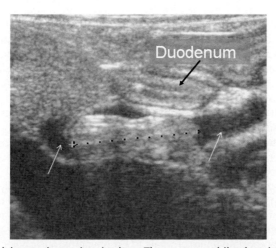

Fig. 10. Ultrasound image in an icteric dog. The common bile duct is dilated. There is a moderately echogenic structure filling its lumen. The structure is homogeneous and does not create acoustic shadowing. During surgery, it could be flushed through the duodenal papilla with saline. The final diagnosis was cholecystitis with a sludge ball causing obstruction of the common bile duct. Thin white arrows show the anechoic lumen of the dilated common bile duct cranial and caudal to the intraluminal structure.

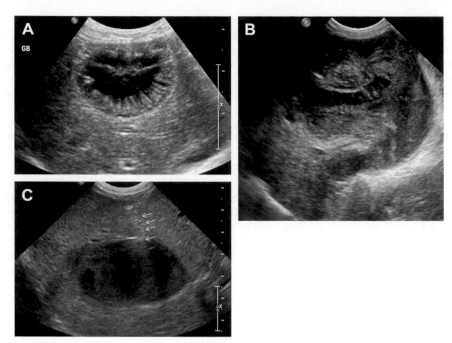

Fig. 11. (A) Ultrasound image of the gallbladder in an icteric dog. The gallbladder contents are hyperechoic and organized into a striated pattern resembling the cut surface of a kiwi fruit. The final diagnosis was gallbladder mucocele. (B) Mucocele in a dog with inspissated material filling the cystic duct and common bile duct and causing obstruction. (C) Mucocele with evidence of free gas. There are hyperechoic foci with dirty shadowing (thin arrows) adjacent to the gallbladder. Gallbladder rupture was diagnosed during surgery.

extrahepatic biliary obstruction.[50–52] Distention of either or both the intrahepatic or extrahepatic bile ducts may be seen. Sonographic signs of rupture include loss of the gallbladder wall continuity, hyperechoic surrounding mesentery, and free peritoneal fluid. The sensitivity of ultrasonography for diagnosing gallbladder rupture is reported as 85%.[51] The therapeutic dilemma as to whether to perform cholecystectomy arises when a gallbladder mucocele is identified sonographically but without signs of rupture. It has been shown that they can transform into an acute clinical condition. A breed predilection has been suggested in cocker spaniels, Shetland sheepdogs and miniature schnauzers.[53] In one study, a significant predisposition for gallbladder mucoceles in Shetland sheepdogs was shown compared with the general hospital population.[53]

Cholecystitis is more frequent in cats than in dogs and is generally associated with bacterial infections. Because bile duct dilation and gallbladder wall changes may not occur in cats that have neutrophilic cholecystitis, bile aspirations for cytologic and bacteriologic examination in cats may be necessary to confirm a suspected diagnosis and administer appropriate antimicrobials.[44] Emphysematous cholecystitis may result from *Escherichia coli and Clostridium perfringens* infections, which are gas-forming bacteria. It has also been associated with diabetes mellitus. Gas within the biliary tract, such as with mineralization, can be identified radiographically and sonographically. Ultrasonographically, it appears as irregular or pinpoint-sized hyperechoic structures that produce reverberation artifacts. The presence of gas in the gallbladder or liver parenchyma should alert the sonographer to the possibility of cholecystitis, cholangitis, choledochitis, or abscess formation.[54]

Endoscopic Retrograde Cholangiopancreatography

Endoscopic retrograde cholangiopancreatography (ERCP) is an established method in people for the diagnosis of biliary obstruction and chronic pancreatitis. It uses a combination of endoscopy and fluoroscopy to image the biliary and pancreatic ducts. Two studies, the first in normal dogs and the second in dogs that had gastrointestinal disease, have been performed using this technique.[55,56] ERCP is technically possible in dogs, and success is influenced by the experience of the investigator. It cannot be performed in dogs with a body weight of 10 kg or less, however. In one study, 20 of 30 dogs that had gastrointestinal disease could be successfully examined using this technique. Abnormal findings compared with a group of healthy dogs included an enlarged common bile duct (n = 2), intraductal filling defects (n = 2), deviated course of the common bile duct (n = 1), and major papilla stenosis (n = 1). In 1 dog with major papilla stenosis and intraductal filling defects, endoscopic-guided sphincterotomy was performed. Endoscopic retrograde pancreatography diagnosed an abnormal course of the accessory pancreatic duct in 2 dogs. Although the use of this technique requires further investigation for validation, the preliminary findings show that changes in the biliary tree of dogs may be going undiagnosed in certain populations of dogs that have gastrointestinal disease.[51,56] The need for special endoscopic equipment, fluoroscopy, and experience likely limits its use to specialty and academic centers.

Nuclear Medical Imaging

Hepatobiliary scintigraphy can be used to quantify liver function, evaluate hepatic morphology, assess biliary tract patency, and diagnosis cholecystitis.[57,58] Cholestasis can also be diagnosed. Hepatic extraction fraction (HEF) is a quantitative measure of hepatocyte function attributable to its ability to extract a radiopharmaceutic agent from the blood by means of a peripheral intravenous injection of ^{99m}Tc-mebrofenin.[59] It also assesses the ability of the hepatocyte to excrete the same radiopharmaceutic agent into the biliary tree. Indications for hepatobiliary scintigraphy include quantification of hepatic function and morphology, biliary tract patency, extrahepatic biliary obstruction, biliary kinetics, gallbladder ejection fraction, and presence of cholecystitis and intra- and extrahepatic cholestasis.[50,57,60]

In healthy animals, the blood pool of the radiopharmaceutic agent clears rapidly, with peak liver radioactivity at 6 to 8 minutes after injection (**Fig. 12A**).[61] It is excreted into the biliary tree with a half-life of 19 minutes. Radioactivity should be observed in the gallbladder and small intestines by 1 hour after injection. For determining patency of the bile duct, hepatobiliary scintigraphy can show abnormalities before they are evident sonographically (**Fig. 12B**).[61] Partial extrahepatic biliary obstruction can still have a normal HEF and prolonged radiopharmaceutic agent clearance from the liver.[61] Complete obstruction is usually associated with a subnormal HEF, prolonged clearance, inability to visualize the biliary tree, and absence of radioactivity in the intestines (**Fig. 12C**).[52,62] Because most studies have been performed in dogs at this time, the role of hepatobiliary scintigraphy in cats is not known.[63]

MRI

Magnetic resonance cholangiopancreatography (MRCP) is a newer technique in human beings for the diagnosis of bile duct obstructions. ERCP is still the "gold standard" for exploration of the biliopancreatic region in people but has a certain

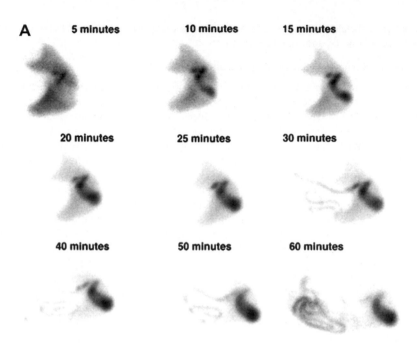

A 5 minutes   10 minutes   15 minutes

20 minutes   25 minutes   30 minutes

40 minutes   50 minutes   60 minutes

Fig. 12. (*A*) Normal hepatobiliary scintigraphy in a dog. These normal images show good liver uptake, early centralization in the gallbladder (already distinct at 10 minutes), normal half-life (the counts in the liver at 20 minutes should be half of the initial counts), and early distinct excretion in the small intestine (already at 30 minutes). (*B*) Hepatobiliary scintigraphy in a dog with liver failure. The liver is enlarged and rounded, and there is a lack of blood pool clearance (by 5 minutes, there should be no heart and body activity), prolonged half-life (the counts at 20 minutes have not dropped to 50% of the initial ones), and alternative route of excretion (kidneys and urinary bladder). The animal is not obstructed, because you can see intestinal activity at 20 hours. (*C*) Example of complete biliary obstruction in a dog; no intestinal activity is seen at 23 hours. This is a chronic obstruction with hepatocellular dysfunction diagnosed by the delayed liver peak uptake, delayed soft tissue clearance and cardiac washout, and alternate excretion by way of the urinary tract. (*Courtesy of* F. Morandi, DVM, MS, Knoxville, TN.)

complication rate associated with it.[64] MRCP is a noninvasive alternative to ERCP and is currently used to diagnose many hepatobiliary and pancreatic diseases in human patients.[65] Although studies in dogs and cats have not been described, this may represent a future imaging modality to diagnose hepatobiliary disease.

VASCULAR DISEASE
Sonography

Venous congestion of the liver occurs secondarily to increased resistance to flow toward the right atrium by way of the vena cava. This may be attributable to a right atrial mass causing obstruction, pericardial effusion, or invasion of the vena cava by a tumor. The hepatic vein is grossly dilated, as is the vena cava, and the liver often becomes enlarged and diffusely hypoechoic. Spectral Doppler analysis of these structures shows high-velocity retrograde flow indicating high resistance to flow toward the right heart (**Fig. 13**). Ascites is usually also present.

B

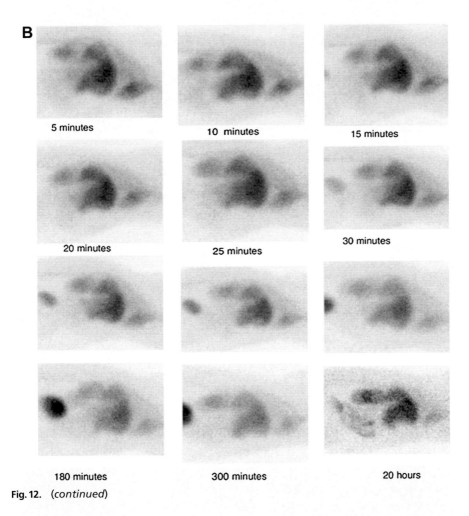

5 minutes   10 minutes   15 minutes

20 minutes   25 minutes   30 minutes

180 minutes   300 minutes   20 hours

Fig. 12. (*continued*)

In veterinary medicine, operative mesenteric portography, splenoportography, and cranial mesenteric angiography are the currently well-established gold standards for depicting the anatomic details of PSSs. The reader is referred to several descriptions of the radiographic techniques.[2,66,67] Congenital PSSs are abnormal vascular communications that allow blood from the intestine to bypass the liver and are classified as intrahepatic or extrahepatic. Diagnostic tests include serum bile acid concentrations, the ammonia tolerance test, portography, ultrasonography, and scintigraphy.[2] Microhepatica is a common sonographic finding in dogs that have extrahepatic PSSs. In addition, bilateral renomegaly, nephrocalcinosis, nephroliths, and cystoliths attributable to urate crystals or stones may be identified. If portal hypertension is present, free fluid may be detected.

The sensitivity and specificity of sonography for the detection of extrahepatic PSSs have been reported to be 80.5% and 66.7%, respectfully.[68] A greater sensitivity of 100% was seen for intrahepatic PSSs alone. In a second study using sonography for the diagnosis of congenital PSSs, results were improved by demonstrating a specificity of 98%, sensitivity of 95%, and accuracy of 94% in 38 dogs.[69,70] Extrahepatic

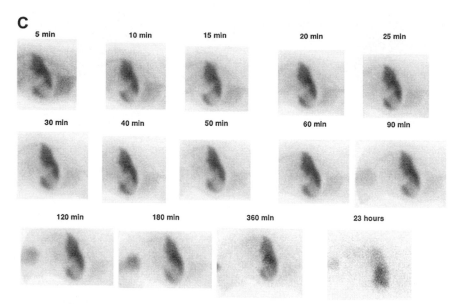

Fig. 12. (*continued*)

shunting vessels generally originate from the portal, splenic, right or left gastric, or gastroepiploic vein in small-breed dogs.[69,71] They are usually identified as tortuous-appearing vessels with hepatofugal flow. The vena cava, portal vein, and porta hepatis region should be scanned from the diaphragm to the level of the kidneys in search of an anomalous branching vessel entering the vena cava or traveling dorsally through the diaphragm toward the azygous vein adjacent to the aorta. Portocaval shunts

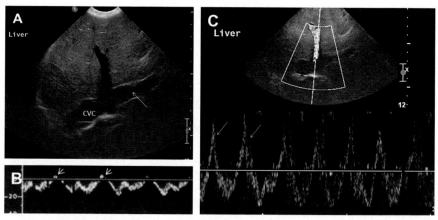

Fig. 13. (*A*) Enlarged liver with distended hepatic veins and vena cava (*arrow*). (*B*) Spectral Doppler image of a normal vena cava waveform. The waveform is triphasic, with low-velocity retrograde flow during atrial systole (*arrows*). (*C*) Spectral Doppler image with sample volume placement in the distended hepatic vein. There is high-velocity flow greater than and less than baseline, indicating high resistance to blood flow toward the vena cava, which also creates higher velocity retrograde flow (*arrows*). The final diagnosis was right heart failure.

terminate in the caudal vena cava, and their entrance is characterized by turbulent flow with color and spectral Doppler (**Fig. 14**). The size of the portal vein cranial to the shunt is generally reduced in diameter.[70,72] A portal vein/aortic ratio of 0.65 or less is predictive for the presence of an extrahepatic shunt, and a value of 0.8 or greater excludes it.[70] If the ratio is 0.80 or greater, other types of disease, such as microvascular dysplasia, intrahepatic shunt, and portal hypertension attributable to chronic liver disease with secondary shunting, could still be present.

CEHU has also been used to determine perfusion patterns in three dogs with congenital extrahepatic solitary PSSs.[73] It was found that with coded harmonic angiographic ultrasound, the size and tortuosity of the hepatic arteries were subjectively increased. Peak perfusion times of dogs with PSSs were significantly shorter (P = .01; 7.0 ± 2.0 seconds) than reported in normal dogs (22.8 ± 6.8 seconds).[73] Contrast-enhanced ultrasound may be a promising new method of detecting increased arterial blood flow that is an indicator of portosystemic shunting in dogs. Increased hepatic arterial blood flow alone does not confirm a diagnosis of PSS, however. Portal hypertension causes reduced portal blood flow to the liver and leads to secondary increased hepatic arterial blood flow in dogs. Prehepatic causes of chronic reduced portal flow and increased hepatic arterial blood flow include portal vein thrombosis and portal vein compression attributable to a regional primary mass or enlarged lymph node. Most of these disease processes would be easily distinguishable with a thorough sonographic examination.

Causes of portal hypertension include chronic liver disease, diffuse nodular regeneration, infiltrative neoplastic disease, congenital hypoplasia of the portal vein, arteriovenous fistula, and portal vein thrombus or extraluminal compression. Ascites is a common clinical feature and sonographic finding, and portal hypertension is suspected when flow is reduced, such as is detected with spectral Doppler. Mean velocities of 10 cm/s or less in the portal vein are highly suspicious for hypertension, but this is not always present.[70] The midabdomen should be screened well for increased size and number of portal vessels, some of which may have a tortuous course.[74,75] These may develop collateral circulation by way of the renal vein and lead to clinical signs of PSS.

Arteriovenous fistulas can be congenital or acquired and create connections between the portal vein and hepatic arteries.[3] The ensuing high pressure overloads

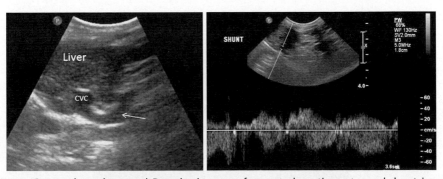

Fig. 14. Gray-scale and spectral Doppler images of an extrahepatic portocaval shunt in an 8-month-old Yorkshire terrier. The left image shows a tortuous vessel between the portal vein and vena cava (CVC) just caudal to the porta hepatis (*arrow*). The right image shows the spectral waveform, with high-velocity bidirectional flow representing turbulence in the shunting vessel.

the venous side, and hypertension occurs. Acquired PSSs form much as with any other cause of portal hypertension, and clinical signs of shunting occur.

Thrombosis of the portal vein occurs with numerous diseases that are associated with the development of coagulopathies (**Fig. 15**). They are recognized sonographically as intraluminal structures of moderate to high echogenicity and the absence of color Doppler signals within the lumen. Thrombosis can be focal or can extend into all branches of the portal venous system and cause acquired shunting.

CT and MRI

Contrast-enhanced helical CT is rapidly becoming one of the more commonly used methods of diagnosing extrahepatic PSSs in dogs at academic institutions and specialty practices. It eliminates the need for invasive radiographic angiography procedures, because the contrast injections can be made by way of a peripheral vein. Other advantages include consistent and superb anatomic depiction of the origin of the anomalous vessel and its entrance into the systemic venous circulation compared with ultrasound, less operator dependency, and the potential for three-dimensional reconstructions.[76,77] It also eliminates variability attributable to operator expertise, such as in sonography. Disadvantages include the need for anesthesia and possible motion artifacts requiring repeat scanning. Furthermore, access to CT scanners may be a limiting factor. Rapid scanning as afforded by helical single- or multislice scanners is critical for the procedure so that it can be done rapidly during a breath-hold procedure. It may be of great value in extra- and intrahepatic shunt detection, when multiple shunts may be present, and in unclear cases after other imaging procedures, such as ultrasonography, contrast radiographic studies, or nuclear medicine portography.

Standard protocols have been established and involve a single scan or dual-phase scanning. In both methods, a test bolus of non-ionic iodinated contrast medium (iodine, ~185 mg/kg of body weight) is made through a cephalic vein catheter to determine maximum opacification of the portal vein after injection of iodinated contrast medium.[78,79] Serial axial images are made at T12 to T13 (approximate location of the porta hepatis) every second or at the shortest interval possible with a given unit's capabilities from the onset of injection in non-helical mode. The time of maximum opacification is used to plan the helical CT study based on time-attenuation graphs. The second injection is performed

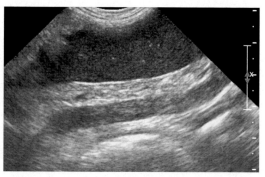

Fig. 15. Portal vein thrombus in a dog with disseminated intravascular coagulation. The main portal vein just caudal to the liver is dilated and filled with heterogeneous material of mixed echogenicities. No flow could be detected around or within the thromboembolic material, and ascites was also present.

with contrast medium (iodine, ~800 mg/kg), and acquisitions are made in helical mode after a breath hold and from the diaphragm to the midlumbar area. Collimation is generally set at a 3- to 5-mm slice thickness with an interval of approximately half of that.

In dual-phase computed tomographic angiography of the portal and hepatic vasculature, the test injection for timing is performed as for the single phase, but the patient is scanned twice during the second injection: first, from caudal to cranial to observe the hepatic arterial phase and then from cranial to caudal to observe the portal phase.[79] Portal phase scanning is initiated shortly before the time of its peak enhancement based on the initial injection for determining maximal enhancement time. Median time delay for peak aortic enhancement has been shown to be 12.0 seconds after injection and 33.0 seconds after injection for the portal vein. There is an approximate 5-second delay between peak contrast attenuation in the aorta and portal vein. The portal phase of the scan is initiated with a median time of 28 seconds (range: 27.7–34.9 seconds) after injection in the cranial-to-caudal direction from the diaphragm to L5. This minimally invasive method allows complete evaluation of the hepatic arterial, venous, and portal vasculature with exquisite anatomic detail and has the potential to diagnose extrahepatic and intrahepatic shunts, arterioportal fistulas, and portal thromboembolic disease (**Fig. 16**).

A technique for CT splenic portography has recently been described.[80] A 20- to 22-gauge 1.5-in needle is placed in the splenic parenchyma under CT guidance. A preloaded extension set is attached, and iodinated contrast media is administered at a concentration of iodine, 175 mg/mL. One milliliter is administered as a rapid bolus, followed by a steady manual injection of 2 mL over 5 seconds. The CT acquisition is started at the time of contrast medium injection, and images are acquired from the level of the fifth lumbar vertebra to the cranial aspect of the diaphragm. Because hand injections are used during acquisition, radiation protection procedures are important to follow and are a disadvantage of not using automatic injectors with remote activated devices. The degree of opacification of the splenic vein in all locations, and that of the main portal vein, is significantly higher in transsplenic computed tomographic portography compared with computed tomographic angiography.[80] Benefits include the simple technique, low dosage of contrast medium required compared with conventional computed tomographic angiography, and much better opacification of the portal system. Disadvantages include inconsistent depiction of the intrahepatic portal vasculature and parenchymal opacification attributable to streamlining and presence of streak artifacts in addition to radiation protection. Streamlining has also been described as a cause for nonuniform distribution of radiopharmaceutic agents during per-rectal scintigraphy in dogs. These artifacts lead to preferential ventrolateral contrast medium distribution into the left divisional branch. In addition, preferential left and ventral streamlining allows fewer arborizations to be detected from the right divisional branch compared with the left divisional branch. Despite these limitations, contrast medium should preferentially distribute into the shunting vessel because of hepatofugal blood flow; further studies require testing this hypothesis in dogs that have PSSs.[80]

MRI has only rarely been reported for diagnosing PSSs in dogs. Magnetic resonance angiography (MRA) is a described method for assessment of the portal vein.[81] MRA is a noninvasive technique that provides functional representation of blood vessels without the use of contrast. Two techniques, time-of-flight and phase contrast, can be used. At this time, MRA has not been well validated in veterinary medicine for diagnosis of PSSs and requires further investigation.

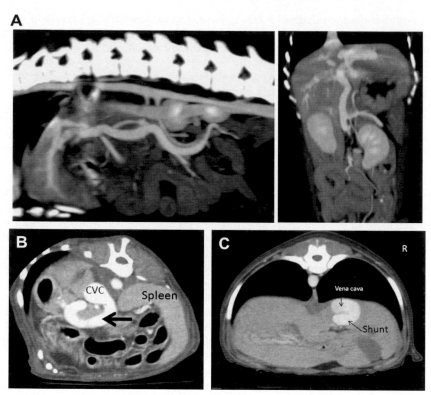

Fig. 16. (A) Reconstructed postcontrast CT images of a normal portal vein and branches in a Yorkshire terrier. The sagittal (*left*) and dorsal (*right*) planes are shown. The portal vein is large and branches out in a normal pattern into the liver, which shows diffuse enhancement of intrahepatic portal vein branches. (B) Single-phase helical scan shows an extrahepatic shunting vessel (*arrow*). CVC, caudal vena cava. (*Courtesy of* G. Seiler, Dr.med.vet., Philadelphia, PA.) (C) Dual-phase helical scan shows an intrahepatic right divisional shunt. (*Courtesy of* A. Zwingenberger, DVM, Davis, CA.)

Nuclear Medical Imaging

Nuclear portal scintigraphy is a highly sensitive and minimally invasive screening method for diagnosing the presence or absence of a PSS. It does require certification for the use of radioisotopes and specialized equipment and software programs, however. Patients must also be held in isolation, generally overnight, until their radiation levels are low enough to return home or to have the shunt surgically repaired. Nuclear portal scintigraphy allows shunt fractions to be assessed before and after surgery to monitor the degree of closure of the shunt but does not allow exact anatomic descriptions to be made.

Per-rectal portal scintigraphy (PRPS) methods are performed by administering sodium ^{99m}Tc-pertechnetate into the colon. In dogs, a dose of 5 to 20 mCi is used, whereas a dose of 5 to 10 mCi is administered in cats.[82] The radionuclide is absorbed into the portal venous system in the distal colon, and it is then transported to the liver by way of the portal vein. After administration, dynamic acquisitions at one frame per second for 2 to 3 minutes are performed with the patient in right lateral recumbency using a 128 × 128 matrix and low-energy general-purpose collimator. The start of acquisition is timed with the administration of the radionuclide into the distal colon.

Radioactive markers are placed ventral to the xyphoid and apex of the heart on the gamma camera for later analysis of heart and liver location.[82,83] A region of interest (ROI) is drawn over the liver and heart regions, and calculations of the time-intensity curves of the heart and liver are performed with dedicated software and provide an objective means of assessing the shunt fraction (**Fig. 17**). Disadvantages include lack of sufficient anatomic detail of the shunting vessel. Radiation safety concerns prevent surgical intervention after the procedure, and there is a need for sedation. Disadvantages of the technique include difficulty in identifying the liver and heart in small patients or those with poor colonic absorption or false-positive results because of rectal vein absorption of pertechnetate, which enters the systemic circulation and heart before the liver.

Positive findings for a PSS are based on the arrival of the radiopharmaceutic agent into the heart before the liver based on the time-activity curves of the ROIs drawn over the heart and liver regions. In abnormal animals, the liver is seen 10 to 12 seconds after heart activity is seen. Shunt fraction is based on the total heart counts between 8 and 16 seconds after injection divided by the total counts within the heart and liver ROIs.[83] Dogs that have microvascular dysplasia have a normal study, with the radionuclide entering the liver before the heart. In acquired shunts, the small vessels in the middle to caudal abdomen are often difficult to visualize. Nondiagnostic or poor-quality scans have been reported at rates of 3.6% and 35.8%, respectively.[82] These can result from poor absorption of the radionuclide, rectal administration, poor visualization of the heart and liver, fluid or diarrhea in the colon at the time of administration, or previous administration of colonic cleansing agents (oral or rectal).

Nonuniform distribution of the radionuclide attributable to portal streamlining may also cause difficulties in interpretation of the study if one is not aware of this normal phenomenon.[84] Streamlining is a cause of nonuniform distribution of the radionuclide during portal scintigraphy within discrete channels of portal blood flow, such that they may distribute the radionuclide preferentially into one or more of the branches of the portal vein, giving a nonuniform appearance of the activity in the liver.

Transsplenic portal scintigraphy is a newly described alternative to PRPS. Compared with PRPS, it provides higher count density, consistent nuclear venograms of the splenic and portal vein, and significantly decreased radiation exposures

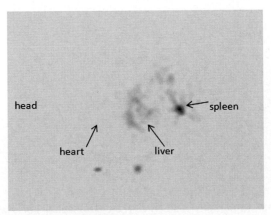

Fig. 17. Normal splenic portal scintigraphy in a dog. This composite image was taken 4 seconds after injection of pertechnetate (2mCi) into the spleen. The activity in the liver ROI appears 12 seconds before the activity of the heart.

(**Fig. 18**). Transsplenic portal scintigraphy was found to be 100% sensitive and specific for diagnosis of congenital portosystemic shunt and significantly ($P<.05$) more likely than PRPS to detect shunt number and termination.[85] The technique is simple to perform and requires a lower dose of sodium ^{99m}Tc-pertechnetate. A small volume (0.2 mL) of 2 mCi is injected by means of a 22-gauge 1.5-in needle into the splenic parenchyma using ultrasound guidance, and dynamic acquisitions at four frames per second for 3 minutes are acquired with the patient in right lateral recumbency.[86] The acquisition must be started immediately before injection because of the more rapid nature of transport to the liver and heart compared with per-rectal methods. In normal animals, the radionuclide passes from the splenic vein to the left gastric vein and then into the main portal vein. One disadvantage of the splenic portal scintigraphic procedure is that shunts entering the vena cava caudal to the splenic vein could be missed.[86] In the future, we may see the use of ^{99m}Tc-mebrofenin applied, which should allow identification of the shunt and assessment of liver function.[82]

TISSUE SAMPLING

A definitive diagnosis of most liver diseases depends on cytology and histopathology and, in some instances, bacteriology. Percutaneous ultrasound-guided aspiration and biopsy of the liver have become routine in dogs and cats. Patient preparation should include fasting for 12 hours before the ultrasound examination and tissue sampling. A coagulation profile is an important screening test before tissue core biopsy procedures, especially considering that several coagulopathies may occur with liver disease. Prothrombin time, activated thromboplastin time, and a platelet count are the minimum tests that should be performed for screening purposes. Cats and dogs should preferably be placed under general anesthesia for biopsy of the liver. Sedation with local anesthesia can also be performed on a case-by-case basis. Depending on the temperament of the dog or cat, sedation may or may not be required for fine-needle aspirations.

For diffuse lesions, the most accessible region of the liver should be sampled. Aspirations are preferred for small (<1 cm)-sized lesions, cystic structures, or lesions with high vascularity.[87] Furthermore, fine-needle aspirations are recommended in diffuse

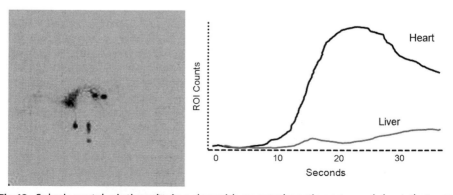

Fig. 18. Splenic portal scintigraphy in a dog with an extrahepatic portocaval shunt that was confirmed and repaired surgically. The graph shows activity in the heart ROI appearing 12 seconds before that of the liver, which shows little activity over time. This is diagnostic for a PSS.

lesions in which lymphoma or mast cell tumors are suspected because they generally result in diagnostic samples. Tissue core biopsies are generally recommended in most diffuse liver diseases and larger masses (>2 cm). Generally, if a tissue core biopsy is being made, fine-needle aspirations can be made at the same time, because a "preliminary" cytologic diagnosis can be made while waiting for the histopathology results, which generally take at least 24 hours or more to obtain. Touch preparations of the core biopsy sample can also be made for cytologic analysis.[87]

A sector, curved, or linear-array transducer may be used depending on where the lesion to be sampled is located.[87] A superficial lesion can be well visualized with a high-frequency curved or linear array, whereas deeper lesions may require a low-frequency curved-array or sector format (phased-array) transducers. Tissue core needles with a 2-cm long sample notch should be used and are typically 16 or 18 gauge depending on the size of the animal. For medium- to large-sized dogs, 16-gauge needles are recommended, whereas 18-gauge needles are best for smaller dog and cats. Manual, semiautomatic, and automatic (spring-loaded gun) can be used depending on the personal preferences of the sonographer. Fine-needle aspiration is generally performed with 20- to 22-gauge 1.5-in needles for diffuse lesions, small nodules, and cystic or highly vascular structures.

After sedation or anesthesia, the skin should be clipped and cleaned in a routine sterile manner. The ultrasound probes should be covered with a sterile sleeve. For focal lesions (masses and nodules), sampling from the lesion and its periphery is recommended. Central lesional aspirations may only yield necrosis, especially with HCC. Two to three samples should be made from the affected region of the liver.

Free-handed or guided techniques can be used. In both situations, the needle should enter the plane of the ultrasound beam so that it can be visualized along its entire length. For free-handed aspirations, the needle is attached to a 3- or 6-mL syringe with the plunger pulled back before needle insertion or with a small amount of negative pressure during the aspiration. The tip of the needle is advanced under the skin and located by observing the ultrasound image and by making small "in and out" excursions under the skin. The needle is advanced until its tip is in the desired location, and in and out excursions are made within the lesion a few times, followed by removal of the needle. This is generally repeated two to three times to ensure adequate sampling for cytology. Nonaspiration techniques result in less blood dilution of the cytologic sample.

Free-handed and guided biopsy procedures may be used to obtain tissue core biopsies of the liver. Needle guidance systems are available for most ultrasound probes but are difficult to use on superficial hepatic lesions. The biopsy guide is attached to the transducer housing once the transducer is cleaned and covered with a sterile covering, such as a fitted sleeve or surgical glove. A number 11 blade should be used to make a small stab incision in the skin where the biopsy needle is to enter. This position is predetermined during the initial scanning of the liver. The needle is advanced as for fine-needle aspirations to the desired depth, taking into account the depth of the lesion and depth of penetration of the biopsy needle.[87] Once the sample is taken, it should be gently removed from the sample notch and placed in formalin.

Complications of ultrasound-guided tissue sampling are rare.[87] After any tissue sampling procedure, the patient should be monitored directly with ultrasound for the presence of free fluid. Small amounts of free fluid at the sampling site are not uncommon with tissue core biopsies but are less frequent with fine-needle aspirations. Small amounts of fluid are generally self-limiting when the patient's coagulation status is normal.

Ultrasound-guided percutaneous cholecystocentesis can be performed safely and can provide valuable cytologic and bacteriologic information to make a diagnosis of cholecystitis and apply appropriate antimicrobial therapy.[88] The best patient position and access to the gallbladder directly through its wall or transhepatically are determined, and this is generally a fairly simple procedure to carry out. One method is to have the patient sedated and in dorsal recumbency, with the skin of the cranioventral abdomen prepared aseptically. A 22-gauge 1.5-in needle connected to a 12-mL syringe should be guided sonographically to the gallbladder using a free-hand method. A biopsy guide can be used if preferred by the sonographer. The gallbladder must not be emptied, and depending on its size, this procedure may not be possible.

ACKNOWLEDGMENTS

The author acknowledges David Schur for his efforts in researching the current literature, creating reference databases, and collecting journal articles in preparation for the writing of this article.

REFERENCES

1. Smith SA, Biller DS, Kraft SL, et al. Diagnostic imaging of biliary obstruction. Compendium on Continuing Education for the Practicing Veterinarian 1998; 20(11):1225–34.
2. Partington BP, Biller DS. Hepatic imaging with radiology and ultrasound. Vet Clin North Am Small Anim Pract 1995;25(2):305–35.
3. d'Anjou MA. Liver. In: Penninck D, d'Anjou MA, editors. Atlas of small animal ultrasonography. Ames (IA): Blackwell Publishing Professional; 2008. p. 217–62.
4. Larson MM. The liver and spleen. In: Thrall DE, editor. Textbook of veterinary diagnostic radiology. 5th edition. St. Louis (MO): Saunders Elsevier; 2007. p. 667–93.
5. Nyland TG, Mattoon JS, Wisner ER, et al. Ultrasonography of the liver. In: Nyland TG, Mattoon JS, editors. Small animal diagnostic ultrasound. 2nd edition. Philadelphia: WB Saunders Co.; 2002. p. 93–127.
6. Rothuizen J. Introduction—background, aims and methods. In: Rothuizen J, Bunch SE, Charles JA, et al. editors. Standards for clinical and histological diagnosis of canine and feline liver diseases—WSAVA Liver Standardization Group. Philadelphia: Saunders Elsevier; 2006. p. 5–14.
7. Nicoll RG, Jackson MW, Knipp BS, et al. Quantitative ultrasonography of the liver in cats during obesity induction and dietary restriction. Res Vet Sci 1998;64(1): 1–6.
8. Feeney DA, Anderson KL, Ziegler LE, et al. Statistical relevance of ultrasonographic criteria in the assessment of diffuse liver disease in dogs and cats. Am J Vet Res 2008;69(2):212–21.
9. Sato AF, Solano M. Ultrasonographic findings in abdominal mast cell disease: a retrospective study of 19 patients. Vet Radiol Ultrasound 2004;45(1):51–7.
10. Beatty JA, Barrs VR, Martin PA, et al. Spontaneous hepatic rupture in six cats with systemic amyloidosis. J Small Anim Pract 2002;43(8):355–63.
11. Drost WT, Henry GA, Meinkoth JH, et al. Quantification of hepatic and renal cortical echogenicity in clinically normal cats. Am J Vet Res 2000;61(9): 1016–20.
12. Robinson DE, Gill RW, Kossoff G. Quantitative sonography. Ultrasound Med Biol 1986;12(7):555–65.

13. Osawa H, Mori Y. Sonographic diagnosis of fatty liver using a histogram technique that compares liver and renal cortical echo amplitudes. J Clin Ultrasound 1996;24(1):25–9.

14. Nyman HT, Kristensen AT, Flagstad A, et al. A review of the sonographic assessment of tumor metastases in liver and superficial lymph nodes. Vet Radiol Ultrasound 2004;45(5):438–48.

15. Nyland TG, Koblik PD, Tellyer SE. Ultrasonographic evaluation of biliary cystadenomas in cats. Vet Radiol Ultrasound 1999;40(3):300–6.

16. Schwarz LA, Penninck DG, Leveille-Webster C. Hepatic abscesses in 13 dogs: a review of the ultrasonographic findings, clinical data and therapeutic options. Vet Radiol Ultrasound 1998;39(4):357–65.

17. Van Winkle T, Cullen JM, van den Ingh T, et al. Morphological classification of parenchymal disorders of the canine and feline liver. In: Rothuizen J, Bunch SE, Charles JA, et al. editors. Standards for clinical and histological diagnosis of canine and feline liver diseases—WSAVA Liver Standardization Group. Philadelphia: Saunders Elsevier; 2006. p. 103–16.

18. Scheck MG. Liver lobe torsion in a dog. Can Vet J 2007;48(4):423–5.

19. von Pfeil DJ, Jutkowitz LA, Hauptman J. Left lateral and left middle liver lobe torsion in a Saint Bernard puppy. J Am Anim Hosp Assoc 2006;42(5):381–5.

20. Schwartz SG, Mitchell SL, Keating JH, et al. Liver lobe torsion in dogs: 13 cases (1995–2004). J Am Vet Med Assoc 2006;228(2):242–7.

21. Sonnenfield JM, Armbrust LJ, Radlinsky MA, et al. Radiographic and ultrasonographic findings of liver lobe torsion in a dog. Vet Radiol Ultrasound 2001; 42(4):344–6.

22. Downs MO, Miller MA, Cross AR, et al. Liver lobe torsion and liver abscess in a dog. J Am Vet Med Assoc 1998;212(5):678–80.

23. Stieger SM, Zwingenberger A, Pollard RE, et al. Hepatic volume estimation using quantitative computed tomography in dogs with portosystemic shunts. Vet Radiol Ultrasound 2007;48(5):409–13.

24. Charles JA, Cullen JM, van den Ingh T, et al. Morphological classification of neoplastic disorders of the canine and feline liver. In: Rothuizen J, Bunch SE, Charles JA, et al, editors. Standards for clinical and histological diagnosis of canine and feline liver diseases—WSAVA Liver Standardization Group. Philadelphia: Saunders Elsevier; 2006. p. 117–24.

25. Cruz A, Wrigley R, Powers B. Sonographic features of histiocytic neoplasms in the canine abdomen. Vet Radiol Ultrasound 2004;45(6):554–8.

26. Whiteley MB, Feeney DA, Whiteley LO, et al. Ultrasonographic appearance of primary and metastatic canine hepatic tumors. a review of 48 cases. J Ultrasound Med 1989;8(11):621–30.

27. Cuccovillo A, Lamb CR. Cellular features of sonographic target lesions of the liver and spleen in 21 dogs and a cat. Vet Radiol Ultrasound 2002;43(3): 275–8.

28. O'Brien RT, Iani M, Matheson J, et al. Contrast harmonic ultrasound of spontaneous liver nodules in 32 dogs. Vet Radiol Ultrasound 2004;45(6):547–53.

29. Albrecht T, Hoffmann CW, Schettler S, et al. B-Mode enhancement at phase-inversion US with air-based microbubble contrast agent: initial experience in humans. Radiology 2000;216(1):273–8.

30. Cosgrove D. Ultrasound contrast agents: an overview. Eur J Radiol 2006;60(3): 324–30.

31. Ziegler LE, O'Brien RT, Waller KR, et al. Quantitative contrast harmonic ultrasound imaging of normal canine liver. Vet Radiol Ultrasound 2003;44(4):451–4.

32. Nyman HT, Kristensen AT, Kjelgaard-Hansen M, et al. Contrast-enhanced ultrasonography in normal canine liver: evaluation of imaging and safety parameters. Vet Radiol Ultrasound 2005;46(3):243–50.
33. Ohlerth S, Ruefli E, Poirier V, et al. Contrast harmonic imaging of the normal canine spleen. Vet Radiol Ultrasound 2007;48(5):451–6.
34. Waller KR, O'Brien RT, Zagzebski JA. Quantitative contrast ultrasound analysis of renal perfusion in normal dogs. Vet Radiol Ultrasound 2007;48(4):373–7.
35. Kenji K. Contrast harmonic imaging of canine hepatic tumors. J Vet Med Sci 2006;68(5):433–8.
36. O'Brien RT. Improved detection of metastatic hepatic hemangiosarcoma nodules with contrast ultrasound in three dogs. Vet Radiol Ultrasound 2007; 48(2):146–8.
37. Wilson SR, Burns PN, Muradali D, et al. Harmonic hepatic US with microbubble contrast agent: initial experience showing improved characterization of hemangioma, hepatocellular carcinoma, and metastasis. Radiology 2000;215(1):153–61.
38. Rettenbacher T. Focal liver lesions: role of contrast-enhanced ultrasound. Eur J Radiol 2007;64(2):173–82.
39. Ohlerth S, O'Brien RT. Contrast ultrasound: general principles and veterinary clinical applications. Vet J 2007;174(3):501–12.
40. Bolondi L, Correas JM, Lencioni R, et al. New perspectives for the use of contrast-enhanced liver ultrasound in clinical practice. Dig Liver Dis 2007; 39(2):187–95.
41. Burns PN, Wilson SR. Focal liver masses: enhancement patterns on contrast-enhanced images: concordance of US scans with CT scans and MR images. Radiology 2006;162–74.
42. Irausquin RA, Scavelli TD, Corti L, et al. Comparative evaluation of the liver in dogs with a splenic mass by using ultrasonography and contrast-enhanced computed tomography. Can Vet J 2008;49(1):46–52.
43. Clifford CA, Pretorius ES, Weisse C, et al. Magnetic resonance imaging of focal splenic and hepatic lesions in the dog. J Vet Intern Med 2004;18(3):330–8.
44. van den Ingh T, Cullen JM, Twedt DC, et al. Morphological classification of biliary disorders of the canine and feline liver. In: Rothuizen J, Bunch SE, Charles JA, et al. editors. Standards for clinical and histological diagnosis of canine and feline liver diseases—WSAVA Liver Standardization Group. Philadelphia: Saunders Elsevier; 2006. p. 61–76.
45. Zeman RK, Taylor KJ, Rosenfield AT, et al. Acute experimental biliary obstruction in the dog: sonographic findings and clinical implications. AJR Am J Roentgenol 1981;136(5):965–7.
46. Leveille R, Biller DS, Shiroma JT. Sonographic evaluation of the common bile duct in cats. J Vet Intern Med 1996;10(5):296–9.
47. Nyland TG, Gillett NA. Sonographic evaluation of extrahepatic bile duct ligation in the dog. Vet Radiol 1982;23:252–60.
48. Newell SM, Selcer BA, Girard E, et al. Correlations between ultrasonographic findings and specific hepatic diseases in cats: 72 cases (1985–1997). J Am Vet Med Assoc 1998;213(1):94–8.
49. Besso JG, Wrigley RH, Gliatto JM, et al. Ultrasonographic appearance and clinical findings in 14 dogs with gallbladder mucocele. Vet Radiol Ultrasound 2000; 41(3):261–71.
50. Pike FS, Berg J, King NW, et al. Gallbladder mucocele causing biliary obstruction in two dogs: ultrasonographic, scintigraphic, and pathological findings. J Am Vet Med Assoc 2004;224(10):1615–22.

51. Pike FS, Berg J, King NW, et al. Gallbladder mucocele in dogs: 30 cases (2000–2002). J Am Vet Med Assoc 2004;224(10):1615–22.
52. Newell SM, Selcer BA, Mahaffey MB, et al. Gallbladder mucocele causing biliary obstruction in two dogs: ultrasonographic, scintigraphic, and pathological findings. J Am Anim Hosp Assoc 1995;31(6):467–72.
53. Aguirre AL, Center SA, Randolph JE, et al. Gallbladder disease in Shetland Sheepdogs: 38 cases (1995–2005). J Am Vet Med Assoc 2007;231(1):79–88.
54. Mehler SJ, Bennett RA. Canine extrahepatic biliary tract disease and surgery. Compendium on Continuing Education for the Practicing Veterinarian 2006; 28(4):302–14.
55. Spillmann T, Happonen I, Kähkönen T, et al. Endoscopic retrograde cholangiopancreatography in healthy Beagles. Vet Radiol Ultrasound 2005;46(2): 97–104.
56. Spillmann T, Schnell-Kretschmer H, Dick M, et al. Endoscopic retrograde cholangio-pancreatography in dogs with chronic gastrointestinal problems. Vet Radiol Ultrasound 2005;46(4):293–9.
57. Daniel GB. Hepatic scintigraphy. In: Daniel GB, Berry CR, editors. Textbook of veterinary nuclear medicine. 2nd edition. Knoxville (TN): American College of Veterinary Radiology; 2006. p. 208–28.
58. van den Brom WE, Rothuizen J. Quantitation of the hepatobiliary dynamics in clinically normal dogs by use of 99mTc-iminodiacetate excretory scintigraphy. Am J Vet Res 1990;51(2):249–52.
59. Bahr A, Daniel GB, DeNovo R, et al. Quantitative hepatobiliary scintigraphy with deconvolutional analysis for the measurement of hepatic function in dogs. Vet Radiol Ultrasound 1996;37(3):214–20.
60. Rothuizen J, van den Brom WE. Quantitative hepatobiliary scintigraphy as a measure of bile flow in dogs with cholestatic disease. Am J Vet Res 1990; 51(2):253–6.
61. Head LL, Daniel GB. Correlation between hepatobiliary scintigraphy and surgery or postmortem examination findings in dogs and cats with extrahepatic biliary obstruction, partial obstruction, or patency of the biliary system: 18 cases (1995–2004). J Am Vet Med Assoc 2005;227(10):1618–24.
62. Boothe HW, Boothe DM, Komkov A, et al. Use of hepatobiliary scintigraphy in the diagnosis of extrahepatic biliary obstruction in dogs and cats: 25 cases (1982–1989). J Am Vet Med Assoc 1992;201(1):134–41.
63. Newell SM, Graham JP, Roberts GD, et al. Quantitative hepatobiliary scintigraphy in normal cats and in cats with experimental cholangiohepatitis. Vet Radiol Ultrasound 2001;42(1):70–6.
64. Adamek HE, Albert J, Weitz M, et al. A prospective evaluation of magnetic resonance cholangiopancreatography in patients with suspected bile duct obstruction. Gut 1998;43(5):680–3.
65. Mesrur Halefoglu A. Magnetic resonance cholangiopancreatography. Semin Roentgenol 2008;43(4):282–9.
66. Lamb CR, Daniel GB. Diagnostic imaging of dogs with suspected portosystemic shunting. Compendium on Continuing Education for the Practicing Veterinarian 2002;24(8):626–35.
67. Schmidt S, Suter PF. Angiography of the hepatic and portal venous system in the dog and cat: an investigative method. Vet Radiol Ultrasound 1980;21:57–77.
68. Holt DE, Schelling CG, Saunders HM, et al. Correlation of ultrasonographic findings with surgical, portographic, and necropsy findings in dogs and cats with portosystemic shunts: 63 cases (1987–1993). J Am Vet Med Assoc 1995;207(9):1190–3.

69. Lamb CR. Ultrasonographic diagnosis of congenital portosystemic shunts in dogs: results of a prospective study. Vet Radiol Ultrasound 1996;37(4):281–8.
70. d'Anjou MA, Penninck D, Cornejo L, et al. Ultrasonographic diagnosis of portosystemic shunting in dogs and cats. Vet Radiol Ultrasound 2004;45(5): 424–37.
71. Szatmari V, Rothuizen J, Voorhout G. Standard planes for ultrasonographic examination of the portal system in dogs. J Am Vet Med Assoc 2004;224(5):713–9.
72. Szatmari V, Rothuizen J, van Sluijs FJ, et al. Ultrasonographic evaluation of partially attenuated congenital extrahepatic portosystemic shunts in 14 dogs. Vet Rec 2004;155(15):448–56.
73. Salwei RM, O'Brien RT, Matheson JS. Use of contrast harmonic ultrasound for the diagnosis of congenital portosystemic shunts in three dogs. Vet Radiol Ultrasound 2003;44(3):301–5.
74. Szatmari V. Simultaneous congenital and acquired extrahepatic portosystemic shunts in two dogs. Vet Radiol Ultrasound 2003;44(4):486–7.
75. Szatmari V, Rothuizen J. Ultrasonographic identification and characterization of congenital portosystemic shunts and portal hypertensive disorders in dogs and cats. In: Rothuizen J, Bunch SE, Charles JA, et al, editors. Standards for clinical and histological diagnosis of canine and feline liver diseases—WSAVA Liver Standardization Group. Philadelphia: Saunders Elsevier; 2006. p. 15–39.
76. Thompson MS, Graham JP, Mariani CL. Diagnosis of a porto-azygous shunt using helical computed tomography angiography. Vet Radiol Ultrasound 2003;44(3): 287–91.
77. Frank P, Mahaffey M, Egger C, et al. Helical computed tomographic portography in ten normal dogs and ten dogs with a portosystemic shunt. Vet Radiol Ultrasound 2003;44(4):392–400.
78. Winter MD, Kinney LM, Kleine LJ. Three-dimensional helical computed tomographic angiography of the liver in five dogs. Vet Radiol Ultrasound 2005;46(6):494–9.
79. Zwingenberger AL, Schwarz T. Dual-phase CT angiography of the normal canine portal and hepatic vasculature. Vet Radiol Ultrasound 2004;45(2):117–24.
80. Echandi RL, Morandi F, Daniel WT, et al. Comparison of transsplenic multidetector CT portography to multidetector CT-angiography in normal dogs. Vet Radiol Ultrasound 2007;48(1):38–44.
81. Seguin B, Tobias KM, Gavin PR, et al. Use of magnetic resonance angiography for diagnosis of portosystemic shunts in dogs. Vet Radiol Ultrasound 1999; 40(3):251–8.
82. Daniel GB, Berry CR. Scintigraphic detection of portosystemic shunts. In: Daniel GB, Berry CR, editors. Textbook of veterinary nuclear medicine. 2nd edition. Knoxville (TN): American College of Veterinary Radiology; 2006. p. 232–53.
83. Daniel GB, Bright R, Ollis P, et al. Per rectal portal scintigraphy using 99mtechnetium pertechnetate to diagnose portosystemic shunts in dogs and cats. J Vet Intern Med 1991;5(1):23–7.
84. Daniel GB, DeNovo RC, Sharp DS, et al. Portal streamlining as a cause of nonuniform hepatic distribution of sodium pertechnetate during per-rectal portal scintigraphy in the dog. Vet Radiol Ultrasound 2004;45(1):78–84.
85. Sura PA, Tobias KM, Morandi F, et al. Comparison of 99mTcO4(−) trans-splenic portal scintigraphy with per-rectal portal scintigraphy for diagnosis of portosystemic shunts in dogs. Vet Surg 2007;36(7):654–60.

86. Morandi F, Cole RC, Tobias KM, et al. Use of 99mTCO4(−) trans-splenic portal scintigraphy for diagnosis of portosystemic shunts in 28 dogs. Vet Radiol Ultrasound 2005;46(2):153–61.
87. Nyland TG, Mattoon JS, Herrgesell EJ, et al. Ultrasound-guided biopsy. In: Nyland TG, Mattoon JS, editors. Small animal diagnostic ultrasound. 2nd edition. Philadelphia: WB Saunders Co.; 2002. p. 30–48.
88. Savary-Bataille KCM, Bunch SE, Spaulding KA, et al. Percutaneous ultrasound-guided cholecystocentesis in healthy cats. J Vet Intern Med 2003;17(3): 298–303.

Liver Biopsy Techniques

Jan Rothuizen, DVM, PhD[a],*, David C. Twedt, DVM, PhD[b]

KEYWORDS

- Liver biopsy • True cut needle • Menghini needle
- Laparoscopy • Wedge biopsy • Fine needle aspiration
- Gall bladder punction • Coagulation

Liver biopsy is an important step in the evaluation of a patient with hepatic disease and is required to formulate a diagnosis, direct therapy, and provide an accurate prognosis. However, a liver biopsy evaluates only a small percentage of the liver and may not represent the entire liver. Consequently, the results should always be combined with the clinical information, laboratory data, and imaging procedures to formulate a diagnosis.[1] There are advantages and disadvantages of each method of obtaining a liver biopsy. This article presents the indications, technique, and diagnostic accuracy of the various biopsy methods, including fine-needle liver aspiration, needle biopsy, laparoscopic-assisted biopsy, and surgical biopsy. Descriptions of many of the surgical techniques are beyond the scope of this article; specific details are available in most surgical texts.

The diagnosis of most liver diseases requires a histopathologic examination of liver tissue. Histology is especially important for parenchymal liver diseases such as hepatitis occurring in dogs and inflammatory biliary tract disease common to the cat. Of the circulatory diseases of the liver, portal vein hypoplasia (microvascular dysplasia) can only be diagnosed by a combination of histopathology and imaging (eg, ultrasonography) techniques. Diffuse liver diseases may be sampled randomly, but focal lesions require careful selective sampling using ultrasound-guided needle biopsy, laparoscopic guidance, or surgically. Large focal lesions should be sampled in the periphery of the lesion because a neoplastic mass may have a necrotic center and the malignant characteristics are best observed in the periphery of the mass.

Neoplasia and diffuse vacuolar disorders (eg, lipidosis, steroid hepatopathy) of the liver can often be diagnosed by cytologic examination obtained using fine-needle aspiration. However, cytology does not show the architectural changes of the liver that can be seen with histopathology. For example, differentiation of liver cell adenomas and carcinomas often cannot be distinguished without evaluating the histopathology. Needle biopsies also have limitations due to their small sample size; for

[a] Department of Clinical Sciences of Companion Animals, University Utrecht, Yalelaan 108, P.O. Box 80.154, 3508 TD Utrecht, The Netherlands
[b] Department of Clinical Sciences, College of Veterinary Medicine and Biomedical Sciences, Colorado State University, Fort Collins, CO 80523, USA
* Corresponding author.
E-mail address: j.rothuizen@uu.nl (J. Rothuizen).

Vet Clin Small Anim 39 (2009) 469–480
doi:10.1016/j.cvsm.2009.02.006
vetsmall.theclinics.com

example, with macronodular cirrhosis, needle aspirates may only sample a hyperplastic nodule and inflammatory and fibrotic areas may be missed.

In every case, all available information must be considered before reaching the final diagnosis, and this implies selecting the proper techniques for obtaining tissue samples (representative and big enough), adhering to the important requirements of tissue handling, and providing the pathologist with all available essential clinical information. The clinician should then consider the information from the history, physical examination, clinical pathology, and ultrasonography or other imaging procedures with the histologic results of the liver biopsy before making the diagnosis.

GENERAL CONSIDERATIONS

The risk/benefit ratio of performing a liver biopsy must be weighed for every case. Although the chance of serious complications is low for a specific case or procedure, there is always the potential for complications to occur. Operator experience also has a significant influence on the complication rate. However, most diseases of the liver are best defined and treated following a liver biopsy with histologic examination.

It is important that the patient fasts for approximately 12 hours to ensure that the stomach is small. Fasting aids the ultrasonographic examination and is required before sedation or anesthesia. The stomach covers the caudal visceral surface of the liver and a distended stomach may prevent the biopsy needle reaching the liver. Anesthesia is required for surgery and laparoscopy, and possibly for some dogs and all cats undergoing a needle biopsy. Needle biopsies can be obtained in cooperative dogs using local anesthesia of the skin and abdominal wall. Fine-needle aspiration is usually performed using minimal or no sedation and without local anesthesia.

Coagulation Testing

As the liver produces all the clotting factors except Factor VIII, bleeding from a liver biopsy is reported to be the most frequent complication. With every liver biopsy there is always a small amount of blood loss, which can be seen by ultrasonography or during laparoscopy or surgery. The average amount of blood loss from a liver biopsy is reported to be around 2 mL in normal dogs. [2,3] Fine-needle aspirates are generally considered safe and there are few reports of serious bleeding following a needle aspirate.[4] If the coagulation tests are normal, bleeding becomes less of a concern.[5] The reserve capacity of the liver in producing clotting factors is so huge that, for most liver diseases, factor production is rarely decreased to the point whereby it becomes a limiting factor. Abnormalities in coagulation tests may also not preclude a liver biopsy but may increase the likelihood of bleeding. The results of routine coagulation tests have shown the degree of bleeding from a biopsy does not correlate with the patient's clotting times.[6] However, a liver biopsy should be avoided if there is clinical evidence of bleeding or marked abnormalities in the coagulation tests. Thrombocytopenia (<80,000 platelets) or prolongation of the coagulation times increases the risk of bleeding following a liver biopsy. The presence of marked abnormalities in coagulation in a patient with liver disease becomes prognostic and suggests significant hepatic dysfunction.[7]

Ideally, before a liver biopsy the coagulation status should be assessed by evaluating the intrinsic pathway (activated partial thromboplastin time [APTT]), the extrinsic pathway prothrombin time (PT), fibrinogen content, and platelet count. A buccal mucosal bleeding time (BMBT) is also recommended especially in breeds associated with von Willebrand's disease. Patients with von Willebrand's disease usually have normal coagulation tests and platelet numbers but have significantly decreased platelet function, which increases the BMBT. Disease of the liver can also lead to an increased consumption of fibrinogen and other clotting factors with a significant effect on coagulation.[8] This situation occurs in diffuse diseases of the liver associated with pronounced hepatocyte necrosis/apoptosis leading to subclinical diffuse intravascular coagulation (DIC). Associated diseases are active forms of hepatitis and malignant lymphoma in the liver. In such cases, fine-needle aspiration of the liver is still possible, allowing identification or exclusion of malignant lymphoma. A fibrinogen concentration less than 50% of the lower reference level can be used as an absolute contraindication for taking a liver biopsy. The activation of factors II, VII, IX, and X depends on the availability of vitamin K_1. In prolonged and complete obstruction of the bile flow, the intestinal absorption of fat-soluble vitamins K_1 may be severely impaired due to the lack of bile acids entering the intestine. In these cases, it is useful to administer vitamin K_1 (1–5 mg/kg subcutaneously daily for several days) and then re-evaluating the effect on the clotting times before biopsy. Some investigators recommend administering vitamin K_1 to all patients if the clotting times are at all abnormal. However, unless there is vitamin K deficiency, there will likely be little improvement. With abnormalities in PT, APTT, or BMBT fresh frozen plasma should be administered 2 hours before the procedure and the patient should be monitored closely following the biopsy. Suspected bleeding following biopsy should be evaluated with abdominocentesis or ultrasonography, and is evident within 0.5 to 1 hour after the procedure. Life-threatening bleeding following biopsy is treated with fresh frozen plasma, fresh whole blood, or, rarely and as a last resort, surgery to stop the source of the bleeding. Bleeding, with a dropping hematocrit level, is usually evident within the first 5 hours following the biopsy.[6]

Ultrasound Examination

It is important to evaluate the structure of the liver, biliary tract, and portal vein in preparation for a liver biopsy. This evaluation is usually done with ultrasonography, but may also be performed by laparoscopy or surgical inspection. Systematic evaluation should be performed to determine: (1) the size of the liver; (2) the presence of focal lesions; (3) the liver architecture and structure; (4) the diameter of the lumen and the thickness of the wall of the extrahepatic and intrahepatic bile ducts and the gallbladder; (5) vascular changes, especially of the portal vein but also the presence of arteriovenous fistulas; (6) the presence of free abdominal fluid; and (7) echo Doppler evaluation of the portal blood flow velocity and direction. These evaluations provide important information for the clinician and the pathologist. Histologic findings become optimally meaningful when combined with the relevant clinical, clinicopathologic, and imaging findings.

Risk Factors

Precautions with respect to the coagulation process are not the only factors associated with complications of a liver biopsy. The experience of the operator must also be considered. With an experienced operator most techniques are safe and have a low complication rate. A third complication associated with a needle biopsy is the induction of vagotonic shock immediately following the procedure.[9] Rapid-firing automatic biopsy needles increase the risk for this complication. The automatic spring-loaded biopsy guns have been reported to produce such a strong impulse to the liver that it causes a lethal shock reaction in cats but this has not been observed in dogs. The larger bile ducts and the gallbladder have a dense autonomic innervation and trauma induced by penetration with a wide core biopsy needle may also induce an autonomic reaction with bradycardia and deep shock within 30 minutes of the procedure, which may be especially relevant if dilated bile ducts of an extrahepatic bile duct obstruction (EHBDO) have been hit. Other biopsy techniques are recommended if an obstruction associated with duct dilation is present. The authors have also observed biopsy-induced shock following liver biopsy when large liver cell carcinomas are sampled. A small percentage of these cases may develop severe shock requiring intensive care treatment, but this is not a reason for avoiding the procedure. The owner should be informed in advance of a potential higher risk. In these situations, it may be better to avoid ultrasound-directed needle biopsy.

What Constitutes a Good Liver Biopsy

An ideal liver biopsy should be of proper size and taken from a location that represents the primary liver pathology. In diffuse liver disease, the biopsy will likely represent the entire liver but focal or regional disease becomes more problematic. Ultrasound examination or visual inspection is important to determine the presence of focal disease. Ideally, at least 2 and preferably 3 biopsies should be obtained from separate liver lobes.[1] If one area seems normal and other areas seem abnormal, representative samples from each area should be taken. Occasionally the normal looking areas may actually be abnormal. Because of the smaller sample size obtained from needle biopsies, there is greater potential for the needle sample not to represent the entire liver. It is stated that 1 good core needle biopsy represents only a 50,000th of the entire liver.[10] The authors believe that 18G needle biopsies are generally too small, fragment easily, and do not contain enough portal areas to be of diagnostic value. Good samples can be obtained with 14G needle diameter for dogs and 16G for small dogs and cats. Laparoscopic wedge and surgical wedge biopsies generally provide larger samples but the procedure is more invasive. Samples from laparoscopic biopsy forceps are usually approximately 5 mm in diameter. Surgical wedge samples should be at least 1 cm, preferably 2 cm deep. Subcapsular tissue contains more fibrous tissue and may have nonspecific inflammatory changes that could be misleadingly interpreted as representing the entire liver. With the larger wedge samples, this may be less of a concern and the pathologist should interpret subcapsular change with caution.

Appropriate tissue handling and histologic interpretation is critical for a correct diagnosis. **Box 1** provides guidelines for tissue handling of liver samples. An accurate interpretation of the biopsy requires the presence of a sufficient number of portal and central areas because different diseases are associated with different sublobular zones. Many pathologists believe that 6 portal areas are necessary to make an adequate diagnosis of inflammatory liver disease.[11,12] The quality of a clinical diagnosis of liver disease depends largely on the histologic description. There is often confusion about which criteria are essential to diagnose a certain disease, and individual pathologists may have different interpretations or even different diagnoses on the same sample. The World Small Animal Veterinary Association (WSAVA) has initiated standards for unification of diagnostic criteria and nomenclature of liver diseases. A team of leading specialists, clinicians and pathologists, have reviewed most known liver diseases of companion animals and have described clear-cut and well-illustrated criteria in the publication, WSAVA Standards for Clinical and Histologic Diagnosis of Canine and Feline Liver Diseases in 2006.[13] The clinician should expect a detailed description according to these international guidelines from their pathologist.

In addition to tissue for histopathology, samples may also be procured for culture or quantitation of copper or other metals. Ideally, approximately 20 to 40 mg of liver (wet weight) is required for copper quantitation using atomic absorption spectrophotometry methods. This amount equates to a sample of approximately 2.5 mm diameter or one full 14G (2-cm long) needle biopsy sample. Smaller samples may decrease

---

Box 1
Guidelines for proper handling of liver tissue

1. Verify the quality of the tissue; it should be unfragmented and at least 1 cm, preferably 2 cm in length. Samples obtained surgically should be cut into thin slices <5 mm thick. The center of thicker pieces will not be fixated adequately in formalin or another fixative.

2. The tissue should be put into the fixative within 5 minutes; 10% neutral buffered formalin is used routinely.

3. The fixation time should not be too long; after long formalin fixation immunohistochemistry becomes impossible with many antibodies.

4. Think in advance about the specific requirements. It may be necessary to perform electron microscopy, specific stains for metabolic diseases, and so forth. In case of doubt, the pathologist should be contacted about the best way to preserve the tissue.

5. For quantitative measurement of metals in liver such as copper, avoid saline if using neutron activation analysis for measurement of small amounts in biopsy samples because the analysis is affected by the presence of sodium. Tissue should be sampled in a metal-free plastic container and freeze-dried; thereafter closed containers can be stored at room temperature.

6. Fill the container completely with fixative so that the sample is not stirred and broken during transportation.

---

the accuracy of the metal analysis. Laparoscopic cup biopsy forceps provide 45 mg of liver tissue, a 14G Tru-Cut–type biopsy needle provides 15 to 20 mg, whereas an 18G needle biopsy provides only 3 to 5 mg of liver tissue. Liver tissue taken for culture should be approximately 5 mg in size and placed in appropriate transport broth or medium that preserves aerobic and anaerobic bacteria.

FINE-NEEDLE ASPIRATION

Fine-needle aspiration (FNA) with cytologic examination is commonly performed in small animals with liver disease because it is cheap and easy to do. FNA can be performed at low risk to the patient and usually without the need for sedation or local anesthesia.[4,14] It is best suited for diffuse hepatic disease. If focal lesions are present ultrasound direction becomes necessary. Bleeding complications from FNA of the liver are uncommon and there is rarely a need to perform coagulation tests unless overt hemorrhage is identified before the aspiration. However, there are limitations to FNA and examination of the liver cytology. These include failure to correctly identify the primary disease due to the small sample size and the cytology does not reflect the morphology of the parenchymal architecture. Several studies have compared liver aspirates and their cytologic interpretation with the histopathologic diagnosis from a biopsy. In a large study of 97 cases involving dogs and cats, only 30% of the canine cases and 51% of the feline cases had overall agreement between the histopathologic diagnosis and the cytologic diagnosis.[15] In this study, the diagnosis of vacuolar hepatopathy was the category with the highest percentage of agreement, whereas inflammatory disease was correctly diagnosed only 25% of the time when dogs and cats were grouped together. Other similar studies also point out the low correlation of cytology with histopathology. Although FNA is frequently used by clinicians to support the diagnosis of hepatic lipidosis in cats, there is a report of 4 cats incorrectly diagnosed as having hepatic lipidosis instead of lymphoma.[16] A multistep approach to cytologic evaluation of nonvacuolar diseases may provide useful standardization for cytologic evaluation and improve the diagnostic accuracy.[17]

The location of the entry site for most FNAs is determined using ultrasound to direct the needle to focal lesions or to certain areas in the liver. Alternatively a blind method, in which a random sample of the liver is obtained, may be adequate if a palpable large liver is present and diffuse disease such as malignant lymphoma or diffuse vacuolar hepatopathies (lipidosis) of the liver is suspected. If a large palpable liver is present and if using a blind technique, the usual entry point is caudal to the costal arch. The liver can also be approached on the right side at the 10th intercostal space at the level of the rib-cartilage junction. For either approach there is no need for local or general anesthesia in dogs or cats if using thin needle sampling. Most FNAs are performed using a 20G to 22G needle. A 3-inch disposable injection needle is usually sufficient, but longer needles may be required for deep-lying lesions. The tissue is aspirated in an identical procedure to that used for peripheral structures such as lymph nodes. The needle attached to a 5 or 12 mL syringe is advanced under ultrasound guidance into the liver. At the site of aspiration the needle is quickly advanced and withdrawn 0.5 to 1 cm several times. Cells within the needle are then blown on the microscope slide with the syringe. Others prefer to apply negative pressure on the syringe plunger while aspirating the liver. Pressure on the plunger is released and the needle withdrawn. This technique collects more cells but also results in more blood contamination, which must be considered in the cytologic interpretation. Liver aspirates are placed on a glass microscope slide, air-dried and routine cytologic staining used. It is also possible to use specific staining methods such as copper stains (rubeanic acid or rhodanine stain) for intracellular copper granules, Sudan stain for lipids, and periodic acid-Schiff stain for the presence of glycogen.

NEEDLE BIOPSY

Several different needles and biopsy techniques are used to obtain liver tissue for examination, each with advantages and disadvantages. The Menghini technique involves tissue aspiration (using saline) with a syringe attached to a large bore hollow needle. The tip of the needle is convex and is sharp around the circumference. Most needles have a blocking device in the shaft to prevent liver tissue going into the syringe. The Menghini or blind technique is not suitable for ultrasound guidance and is almost always performed using the needle tip as a probe to palpate the appropriate location.[1] When the site is determined, suction is applied to the syringe and the needle is quickly thrust into the liver and then rapidly retrieved. A core of liver is then sucked into the needle. The samples are larger than those obtained with Tru-Cut needles because the entire lumen is filled with tissue and the length of the sample can be predetermined. The Menghini technique is not suitable for cats.

The Tru-Cut–type needle is generally performed using ultrasound guidance, but may also be done under visual control during laparoscopy or surgery. This technique is the most widely used. The Tru-Cut–type needle has an outer cannula and an inner notched shaft in which a tissue specimen is retained. The notched portion has a 2-cm long indentation which is first advanced into the liver, so that the tissue can fall in the indentation. Then, the outer cutting cannula slides over the inner notched shaft so that the tissue is sliced off. The entire instrument is finally withdrawn and the tissue slice retrieved. Tru-Cut needles have a sharp tip and should therefore only be used under visual control such as ultrasound guidance or during surgery. There are 3 types of Tru-Cut needles: manual, semi-automatic, and those used in a biopsy gun device.[18] Manual devices are cheap but they are the most difficult to handle and their use is not advised other than during surgery under direct visual control. Semi-automatic needles are the most expensive but easy to use. These needles are recommended for cats. Biopsy gun devices require a larger financial investment, but the Tru-Cut needles used with them are inexpensive. The gun-driven needles are recommended for centers where biopsies (not only of the liver but also of kidneys and other structures) are routinely taken under ultrasound guidance.[19] An advantage of Tru-Cut guns is that they operate so quickly that a firm, fibrotic liver or a liver with concurrent ascites tissue is more easily sampled. In these situations, the liver may be hard to puncture using conventional needles. As a rule, most semi-automatic and gun-driven Tru-Cut needles advance 2 cm into the liver so it is important to note the amount of liver tissue available in front of the needle before advancement so that no structures other than the liver are hit with the needle.

LAPAROSCOPIC LIVER BIOPSY

Diagnostic laparoscopy is a technique used to view and biopsy the organs in the abdominal cavity.[20] The technique involves distention of the abdominal cavity with gas followed by placement of a rigid telescope through a portal (cannula) in the abdominal wall to examine the contents of the peritoneal cavity. Biopsy forceps or other instruments are then passed into the abdomen through adjacent portals to perform various procedures. Laparoscopy requires general anesthesia but the limited degree of invasiveness, diagnostic accuracy, large biopsy sample size, and rapid patient recovery make laparoscopy a valuable technique for obtaining liver tissue. The excellent view of the liver with magnification is an advantage but limitations include the expense of the equipment, adequate operator training, and increased time over needle biopsy techniques. Laparoscopy is frequently used to obtain biopsies of the liver, pancreas, kidney, spleen, lymph node, and intestine. Laparoscopy may also reveal small (0.5 cm or less) metastatic lesions, peritoneal metastases, or other organ involvement not easily observed by other techniques. One of the ancillary diagnostic techniques using laparoscopic guidance also includes gallbladder aspiration (choleocystocentesis).

Laparoscopy is a step between needle liver biopsy and surgical laparotomy for obtaining tissue for histopathology. Because most liver diseases are nonsurgical, laparoscopy is often the preferred technique over laparotomy. The advantages of laparoscopy over conventional surgical laparotomy include improved patient recovery because of smaller surgical sites, lower postoperative morbidity, and decreased infection rate, postoperative pain, and hospitalization time. Other less obvious benefits of laparoscopy are related to fewer stress-mediated factors than are reported to occur with surgery.

Discussion of basic laparoscopic equipment and a detailed description of the techniques for laparoscopy are beyond the scope of this article and the reader should consult specific texts or articles on laparoscopy. For most diagnostic laparoscopic procedures a 5-mm diameter 0° field of view telescope is recommended. The 0° designation means that the telescope views the visual field directly in front of the telescope in a 180° circumference. Angled viewing scopes such as the 30° telescope enable the operator to see into areas with a small field of view. However, angled telescopes make the orientation more difficult for the inexperienced operator. Five-millimeter diameter forceps with oval biopsy cups are most often used for liver biopsy.[21]

The patient should be fasted for at least 12 hours. Under general anesthesia 2 cannula portals are placed through the abdominal wall, one for the telescope and the other for the biopsy forceps. There are 2 basic entry sites for liver biopsy. The first uses dorsal recumbency in which the telescope is placed on the midline behind the umbilicus. This position provides a view of the entire surface of the liver, however the falciform ligament is often a nuisance and the pancreas is more difficult to identify. The second entry site requires placement of the animal in left lateral recumbency with the telescope portal in the right mid-abdominal wall. This lateral approach is preferred by the authors because the falciform ligament is not in the way, the right limb of the pancreas is easily seen, and the extrahepatic biliary system can be easily followed to where it enters the duodenum. Using this approach the left lateral lobe of the liver is difficult to examine completely.

The liver, extrahepatic biliary system, and other abdominal structures are examined and can be palpated using a specialized palpation probe. The palpation probe is used to move or elevate lobes of the liver for complete inspection and to aid in selecting representative areas of the liver to be sampled. Using the oval biopsy cups either an edge of the liver or the surface of the liver is sampled. To take a biopsy of the surface of the liver, the forceps are directed at approximately 90° angle to the liver, opened and pushed into the liver, and then closed. Sample size will vary with the operator's technique and depth of penetration. With either sampling technique the forceps are closed tightly for 15 to 30 seconds and then gently tugged away from the liver. The biopsy site is then examined for bleeding which usually subsides quickly. Because of the magnification of the telescope, 1 to 2 milliliters of blood may seem excessive. Abnormal hemorrhage rarely occurs but if present can be controlled by several methods. Some prefer using monopolar electrocautery while compressing the liver tissue with the biopsy forceps. Electrocautery is reported to affect only the periphery of the biopsy sample.[2] A second technique is to place absorbable gelatin coagulation material in the biopsy site. It is also possible to apply compression over the bleeding area with forceps or the palpation probe.

Intrahepatic lesions observed using ultrasound may be more difficult to identify. Deeper samples of the liver can be obtained using laparoscopic direction of a biopsy needle. Needles are passed directly through the abdominal wall and can be guided to the area to be sampled without the need for a cannula. Laparoscopic-guided chole-cystocentesis can also be performed if inflammatory or infectious biliary tract disease is suspected. A 22G long needle is used to collect bile for culture and cytology. The needle is directed through the abdominal wall behind the diaphragm into the gallbladder and the contents aspirated. It is important to remove as much bile as possible to empty the gallbladder and prevent leakage when the needle is removed.

As previously stated it is important to biopsy areas that seem normal as well as those that seem abnormal. Some investigators suggest that biopsies taken at the edge of the liver often do not reflect deeper lesions and that the histopathology at the subcapsular edge of the liver is usually more reactive.[22] Others suggest that the samples collected by laparoscopic cup biopsy are so large that this should not be considered a major concern.

The complication rate of laparoscopy is low. In an unpublished review of a series of cases involving diagnostic laparoscopy, the complication rate was less than 2%. Serious complications include anesthetic- or cardiovascular-related death, bleeding, or air embolism. Minor complications are generally operative and are associated with inexperience or failure to understand the limitations and potential complications.

SURGICAL LIVER BIOPSY

Liver biopsy alone is rarely an indication for a laparotomy. However, there are indications for surgical procedures such as investigation of an extrahepatic biliary obstruction or for correction of a vascular anomaly. In these cases, a liver biopsy is always indicated. Liver biopsies are also often obtained in conjunction with other surgical procedures. A biopsy should be performed if the liver looks abnormal or abnormal liver enzyme levels are discovered before surgery. It is recommended that a surgical liver biopsy be taken early during the laparotomy because hepatocellular changes can result from prolonged anesthesia, vascular changes, and manipulation of the bowel.[2,23]

There are several techniques for obtaining liver tissue during a laparotomy. The most commonly used method is the suture fracture technique. With this method, samples are generally obtained from the tip of a liver lobe. A 5- to 6-mm skin biopsy punch has also been described to sample focal superficial lesions. Once the core sample is obtained with the punch, gelatin coagulation material is placed in the biopsy site. Readers should refer to surgical texts for details of surgical methods of liver biopsy.

The advantage of surgery is the exposure, ability to manipulate the tissues, and ability to monitor the biopsy site for bleeding. A review comparing two 18G needle Tru-Cut biopsy samples with a larger wedge biopsy found poor histologic correlation, pointing out the advantage of larger surgical or laparoscopic biopsies.[20] The extrahepatic biliary system can also be completely investigated with surgery and bile is easily sampled through directed aspiration. The disadvantage of surgical biopsy is the need for general anesthesia, the large abdominal incision, and the postoperative recovery

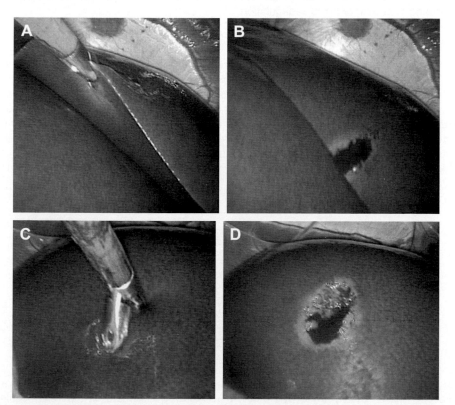

Fig. 1. Laparoscopic liver biopsy. Liver biopsies are taken with 5-mm oval biopsy forceps. (A) View of a liver biopsy taken from the edge of a liver lobe; (B) view showing the liver following the biopsy; (C) view showing a liver biopsy taken from the surface of the liver; and (D) view showing the liver following the biopsy.

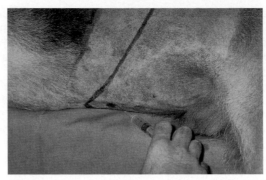

Fig. 2. Local anesthesia given for Menghini needle liver biopsy. The incision is made through the skin and abdominal wall just 1 to 2 cm caudal to the xyphoid in the midline. The position of the last rib is indicated.

time. The sample size of a biopsy obtained through surgery is the largest of any of the methods described, providing more than adequate tissue for histopathology, copper analysis, and culture. Bleeding can also be controlled easily using focal pressure, suturing methods, or electrocoagulation.

GALLBLADDER PUNCTURE

Although this is not strictly a liver-sampling procedure, sampling of bile in all cases in which inflammatory/infectious biliary disease is suspected, is an essential diagnostic step.[24,25] Puncture of the gallbladder can be performed safely using the ultrasound-guided thin needle technique. There is no need to approach the gallbladder transhepatically; any approach is safe. Thin needle sampling does not lead to vagal reactions and shock. Puncture of the gallbladder should be avoided in cases of extrahepatic bile duct obstruction because of the risk of inducing rupture or bile leakage. Sampling of bile for cytology and culture is especially important in cats, in which cholangitis is a major hepatobiliary disorder.

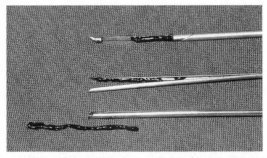

Fig. 3. Typical liver tissue samples obtained with different biopsy devices. Top: a Tru-Cut needle, which is usually driven by a biopsy gun. Half of the diameter of the inner needle is available to collect the biopsy. Bottom: Menghini needle tip with the tissue sample aspirated. The entire lumen of the needle is available to collect tissue; the sample is caught by aspiration with saline while advancing the needle into the liver. Middle: a Vim-Silverman needle, no longer in use.

SUMMARY

A liver biopsy is generally safe and provides useful information about the liver. However, the importance of the information to be obtained from a biopsy must be weighed against the risk to the patient. A liver biopsy provides important information on the status of the liver. Only after the clinical information, liver biopsy, and histopathology are obtained can a diagnosis and prognosis be made. With proper training and adequate operator experience liver biopsy is an important diagnostic tool (**Figs. 1–3**).

REFERENCES

1. Rothuizen J. Diseases of the liver and biliary tract. In: Dunn J, editor. Textbook of small animal medicine. London: Saunders; 1999. p. 448–97.
2. Rawlings CA, Howerth EW. Obtaining quality biopsies of the liver and kidney. J Am Anim Hosp Assoc 2004;40:352–8.
3. Vasanjee SC, Bubenik LJ, Hosgood G, et al. Evaluation of hemorrhage, sample size, and collateral damage for five hepatic biopsy methods in dogs. Vet Surg 2006;35(1):86–93.
4. Weiss DJ, Moritz A. Liver cytology. Vet Clin North Am Small Anim Pract 2002; 32(6):1267–91.
5. Hitt ME, Hanna P, Singh A. Percutaneous transabdominal hepatic needle biopsies in dogs. Am J Vet Res 1992;53:785–7.
6. Bigge LA, Brown DJ, Penninck DG. Correlation between coagulation profile findings and bleeding complications after ultrasound-guided biopsies: 434 cases (1993–1996). J Am Anim Hosp Assoc 2001;37(3):228–33.
7. Badylak SF, Dodds WJ, Van Vleet JF. Plasma coagulation factor abnormalities in dogs with naturally occurring hepatic disease. Am J Vet Res 1983;44(12): 2336–40.
8. Badylak SF, Van Vleet JF. Alterations of prothrombin time and activated partial thromboplastin time in dogs with hepatic disease. Am J Vet Res 1981;42(12): 2053–6.
9. Smith S. Ultrasound guided biopsy. Semin Vet Med Surg 1989;4:95–104.
10. Geller SA. Liver biopsy for the nonpathologist. In: Gitnick G, editor. Principles and practice of gastroenterology and hepatology. 2nd edition. Norwalk (CT): Appleton & Lange; 1994. p. 1023–36.
11. Desmet V, Fevery J. Liver biopsy. In: Hayes PC, editor, Investigations in Hepatology. Baillière's Clinical Gastroenterology, vol 9, nr 4. London: Baillière Tindall; 1995. p. 811-28.
12. Crawford AR, Xi-Zhang L, Crawford JM. The normal adult human liver biopsy: a quantitative reference standard. Hepatology 1998;28(2):323–31.
13. Rothuizen J, Bunch SE, Cullen JM, et al. WSAVA standards for clinical and histological diagnosis of canine and feline liver diseases. Edinburgh: Saunders; 2006.
14. Kerwin SC. Hepatic aspiration and biopsy techniques. Vet Clin North Am Small Anim Pract 1995;25:275–91.
15. Wang KY, Panciera DL, Al Rukivat RK, et al. Accuracy of ultrasound-guided fine-needle aspiration of the liver and cytologic findings in dogs and cats: 97 cases (1990–2000). J Am Vet Med Assoc 2004;224:75–8.
16. Willard M. Fine-needle aspirate cytology suggesting hepatic lipidosis in four cats with infiltrative hepatic disease. J Feline Med Surg 1999;1(4):215–20.
17. Stockhaus C, Van Den Ingh T, Rothuizen J, et al. A multistep approach in the cytologic evaluation of liver biopsy samples of dogs with hepatic diseases. Vet Pathol 2004;41:461–70.

18. de Rycke LM, van Bree HJ, Simoens PJ. Ultrasound-guided tissue-core biopsy of liver, spleen and kidney in normal dogs. Vet Radiol Ultrasound 1999;40(3):294–9.
19. Hoppe FE, Hager DA, Poulos PW, et al. A comparison of manual and automatic ultrasound-guided biopsy techniques. Vet Radiol 1986;27:99–101.
20. Monnet E, Twedt DC. Laparoscopy. Vet Clin North Am Small Anim Pract 2003;33: 1147–63.
21. Twedt DC. Laparoscopy of the liver and pancreas. In: Tams TR, editor. Small animal endoscopy. 2nd edition. St. Louis (MO): CV Mosby Co; 1999. p. 44–60.
22. Patrelli M, Scheuer PA. Variation in subcapsular liver structure and its significance in the interpretation of wedge biopsies. J Clin Pathol 1967;20:743–8.
23. Fossum TW, Hedlund CS. Surgery of the liver. In: Fossum TW, editor. Small animal surgery. St. Louis (MO): Mosby; 1997. p. 367–99.
24. Cole TC, Center SA, Flood SN, et al. Diagnostic comparison of needle and wedge biopsy specimens of the liver in dogs and cats. J Am Anim Hosp Assoc 2002; 220:1483–90.
25. Savary-Bataille KC, Bunch SE, Spaulding KA, et al. Percutaneous ultrasound-guided cholecystocentesis in healthy cats. J Vet Intern Med 2003;17(3):298–303.

Idiopathic Hepatitis and Cirrhosis in Dogs

Robert P. Favier, DVM

KEYWORDS

• Hepatitis • Cirrhosis • Dog • Treatment • Prognosis

INCIDENCE AND PATHOGENESIS

Primary hepatitis (PH) is the most frequently occurring liver disease in dogs and should be distinguished from nonspecific reactive hepatitis (NSRH). A previous study found that 1% of all referred patients that presented to the author's university clinic had a form of canine PH. In contrast to human hepatology, the diagnosis of canine hepatitis is based mainly on histologic morphology, and the term, *hepatitis*, often is used regardless of cause. Regularly encountered forms of PH in dogs include acute hepatitis (AH) and chronic hepatitis (CH) (with or without cirrhosis); less frequently encountered forms are lobular dissecting hepatitis (LDH), granulomatous hepatitis (GH), and eosinophilic hepatitis (EH). For each of these forms, the World Small Animal Veterinary Association (WSAVA) Liver Standardization Group has published standards for diagnosis.[1] Of 101 cases of PH referred to the author's clinic between 2002 and 2006 (Department of Clinical Sciences of Companion Animals, Utrecht University), 21 (21%) had AH (of which CH developed in at least five at a later date), 67 (66%) CH, seven (7%) LDH, one (1%) GH, and one (1%) EH. Of the CH cases, after re-evaluation of the biopsies with copper staining, 36% seemed copper associated (CH[ca]), higher than expected, and 64% of the CH cases had an unknown cause and were considered idiopathic (CH[i]). Among dogs with CH(i) and CH(ca), approximately 50% had cirrhosis at initial diagnosis, and both groups contained several female Labrador retriever dogs (seven and five, respectively).

In different publications and case reports, a wide variety of causes for hepatopathy in general has been documented, including microorganisms, toxins and drugs, immune-mediated reactions, and breed-associated metabolic errors.[2] The inherited disorders of copper metabolism, in particular, have received much attention in the last few decades.[3–9] In spite of a large effort, however, the majority of PH cases remain of idiopathic origin. Although hepatitis in dogs has been characterized extensively, there are no data published on the occurrence of the various WSAVA-classified forms of hepatitis in a clinical population, progression between those forms, or occurrence of idiopathic and copper-associated forms of hepatitis.[10–12]

Department of Clinical Sciences of Companion Animals, Faculty of Veterinary Medicine, P.O. Box 80154, 3508 TD Utrecht, The Netherlands
E-mail address: r.p.favier@uu.nl

Vet Clin Small Anim 39 (2009) 481–488
doi:10.1016/j.cvsm.2009.01.002
0195-5616/09/$ – see front matter © 2009 Elsevier Inc. All rights reserved.

vetsmall.theclinics.com

ACUTE HEPATITIS

In the field, most cases of AH probably are missed. Dogs with AH are ill for a couple days, after which they recover spontaneously with or without supportive care without knowing what has happened. The most aggressive form of AH, fulminant hepatitis, is rapidly progressive within hours or days. In the author's referral clinic, these patients are not often seen (alive), probably because the time to get to the clinic via the referring veterinarian is too long. Canine adenovirus-1 (CAV1) is a known cause for the development of AH (sometimes fulminant). Because of vaccination, AH caused by CAV1 has been controlled effectively and practically eliminated from the domestic dog population.

There is an impression that, although initially diagnosed as acute, some cases remain acute for months on histopathology and might be considered more or less CH, although fibrosis is lacking. This form of hepatitis, although not a WSAVA-classified form, might be considered subacute hepatitis. When starting with prednisone treatment of subacute hepatitis in the clinically chronic stage, this hepatitis does not seem to respond clinically or histopathologically.

Twenty-five percent of the dogs with AH had AH(ca). Hepatitis resulting from primary copper accumulation starts somewhere in the process of developing hepatitis and, depending on the stage at which the diagnosis is made, can be acute or chronic. This finding suggests that even when dealing with a dog that has hepatitis with a history of sudden onset, suggesting an acute inflammation, copper may be the cause, and it is advisable to ask for a routine copper staining in this type of patient. From 21 dogs with AH initially diagnosed, at least five had CH when a second liver biopsy was taken 6 weeks later.

CHRONIC HEPATITIS AND CIRRHOSIS

CH is a frequently occurring disease in dogs. Approximately two thirds of the patients with PH referred to the author's university clinic had CH at initial diagnosis, and several more patients with AH progressed histologically to CH. In humans, the diagnosis of CH is based on patient history and results of histopathologic examination of liver biopsies. Because the diagnosis is etiology-based, a specific etiology-focused treatment approach is possible. In contrast, diagnosis in dogs is mainly morphology based with severity based on the type and distribution of inflammatory cells, hepatocellular apoptosis and necrosis, and the abundance and localization of fibrosis.[1] In most cases, there is no evidence of a cause, resulting in a large proportion of CH(i) cases.[2] This poor understanding of the cause of CH(i) results in limited options for adequate treatment and in variable results. Although probably not the initial cause, oxidative stress plays an important role in the maintenance and progression of disease, and, for this reason, antioxidants might play a beneficial role in the treatment of CH, at least. For decades, canine CH(i) patients have been treated mainly with orally administered immunosuppressive medication, of which prednisone is most commonly used. The efficacy of prednisone has been described in one publication.[10] In this retrospective study, a prolonged survival time was demonstrated for prednisone-treated canine CH patients in comparison with untreated patients. These results indicate a positive long-term effect of prednisone in the treatment of CH(i). In addition to anti-inflammatory effects, corticosteroids have (weak) antifibrotic properties. A retrospective histopathologic evaluation of inflammatory activity and fibrosis formation in dogs with CH(i) before and after a 6-week treatment with prednisone, although not double-blind or placebo controlled, found a reduced inflammatory activity and a stable fibrotic situation, the latter suggesting a fibrosis inhibitory effect of prednisone (Poldervaart, in preparation).

CIRRHOSIS

Fibrosis, a hallmark of CH, is defined as a detectable deposit of extracellular matrix (ECM). Cirrhosis is the end stage of CH and is defined as a diffuse process character-ized by fibrosis of the liver and the conversion of normal liver architecture into structurally abnormal nodules, micro- or macronodular.[1] Cirrhosis is the result of an accumulation of ECM materials, which is the resultant of increased synthesis or decreased breakdown. The bulk of ECM in the fibrotic liver is produced by myofibro-blast (MF)-like cells. Three different MF-like cells are described based on location and immunohistochemical profile.[13] These comprise portal or septal MF; interface MF; and perisinusoidally located hepatic stellate cells, which are nonparenchymal, quiescent cells that are activated by hepatic injury and produce most of the factors that lead to hepatic fibrosis. One of the most important of these factors is transforming growth factor-beta (TGF-β), which acts via its two receptors, TGF-β receptor type I (TGF-β RI) and TGF-β receptor type II (TGF-β RII), at the cell surface and the intracellular substrates, the Smad proteins. TGF-β stimulates fibrosis by inducing the up-regula-tion and the release of many of the ECM components (collagens and glycoaminogly-cans) and inhibitors of the metalloproteinases, preventing the breakdown of the ECM.

Important regulators of ECM turnover and breakdown are plasminogen activator–plasmin system components. Urokinase-type plasminogen activator (uPA) generates plasmin from circulating plasminogen by proteolytic cleavage. This plasmin is capable of degrading ECM components directly by proteolysis and indirectly by inhibiting deposition of ECM by activation of matrix metalloproteinases. In this way, an up-regu-lation of uPA in the liver might inhibit the deposition of ECM and reverse hepatic fibrosis. Overall, matrix remodelling is an important component of liver regeneration.

Cirrhosis is considered irreversible, although the point at which this happens is not well defined. Until now, no antifibrotic therapy has been clinically available, and in humans, liver transplantation remains the only treatment option in cases of hepatic dysfunction resulting from cirrhosis. Recent evidence suggests that the process of fibrogenesis might be reversible,[14,15] opening possibilities for evaluation of newly designed antifibrotic therapies.

LOBULAR DISSECTING HEPATITIS

The clinical symptoms in dogs with LDH are more or less acute, but on histopathology, they are diagnosed as having a CH with cirrhosis based on a massive deposition of fibrous tissue around individual or small groups of hepatocytes. The cause of this form of hepatitis is unknown. In most cases, patients with LDH are young animals (average age 2.3 years in the author's clinic) and die shortly after diagnosis, with an estimated median survival time of 0.7 $\pm$ 01 months (n = 7, 2002–2006) despite treat-ment consisting mostly of prednisone and sometimes diuretics because of the devel-opment of severe ascites resulting from portal hypertension.

NONSPECIFIC REACTIVE HEPATITIS

Nonspecific reactive hepatitis (NSRH) is an aspecific response to extrahepatic disease processes, especially inflammation somewhere in the splanchnic bed (gastrointestinal tract or pancreas) or a systemic illness with fever. It also can be found as a residual lesion of a previous inflammatory primary intrahepatic disease. NSRH, a secondary problem, does not have to be treated. It is essential to look for the primary cause (gastrointestinal tract or systemic illnesses) and to treat that underlying cause.

CLINICAL PRESENTATION

Patients with PH seen in the author's clinic present, in most cases, with nonspecific clinical signs. The most noticed symptoms mentioned by owners are decreased appetite (50%), vomiting (48%), polyuria-polydipsia (47%), reduced activity (39%), weight loss (28%), jaundice (24%), diarrhea (23%), and abdominal distension (21%). Episodic neurologic symptoms resulting from hepatic encephalopathy rarely are mentioned. Acholic feces, a specific indicator for extrahepatic biliary obstruction, are not seen in cases of PH. Depending on the form of hepatitis, signs can be obvious from hours (acute fulminant hepatitis) to months (CH).

DIAGNOSTIC EVALUATION
Physical Examination

At general appearance, dogs with CH, but not AH, have a slight to moderate muscle atrophy. Dogs with ascites resulting from portal hypertension show abdominal distension.

Physical examination related to liver diseases concentrates on the mucous membranes and abdominal palpation. In cases of hepatomegaly, examination of the circulation is indicated to detect or exclude cardiac disease. The mucous membranes are normal in most patients with liver disease. Abnormalities may include icterus, pallor, and indications for coagulopathy. Very pale mucous membranes in the presence of icterus indicate that the liver dysfunction is secondary to hemolytic anemia, and a further workup should focus on this problem. Petechiae, an indicator for thrombocytopenia or thrombocytopathy, although rarely seen in patients with PH, can be found as a result of disseminated intravascular coagulopathy.

Hepatomegaly, as a finding at abdominal palpation, is rare in dogs with PH. Ascites, leading to abdominal distension, resulting from portal hypertension or hypoproteinemia, also may be an indication for liver disease, but there are many diseases of origins other than hepatic that may induce ascites formation. Abdominal palpation also may reveal splenomegaly in cases of portal hypertension.

In most dogs with hepatitis, physical examination reveals no specific information. Therefore, in the majority of cases that involve symptoms (described previously), laboratory investigation is required to detect or exclude a liver disease.

Blood

Blood work can be used for two purposes: first, to detect or to exclude a (primary) liver problem, and second, to screen for the overall status of a patient. To address the first, blood work should consist of, at minimum, serum bile acids, alkaline phosphatase (AP), and alanine aminotransferase (ALT). In almost all cases of PH, one of these parameters is out of the upper reference range. Liver enzymes are indicators for cellular damage, whereas bile acids are a functional parameter. Of the liver enzymes, ALT is the first to increase when PH is present. Adding more (liver) enzymes to the diagnostic panel does not give more information. When patients with jaundice present to a clinic, this part of the blood workup is not necessary. For the second purpose, a complete blood cell count and a biochemistry and coagulation profile are necessary. The biochemistry profile should include at minimum—in addition to serum bile acids, AP, and ALT—urea, creatinine, total protein, albumin, sodium, and potassium. If further workup liver biopsies are needed, a coagulation profile has to be determined.

This test should be performed shortly before the biopsy procedure because coagulation parameters may change quickly in patients with hepatitis (inadequate vitamin K absorption, reduced production of coagulation factors, or increased consumption [disseminated intravascular coagulopathy]). In the author's clinic, prothrombin time, activated thromboplastin time, fibrinogen concentration, and platelet count are measured. Fibrinogen concentration, in particular, is a critical indicator, and a concentration less than 1 g/L is a contraindication for taking a liver biopsy, which happens in approximately 8% of cases of PH. This lowered fibrinogen concentration increases in more than 90% of these cases above the critical level after a 1-week treatment with prednisone/prednisolone so that a liver biopsy can be taken safely at that time.

There is some debate on what type of liver function tests to use for a functional evaluation. Worldwide, the serum bile acid tolerance test (comparison of pre- and postprandial serum bile acids) commonly is used. A major reason for this is that it is easily accessible for private clinics because samples can be sent to laboratories for measurement. The serum bile acid tolerance test does not give much additional information regarding the liver function above only preprandial serum bile acid concentration; for screening for portosystemic shunting, determination of the basal plasma NH_3 concentration is a better test.[16] When the basal plasma NH_3 measurement is not informative, the rectally applied NH_3 tolerance test confirms or excludes the presence of portosystemic shunting. Measurement of plasma NH_3, which should be done immediately after sampling, can be more problematic in private clinics, although in recent years equipment for ammonia measurement has become more accessible for private clinics.

Ultrasound scan
For further diagnostic workup, ultrasound scan is needed. With ultrasonography, the liver parenchyma, gallbladder/biliary tree, portal vein, acquired shunting (when present), and ascites can be evaluated. In a recently performed evaluation of patients with PH, in 20% of the cases no abnormalities were found at abdominal ultrasonography. In approximately 25% of the cases, the liver was enlarged, irrespective of type of hepatitis. Ascites, in cases of liver disease, resulting from portal hypertension, often combined with a slightly to moderately decreased plasma albumin concentration, was found mainly in dogs with CH and LDH. In cases of ascites resulting from liver failure, there also is a high chance of finding acquired portosystemic collaterals. The best place to look is the region caudal to the left kidney. The finding of enlarged portal lymph nodes, ascites, or a decreased liver size has a negative prognostic value.

Finally, ultrasonography is necessary for guiding liver biopsies with Tru-Cut needles (Manan Medical Products, PBN Medicals, Stenlose, Denmark).

CT/MRI
For a further workup of patients with hepatitis, CT or MRI normally is not necessary. In cases in which a primary liver tumor is suspected, based on ultrasonography, and surgical intervention is needed, preoperative screening with CT or MRI with contrast is helpful in estimating size and localization of the tumor and visualizing the presence of tumor metastasis.

Liver Biopsy: Pathology
A liver biopsy is considered the gold standard for establishing a diagnosis of PH and to differentiate, when necessary, PH from NRSH. Fine-needle aspiration is not sufficient for diagnosing any form of hepatitis (primary or secondary). Liver biopsies can be ultrasound guided with a True-Cut needle or blind by aspiration using a syringe attached to

the needle (Menghini technique). At least two or more samples are advisable to mini-mize sampling errors. Because approximately one third of the cases of PH referred to the author's clinic are copper associated, the author advocates routine staining for copper (eg, with rubeanic acid) in addition to hematoxylin-eosin staining as standard procedure for liver histology in dogs.

TREATMENT AND PROGNOSIS

Most cases of idiopathic AH do not need treatment, but, depending on the severity of vomiting and presence of dehydration, antiemetic treatment and fluid therapy are indi-cated. Most dogs with AH recover after several days without medical interference. Progression from (initial) AH to its chronic counterpart may occur, resulting in recur-rence of clinical signs.[2] It is advisable to repeat the liver biopsy 6 to 8 weeks after the initial diagnosis to control if the hepatitis has been solved or has progressed to CH. CH(i) is treated as an immune-mediated disease with oral submission of predni-sone or prednisolone combined with supportive therapy (eg, antiemetic, antidiuretic, fluid therapy, and dietary adjustments). As discussed previously, only one publication (a retrospective evaluation) is available on the efficacy of prednisone in the treatment of CH in dogs, which showed a prolonged survival time for dogs with CH when treated with prednisone (0.6–1.1 mg/kg per day).[10] The response to prednisone therapy is controlled on a regular basis by liver biopsy, usually at a 6-week interval, and therapy is continued until histologically no hepatocellular death and inflammation are observed. In humans, the application of glucocorticoid treatment is indicated in alcohol-induced cirrhosis and autoimmune hepatitis in contrast to virally induced hepatitis, where it is contraindicated. Histologic similarities between human virally induced hepatitis and canine CH could indicate a reverse effect of prednisone efficacy. The majority of dogs with CH(i) referred to the author's clinic (2002–2006, n = 36) treated with prednisone (1 mg/kg per day), initially aimed at a 6-week treat-ment period, showed an estimated median survival time of 9.9 months. When only the CH(i) with cirrhosis cases treated with prednisone (n = 19) were included, the median survival time was 1.3 months, stressing that the presence of cirrhosis is a strong negative prognostic indicator. In the past, when unacceptable side effects (extreme polyuria-polydipsia, severely increased appetite, and reduced exercise toler-ance) resulting from prednisone/prednisolone medication occurred, the author and colleagues tapered the dosage of prednisone/prednisolone and started a combined therapy with azathioprine (1 mg/kg per day) for 6 weeks. Because of increased aware-ness of toxic side effects of cytostatic drugs in households (young children and preg-nant women), however, and because treatment of CH(i) has no proved benefit, the author does not advocate this combination therapy any longer.

Other than immunosuppressive medication, proposed medicinal options for treat-ment of CH(i), based mainly on extrapolated human data and personal experiences, are ursodeoxycholic acid (UDCA) (7.5 mg/kg twice a day); antioxidants, such as S-ad-enosyl-L-methionine (SAMe) (10 mg/kg twice a day)[17]; silymarin (100–200 mg/dog single oral administration); vitamin E (100–400 IU/day); and the antifibrotic drug, colchicine (0.025 mg/kg/day). UDCA is a synthetic nontoxic hydrophilic bile acid that provides a few positive actions. First, UDCA enhances the bile flow, and in this way it stimulates the excretion of inflammatory products. Second, UDCA decreases by dilution the concentration of the endogenous, more toxic bile acids. Third, it modu-lates the immune system, resulting in a reduction of the immune response, and fourth, there is proof that UDCA has antioxidative properties. The author's clinic recently started a trial with UDCA to evaluate if this drug might be a fair alternative for prednisone as a treatment of CH(i). SAMe is a natural metabolite in hepatocytes and is a precursor of glutathione. It is important in the defense against oxidative stress, and exhaustion might occur as a result of exposure to toxic substances in patients with CH. Silymarin seems to act as a strong free-radical scavenger by increasing cellular levels of superoxidedismutase, important in enzymatic defenses against oxidative stress—it regulates cell membrane permeability and has been shown to inhibit leukotriene synthesis and the effects of tumor necrosis factor alpha. Evidence from many human and veterinary reports underlines the protective effects of silymarin in patients with mushroom or acetaminophen intoxications.[18,19] Vitamin E is a nutritional antioxidant that protects against different routes of membrane peroxidation.

Colchicine has been proposed for treating CH fibrosis presumably by decreasing the formation and increasing the breakdown of collagen, but benefit is unproved, and there is little experience with colchicine in dogs. It can be a toxic drug after small overdoses. It is not advisable to use this drug in dogs until it is proved effective.

Many of the medications discussed previously generally are accepted and clinically used for the treatment of liver diseases, mostly as part of a multidrug therapy. Unfortunately, until now, for most of these drugs, critical scientific evaluation of their effectiveness is lacking.

If there is clinical evidence of portal hypertension (ascites or hepatic encephalopathy), treatment with spironolactone, a potassium-sparing diuretic (1–2 mg/kg twice a day), lactulose (0.5 mL/kg 2 to 3 times a day), and dietary adjustments (high-quality protein diets, moderately restricted) can be started. Spironolactone is preferred to furosemide because of the underlying pathophysiology of portal hypertension in which the rennin-angiotensin-aldosterone system is activated. In cases of severe ascites, a combination of spironolactone and furosemide may be effective. Lactulose, a synthetic disaccharide fermented by colonic bacteria into short-chain fatty acids, helps acidify the colonic environment to trap NH_3 (NH_4^+) so that it remains mainly in the feces and does not enter the portal circulation, reducing clinical signs of HE. When the portosystemic collaterals are optimally activated, and plasma albumin concentration is above the edema border (>15 g/L), ascites can disappear, and diuretic treatment might be stopped. This activation of collaterals normally takes 2 to 3 weeks. Symptomatic treatment of gastric erosions and ulceration consists of sucralfate (1 g by mouth 3 times a day) and a H_2-blocker (ranitidine [1 mg/kg twice a day], famotidine, or omeprazole [1 mg/kg once daily] [avoid cimetidine]).

In cases of CH(ca) or AH(ca), an etiology-based specific therapeutic approach is applied by feeding a low-copper diet, submission of a copper chelator (eg, D-penicillamine, 10–15 mg/kg twice a day), or submission of exogenous zinc (10 mg elemental zinc/kg twice a day). Penicillamine has, in addition to metal chelating properties, an immunomodulatory effect and possesses antifibrotic activity via inhibition of collagen crosslinking, causing collagen to be more susceptible to degradation.

SUMMARY

Poor understanding of the causes of PH, especially CH(i), results in limited options for adequate treatment and variable results. Elucidating the causes, aside from the copper-associated form of hepatitis, is of utmost importance to find etiology-based treatments for canine (chronic) hepatitis, when possible, most likely resulting in a better prognosis. The prognosis for patients with CH(i), with developed cirrhosis, is poor. Because many AH and CH cases are concluded to be copper associated (25%–30%), it is advisable to ask for a copper staining (eg, rubeanic acid) in addition to routine hematoxylin-eosin staining when sending liver materials to a pathology department; otherwise, this diagnosis can be missed and patients do not get appropriate treatment with copper-binding agents.

REFERENCES

1. Van den Ingh TSGAM, Van Winkle TJ, Cullen JM, et al. Morphological classification of parenchymal disorders of the canine and feline liver. In: Rothuizen J, Bunch SE, Charles JA, et al, editors. Standards for clinical and histological diagnosis of canine and feline liver diseases. Philadelphia: Saunders Elsevier; 2006. p. 85–101.
2. Watson PJ. Chronic hepatitis in dogs: a review of current understanding of the aetiology, progression, and treatment. Vet J 2004;167:228–41.
3. Twedt DC, Sternlieb I, Gilbertson SR. Clinical, morphologic, and chemical studies on copper toxicosis of Bedlington Terriers. J Am Vet Med Assoc 1979;175:269–75.
4. Thornburg LP, Shaw D, Dolan M, et al. Hereditary copper toxicosis in West Highland white terriers. Vet Pathol 1986;23:148–54.
5. Haywood S, Rutgers HC, Christian MK. Hepatitis and copper accumulation in Skye terriers. Vet Pathol 1988;25:408–14.
6. Mandigers PJ, van den Ingh TS, Bode P, et al. Association between liver copper concentration and subclinical hepatitis in Doberman Pinschers. J Vet Intern Med 2004;18:647–50.
7. Webb CB, Twedt DC, Meyer DJ. Copper-associated liver disease in Dalmatians: a review of 10 dogs (1998–2001). J Vet Intern Med 2002;16:665–8.
8. van de Sluis B, Rothuizen J, Pearson PL, et al. Identification of a new copper metabolism gene by positional cloning in a purebred dog population. Hum Mol Genet 2002;11:165–73.
9. Hoffmann G, van den Ingh TS, Bode P, et al. Copper-associated chronic hepatitis in Labrador Retrievers. J Vet Intern Med 2006;20:856–61.
10. Strombeck DR, Miller LM, Harrold D. Effects of corticosteroid treatment on survival time in dogs with chronic hepatitis: 151 cases (1977–1985). J Am Vet Med Assoc 1988;193:1109–13.
11. Sevelius E. Diagnosis and prognosis of chronic hepatitis and cirrhosis in dogs. J Small Anim Pract 1995;36:521–8.
12. Shih JL, Keating JH, Freeman LM, et al. Chronic hepatitis in Labrador Retrievers: clinical presentation and prognostic factors. J Vet Intern Med 2007;21:33–9.
13. Yzer J, Roskams T, Molenbeek RF, et al. Morphological characterisation of portal myofibroblasts and hepatic stellate cells in the normal dog liver. Comp Hepatol 2006;5:7.
14. Bonis PA, Friedman SL, Kaplan MM. Is liver fibrosis reversible? N Engl J Med 2001;344:452–4.
15. Friedman SL. Reversibility of hepatic fibrosis and cirrhosis—is it all hype? Nat Clin Pract Gastroenterol Hepatol 2007;4(5):236–7.
16. Gerritzen-Bruning MJ, van den Ingh TS, Rothuizen J. Diagnostic value of fasting plasma ammonia and bile acid concentrations in the identification of portosystemic shunting in dogs. J Vet Intern Med 2006;20:13–9.
17. Center SA, Karen LW, McCabe J, et al. Evaluation of the influence of S-adenosylmethionnine on systemic and hepatic effects of prednisolone in dogs. Am J Vet Res 2005;66:330–41.
18. Vogel G, Tuchweber B, Trost W, et al. Protection by silibinin against Amanita phalloides intoxication in beagles. Toxicol Appl Pharmacol 1984;73(3):355–62.
19. Saller R, Brignoli R, Melzer J, et al. An updated systematic review with meta-analysis for the clinical evidence of silymarin. Forsch Komplementmed 2006;15(1):9–20.

Copper-Associated Liver Diseases

Gaby Hoffmann, Dr med vet, PhD

KEYWORDS

- Wilson's disease • Metabolic disease • Centro-lobular copper
- Heritability • Diet

Copper (Cu) is an essential trace element, belonging to the first transition series of elements. Other members of this series include zinc, manganese, cobalt, iron, and chromium. The atomic weight of naturally occurring copper is 63.546.

The liver is essential for copper metabolism because it is the principal recipient of absorbed copper, has the highest stored copper content, delivers copper in protein-bound form to other tissues, and is the principal organ of excessive copper elimination by biliary excretion.[1,2]

Copper transport between organelles and across membranes is much the same for animals, bacteria, fungi, and plants because of the highly conserved cellular copper transport elements (**Fig. 1**).[2]

Trace elements, in general, function as cofactors for antioxidant enzymes. Copper is a transition metal able to cycle between two redox states: oxidized Cu^{2+} (cupric ion, stable) and reduced Cu^+ (cuprous ion, unstable). Copper can therefore function as an electron acceptor/donor for different enzymes.[3] It plays a role as a cofactor in hydrolytic, electron transfer and oxygen-utilization enzymes in the generation of cellular energy (cytochrome-c-oxidase), detoxification of oxygen-derived radicals (superoxide dismutase), iron metabolism (ceruloplasmin), blood coagulation, neuropeptide modification (dopamine-B-hydroxylase), melanin synthesis (tyrosinase), and connective tissue cross-linking (lysyl-oxidase).[1,4–10]

Free copper ions are able to catalyze the formation of hydroxyl radicals via the *Haber-Weiss reaction*:

$$O_2^{\cdot -} + Cu^{2+} \rightarrow O_2 + Cu^+ \tag{1}$$

$$Cu^+ + H_2O_2 \rightarrow Cu^{2+} + OH^- + OH^{\cdot} \tag{2}$$

$$O_2^{\cdot -} + H_2O_2 \rightarrow O_2 + OH^- + \mathbf{OH^{\cdot}}$$

The final outcome of this reaction is the toxic hydroxyl radical (OH·). This radical can directly damage lipids, proteins, and nucleic acids. Oxidative damage can induce

Department of Clinical Sciences of Companion Animals, Utrecht University, Faculty of Veterinary Medicine, P.O. Box 80.154, NL 3508TD Utrecht, The Netherlands
E-mail address: g.hoffmann@uu.nl

Vet Clin Small Anim 39 (2009) 489–511
doi:10.1016/j.cvsm.2009.02.001
0195-5616/09/$ – see front matter © 2009 Elsevier Inc. All rights reserved.

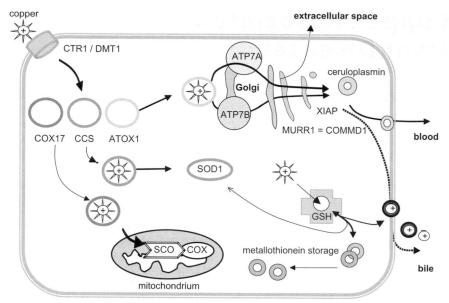

Fig. 1. Copper trafficking within the cell. Several intracellular pathways are involved in normal hepatic copper metabolism. Because of a high potential for oxidative damage, no free copper is present within the cell. Excessive copper is excreted into bile after interaction with COMMD1. CTR1, copper transporter 1; COX17, CCS, ATOX1, SCO, target-specific copper transporters; ATP7A, Menkes disease protein; ATP7B, Wilson's disease protein; SOD1, superoxide-dismutase 1; COX, cytochrome c oxidase; MURR1 = COMMD1, copper metabolism murr1 domain-containing protein 1, associated with copper toxicosis in Bedlington terriers; DMT1, divalent metal transporter 1; XIAP, X-linked inhibitor of apoptosis; GSH, glutathion. (*Data from* Refs.[14,16,22,40,45,73–99]).

inflammation, which ultimately can lead to liver damage. Oxidative stress affects transcription factors, resulting in deregulated gene expressions. In addition, oxidative stress is a major inducer of cytokine production in macrophages and other cells, of which profibrotic cytokines favor the production of collagen.[3,5,11,12]

Normal liver copper concentrations in dogs are higher than in people, mice, and rats.

The daily food intake of copper is about 14 to 15 mg/kg dry weight food in dogs, but considerable variation can be found between brands. Copper is present in vegetables, fruits, grains, nuts, meat, seafood, and drinking water, but to obtain copper concentrations in the above range, copper is commonly added to commercial dog food. Forty percent to 60% of ingested copper is absorbed across the apical membrane of the mucosa of the upper small intestine. The remaining copper leaves the body unabsorbed in feces.[11]

Two proteins are thought to be responsible for the absorption of dietary copper: the divalent metal transporter 1 (DMT1) and the copper transporter 1 (Ctr1). DMT1 transports copper (Cu^{2+}) directly from copper in the diet. Ctr1 is a transporter of Cu^+, which is reduced by endogenous plasma membrane reductases and dietary components such as ascorbate.[3] In the bloodstream, copper is bound to albumin (not specific binding), ceruloplasmin or transcuprein (specific binding). Within 2 to 6 hours of absorption, copper from blood enters the liver and the kidneys. In the liver, copper is immediately bound by intracellular chaperones, which are target-specific transporter proteins. These chaperones deliver copper to specific intracellular target molecules. In a second step, after 4 hours or more, copper is exported from the liver cell by the copper-transporting ATPase, ATP7A, re-enters the blood stream, and is delivered to other organs.[1,3,13–16]

COPPER STORAGE DISORDERS IN HUMANS

Wilson's disease (Online Mendelian Inheritance in Man [OMIM] 277,900) and Menkes disease (OMIM 309,400) are autosomal recessive inherited copper storage disorders. Wilson's disease is the most completely characterized disorder of copper toxicity in humans. Patients with this disorder accumulate copper in various tissues, particularly the liver and brain and, in small amounts, in the cornea and kidney. Reduction or absence of ATP7B-gene expression in these patients reduces the rate of incorporation of copper into ceruloplasmin, and reduces biliary excretion of copper. Progressive hepatic copper accumulation, liver cirrhosis, and basal ganglia degeneration ensue. Ocular accumulation of copper leads to a typical circumferential corneal pigmentation, known as Kayser-Fleisher rings. In the blood, ceruloplasmin concentrations are reduced and nonceruloplasmin-copper is greatly increased.

Other disorders of copper metabolism in humans include Indian childhood cirrhosis and non-Indian childhood cirrhosis (Endemic Tyrolean infantile cirrhosis [OMIM 215,600] and idiopathic copper toxicosis). These disorders of copper toxicity resemble Wilson's disease phenotypically. However, their genetic background is still unsolved, although a complex etiology is suggested, with influencing factors from the environment, such as high copper intake.[1,2,6,9]

Furthermore, copper is involved in a number of diseases without known impact on the pathogenesis, including Parkinson's disease, Alzheimer's disease, and Prion diseases.[17–21]

COPPER STORAGE DISORDERS IN MICE, RAT, AND SHEEP

The toxic milk mouse and the Long-Evans Cinnamon rat (LEC-rat) were the first animal models used to study Wilson's disease with both models having many features in common with their human counterpart. In these animals, mutations in the ATP7B gene lead to copper accumulation in the liver and progressive inflammation and cirrhosis.[12,15]

North Ronaldsay sheep, with an unknown abnormality of copper metabolism, develop liver cirrhosis comparable to idiopathic copper toxicosis in people owing to copper-induced increased lysosomal activity and hepatic stellate cell activation.[22]

COPPER-ASSOCIATED CHRONIC HEPATITIS

Hepatic copper accumulation can result from increased uptake of copper, primary defects in hepatic copper metabolism, or from altered biliary excretion of copper. Toxicity of copper is dependent upon the molecular association and subcellular localization of molecules as well as their total concentration in tissue. In inherited copper storage disorders, copper accumulation is always localized centrolobularly. This is the case in Bedlington terrier copper toxicosis, Wilson's disease in humans, and liver disease in LEC-rats. In contrast to primary copper storage disorders, secondary copper loading of liver cells during cholestasis or cholatestasis, copper is mainly restricted to the periportal parenchyma.[16,23]

Copper-Associated Chronic Hepatitis in Dogs

In the Bedlington terrier, inherited copper toxicosis is a well-described disease. In this breed a deletion of exon 2 in the COMMD1 gene (previously called MURR1) causes accumulation of copper in hepatocytes, resulting in chronic hepatitis.[24–26] Moreover, hepatic copper storage and associated hepatitis are breed associated in the West Highland white terrier, Skye terrier, Doberman pincher, Dalmatian, and Labrador retriever.[12,27–32]

The average canine liver copper concentration is 200 to 400 ppm (ppm = μg/g = mg/kg) per dry weight (dw) of liver tissue.[28–31,33,34] Hepatic copper concentrations in affected dogs of breeds with primary copper storage disease vary between individual animals and between breeds from 600 to above 2200 ppm (**Table 1**).

CLINICAL SIGNS AND LABORATORY RESULTS IN DOGS WITH COPPER-ASSOCIATED CHRONIC HEPATITIS

Dogs with hepatic copper accumulation can appear normal over years before developing clinical signs late in disease, although copper may begin to accumulate by 5 to 6 months of age. One investigator followed dogs with the COMMD1 deletion from birth to 3 years of age, and found excessive copper accumulated in the liver by 1 year of age, although histologic evidence of hepatitis did not occur before affected dogs were 2 years old (R. Favier, 2005, personal communication). Therefore, dogs with inherited copper storage disorders appear to be subject to a prolonged period of several years between severe accumulation of copper and development of histologic signs of inflammation, as well as between the consolidation of histologic signs of inflammation and recognition of clinical signs of disease.

With the exception of hemolysis from copper release into blood, which is only described for Bedlington terriers, symptoms of the disease are all nonspecific, resulting from liver dysfunction. The clinical signs may start with a mild decrease in activity or appetite. In most cases, owners will recognize these intermittent signs only with retrospect. Over weeks to months, dogs may vacillate between periods of decreased activity and periods of normal behavior. After months to years, symptoms become more prominent, and may include salivation with intermittent vomiting and nausea. Polyuria and polydipsia, icterus, diarrhea, and ascites may develop in advanced disease (**Box 1**).

Table 1					
Normal range of liver copper concentrations in dogs					
Range, ppm dw	Reference Range	Dogs	Breed	Method	Reference
120–304	<400	6	Labrador retriever	NAA	28
100–700	197 ± 113	13	Doberman pinschers	NAA	30
91–358	206 ± 56	22	Bedlington terriers	SP	31
94–270	190 ± 56	15	mixed breed dogs	SP	31
60–270	155 ± 66	13	mixed breed dogs	SP	30
38–650	156 ± 119	37	5 mixed breed dogs + 32 pure breed dogs	SP	34

Abbreviations: NAA, neutron activation analysis; ppm, parts per million (ppm equals μg/g, as well as mg/kg); SP, spectroscopy.

> **Box 1**
> **Clinical signs of copper-associated chronic hepatitis in dogs**
>
> Exercise intolerance
>
> Depression
>
> Anorexia
>
> Vomiting
>
> Weight loss
>
> Polyuria/Polydipsia
>
> Icterus
>
> Diarrhea
>
> Ascites
>
> Salivation
>
> Nonspecific clinical signs of copper-associated chronic hepatitis.

Findings on routine serum biochemical analyses include a greater relative increase in ALT (alanine aminotransferase) activity than ALP (alkaline phosphatase), suggesting primary hepatocellular liver disease.

DIAGNOSIS

Histopathologic evaluation of liver tissue is currently the only means of diagnosis of copper-associated hepatitis. Two or more liver biopsies, taken with a large-core needle (14 gauge), are a required minimum to evaluate liver tissue and determine copper toxicosis quantitatively or semi-quantitatively. Liver biopsy samples containing more than 6 to 8 portal triads are considered adequate for histologic diagnosis of human liver disease.[35] From reports comparing different biopsy techniques in dogs, relatively large-sized biopsies of the liver are required for accurate diagnosis (14 gauge, 1.8-mm diameter, 1-cm length).[35–39] To avoid puncture of adjacent organs, such as the gallbladder, stomach or intestine, the patient should be fasted for 12 hours before the procedure. In people with liver disease, significant hemorrhage after biopsy occurs in approximately 0.2% of patients.[16,35]

The typical magnitude and localization of copper within zone 3 within the liver lobule (centrolobular) are characteristics of primary copper storage disease.[28,40,41] Copper accumulates in hepatocytes, and results in hepatocellular inflammation with copper-laden macrophages and chronic hepatitis. The chronic hepatitis is characterized by hepatocellular apoptosis, necrosis, regeneration, and fibrosis, as well as an inflammatory infiltrate, which can be mononuclear or mixed. Fibrosis is part of the histopathologic definition of chronic hepatitis but may appear delayed in the disease process. Cirrhosis results as the end stage of the disease.[42]

COPPER ASSESSMENT

Copper concentrations in liver tissue can be measured quantitatively by irradiation of small biopsies and measurement of the induced Cu radioactivity in small pieces of liver (2 mg of tissue), or by spectrophotometric methods on fresh frozen liver (1 to 2 g of tissue needed). For the latter method, formalin-fixed tissue can be submitted, but measurement of copper concentrations in wet weight liver tissue is not recommended, especially in marginally elevated copper concentrations, because the reference ranges for copper are established on dry tissue basis. Alternatively, histochemical stains, such as rubeanic acid and rhodanine, are recommended to evaluate liver tissue semiquantitatively for copper. These stains consistently detect copper in liver biopsy specimens when amounts exceed the normal limit of 400 µg/g dw. It has been suggested that rhodanine demonstrates the protein to which copper binds rather than the copper itself.[43]

A histochemical grading system for evaluation of liver tissue stained with rhodanine for semiquantitative evaluation of hepatic copper concentrations in Bedlington terriers was developed by Johnson and colleagues.[44] The same grading system was applied for assessment of semiquantitative copper scores in rubeanic acid (dithio-oxamide)–stained liver tissue of Bedlington terriers, Doberman pinchers, and Labrador retrievers.[28,44–46] In a grading scale of 0 to 5, with 0 having no copper, scores above 2 are considered abnormal in both staining methods (**Fig. 2**).

Further staining methods, which have been applied for detection of copper include Timm's silver stain, cresyl-violet, dithizone, and orcein for copper-associated

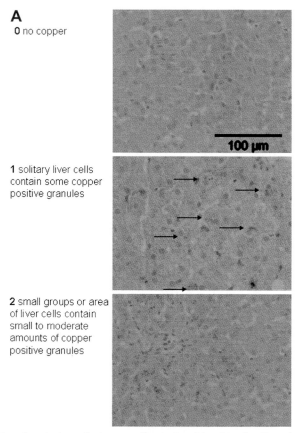

A 0 no copper

100 µm

1 solitary liver cells contain some copper positive granules

2 small groups or area of liver cells contain small to moderate amounts of copper positive granules

Fig. 2. (A, B) A histochemical grading system for evaluation of canine liver tissue stained with rhodanine or rubeanic acid. Copper scores above 2 are considered abnormal. Histology slides of 3-µm thickness of liver tissue from dogs stained with rubeanic acid for copper are shown as example. (Courtesy of T.S.G.A.M van den Ingh, TCCI Consultancy BV, Utrecht, The Netherlands.)

B

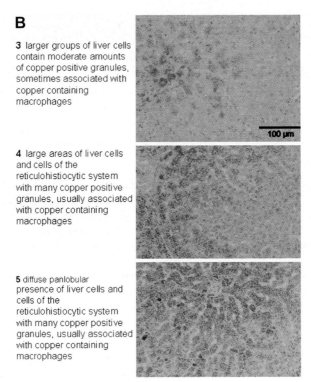

3 larger groups of liver cells contain moderate amounts of copper positive granules, sometimes associated with copper containing macrophages

4 large areas of liver cells and cells of the reticulohistiocytic system with many copper positive granules, usually associated with copper containing macrophages

5 diffuse panlobular presence of liver cells and cells of the reticulohistiocytic system with many copper positive granules, usually associated with copper containing macrophages

Fig. 2. (*continued*)

protein.[47] These staining methods have not been established for detection of copper in pets, and no grading system is available for veterinary use (**Table 2**).

COPPER ACCUMULATION SECONDARY TO CHOLESTASIS IN DOGS

Copper may accumulate in the liver secondary to cholestatic liver diseases. Because of defective copper excretion in the bile, cholestatic liver diseases often result in copper accumulation in the periportal areas. The accumulation occurs in hepatocytes. The magnitude of copper accumulation from cholestasis is not as high as that found in dogs with inherited copper storage disorders. In a review of 17 liver biopsies from breeds not identified to be affected by inherited copper-associated liver disease, the mean copper concentration was 984 μg/g dry weight liver.[34] Another study revealed that 3+ or higher histochemical detection of copper in the central area of the liver lobule indicates a primary copper storage disease.[42,45] In their study, Spee and colleagues[42] were able to find distinction criteria to determine whether copper accumulation is primary or secondary to hepatitis by comparison of liver biopsies from Bedlington terriers with copper toxicosis with those harvested from non–copper-associated breeds diagnosed with severe chronic hepatitis, and dogs with chronic extrahepatic cholestasis. Copper metabolism was analyzed using histochemical staining and quantitative reverse transcriptase polymerase chain reaction (RT-PCR) by comparison of the gene expressions of *ATOX1*, *COX17*, *ATP7A*, *ATP7B*, *CP*, *MT1A*, *COMMD1*, and *XIAP*. Oxidative stress was measured by determining GSH/GSSG ratios and gene-expression (*SOD1*, *CAT*, *GSHS*, *GPX1*, *CCS*, *p27KIP*, *Bcl-2*).

| Table 2 | | |
| Staining methods for copper in liver tissue | | |
Staining Method	Grading System for Veterinary Use	Copper Color
Rhodanine	Yes	Red to red-yellow
Rubeanic acid (dithiooxamide)	Yes	Deep blue to black
Timms silver stain	No	Black
Orcein	No	Black

BEDLINGTON TERRIER

In 1975, hepatic copper toxicity was first described in Bedlington terriers.[48] It was subsequently shown that affected Bedlington terriers have an inherited autosomal recessive defect of the MURR1 gene, which was renamed to COMMD1 (copper metabolism murr1 domain–containing protein 1). The extent of hepatic damage tends to parallel the increasing hepatic copper concentrations, which occur from decreased copper excretion into bile in COMMD1-deficient liver cells. The accumulated copper in liver tissue is seen as dense granules in lysosomes and occurs mainly in the centrolobular region of the liver. The histologic changes extend from focal necrosis to chronic hepatitis, which may ultimately lead to cirrhosis. In some cases, acute hepatic necrosis, copper-associated hemolytic anemia, and acute liver failure may occur. Female and male dogs are equally affected.

Copper toxicosis in Bedlington terriers (**Fig. 3**) can clinically be divided into three stages (**Table 3**). In the first stage, hepatic copper concentrations increase from 400 to 1500 ppm dw. Copper accumulation initially occurs in zone 3 of liver lobule (centrolobular hepatocytes). This stage remains clinically silent. A liver biopsy will reveal increased concentrations of copper but the histologic structure of the liver appears normal.

In the second stage, copper concentrations increase further into a range of 1500 to 2000 ppm dw. Histologically, copper accumulation is also found in zones 2 and 1 (midzonal and periportal hepatocytes). A liver biopsy will reveal inflammation with centrilobular mixed cell foci, containing necrotic hepatocytes, lymphocytes, plasma cells, neutrophils, and copper-laden macrophages. In the most advanced stage, dogs become clinically ill. Copper concentrations may exceed 2000 ppm dw and histology reveals hepatitis and cirrhosis. Cholestasis and bile duct proliferation occur along with fibrosis probably because of compression exerted on bile ducts in a distorted fibrotic liver and/or a cytokine-induced proliferation of bile ducts.[31,48–58]

Homozygous affected dogs have the highest copper concentrations. Heterozygous carrier dogs generally have an increase in copper concentrations until the age of 6 to 9 months before concentrations fall back to within the normal range.

The disease can be diagnosed by copper measurement in liver biopsies, as well as with genetic testing. Estimates of the incidence of copper toxicosis in Bedlington terriers varied from 34% to 66% between countries before genetic testing became available. Genetic assays investigate the presence of a particular microsatellite marker, which is in linkage disequilibrium with the COMMD1 mutation, or they detect the deletion of exon 2 of COMMD1 directly.

DOBERMAN PINSCHER

Copper-associated hepatitis in Dobermans almost exclusively affects female dogs. In young dogs (1 to 3 years), increased serum ALT, centrolobular copper accumulation,

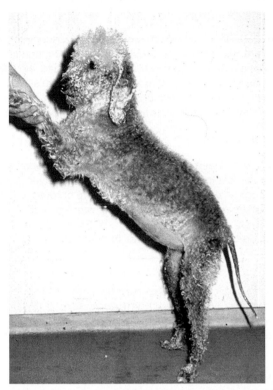

Fig. 3. Bedlington terrier with copper toxicosis. (*Courtesy of* Jan Rothuizen, DVM, PhD, Utrecht, The Netherlands.)

and subclinical hepatitis occur. Clinical evidence of liver disease usually begins around 4 to 7 years of age with chronic hepatitis and cirrhosis. Copper appears to be associated with the disease, because recent studies suggest that copper is often increased before the development of clinical hepatitis. Furthermore, copper excretion studies reveal decreased biliary Cu excretion in affected Doberman pinschers. Moreover, copper chelator (penicillamine) therapy in subclinical dogs normalized copper concentrations with improvement in the grade of histologic damage.[59]

Stage	Clinics	Copper	Liver Histology
1	No clinical signs	Copper in zone 3 (centrolobular) from 400–1500 ppm	Normal liver structure
2	No clinical signs	Copper in all zones 1500–2000 ppm	Inflammation
3	Clinical illness	Copper in all zones >2000 ppm dw	Inflammation + cirrhosis

Table 3
Stages of copper toxicosis in Bedlington terriers

DALMATIAN

In a retrospective study of 10 Dalmatians with copper-associated chronic hepatitis, two of the dogs were related and all presented for gastrointestinal clinical signs.[32] Males were equally affected as females and all dogs had elevated liver enzymes and necro-inflammatory liver changes, as well as centrolobular copper accumulation. In five dogs, hepatic copper concentrations exceeded 2000 μg/d dw liver, with several dogs having copper levels as high as those observed in Bedlington terriers.[32]

WEST HIGHLAND WHITE TERRIER

Affected dogs of this breed were 3 to 7 years of age. Some dogs had elevated hepatic copper concentrations (centrolobular) but no evidence of liver disease, which led to the suspicion that copper was a cause of subsequent chronic hepatitis and cirrhosis. Copper accumulation does not appear to increase with age in the West Highland white terrier, and there is no gender predilection.[34,60] Biliary excretion studies revealed a decreased excretion of radioactive copper in affected dogs.[61]

SKYE TERRIERS

Cholestasis was the suspected etiology of copper-associated chronic hepatitis and cirrhosis in Skye terriers. The 10 described dogs were 1 to 10 years old. Female and male dogs were equally affected, and presented with intermittent signs of anorexia, vomiting, and ascites. At a terminal stage of the disease, the animals developed jaundice and died.[27]

LABRADOR RETRIEVER

Chronic hepatitis is reported to be common in this breed and copper accumulation is associated with about 75%, but not all cases of chronic hepatitis. Females are more commonly affected, and generally are presented at around 7 years of age (range 2 to 10 years). Clinical signs are nonspecific and include anorexia, vomiting, and weight loss. Hepatic copper concentrations generally range from 650 to 3000 μg/g dw (histologically above 2+ with rubeanic acid staining). The histologic localization of copper in the centrolobular region of the liver lobule is an indicator for primary copper accumulation.[23,28,62]

OTHER BREEDS

Publications of other breeds with liver disease (**Table 4**) associated with copper accumulation include reports of an Anatolian shepherd dog, 6 German shepherd dogs, 11 Keeshonden, and a Boxer.

THERAPY
Diet

The goal of medical therapy is to reduce the absorption of copper and to enhance its excretion. Therefore, diets heavily supplemented with copper and copper-containing vitamin/mineral supplements should be avoided. Foods containing large amounts of copper, such as eggs, liver, shellfish, organ meats, beans/legumes, mushrooms, chocolate, nuts, and cereals should be excluded from the diet.

We have investigated the effects of a low-copper diet and zinc gluconate on hepatic copper accumulation in 21 client-owned Labradors that were related to former dogs affected with copper associated chronic hepatitis and that had been diagnosed with elevated hepatic copper concentrations. We found that feeding of low copper diets to Labradors is effective in reducing hepatic copper concentrations. Hepatic copper concentrations were assessed before and following an average of 8 months and 16 months of treatment. During this time, all dogs were fed exclusively on a low copper diet (hepatic, Royal Canin). In addition, the dogs were assigned to one of two groups in a randomized double-blind manner to receive a supplement of zinc gluconate or a placebo. Hepatic copper concentrations decreased significantly in both groups at control examinations.

Chelation

Chelating agents are commonly used to enhance urinary copper excretion. Chelators compete with binding sites for metals and produce a water-soluble complex with copper, which is then excreted into urine or bile. The standard chelating agent for the treatment of copper storage disorders in people and dogs is penicillamine. Another accepted treatment in people is the use of zinc for induction of intestinal metallothionein for chelation of copper and prevention of intestinal uptake of the metal.[55,63–66]

PENICILLAMINE

Recommended dosage: *10 to 15 mg/kg twice a day orally*

Penicillamine can chelate copper and other metals. The drug leads to mobilization of copper from tissues and promotes copper excretion in urine. Penicillamine also may increase the synthesis of metallothionein, and has anti-inflammatory, immunosuppressive, and antifibrotic effects.[59,67–72] Lifelong therapy might be required. The drug is effective for the treatment of chronic hepatitis owing to copper accumulation. Adverse effects occur in about 20% of dogs as inappetence, vomiting, and diarrhea. These adverse effects can generally be adverted by mixing the drug with food, and dividing the daily dosage into frequent applications. Side effects reported in people include vitamin-B deficiency from increased urinary loss of pyridoxine, fever, cutaneous eruptions, lupuslike symptoms, lymphadenopathy, cytopenias, and proteinuria. Penicillamine is potentially teratogenic and its use during pregnancy is not recommended. Pet owners should be informed about the potential risks of handling the drug for pregnant women.

Clinical improvement from penicillamine treatment might take weeks to months, and large interindividual variations are observed with respect to the effectiveness of the drug in people, as well as in dogs. Follow-up liver biopsies are generally required to determine if a patient will need long-term therapy. One author described an average detoxification rate of around 900 ppm copper decrease per year during penicillamine treatment in Bedlington terriers.[55,66]

Penicillamine was effective for treatment of Doberman pinschers with copper-associated subclinical hepatitis.[59] We have tested copper chelation therapy with penicillamine (10 to 15 mg/kg twice daily orally for 3 to 6 months) in Labrador retrievers in a randomized, double blind, placebo-controlled study and found the drug to be effective for the treatment of hepatic copper accumulation in this breed.

ZINC

Recommended dosage: *200 mg of elemental zinc daily per dog (in divided doses) or 7.5 mg elemental zinc/kg twice a day orally*.

Oral zinc is given to reduce copper absorption from the diet. Zinc induces the production of metallothionein in intestinal mucosal cells. Metallothionein is

Table 4
Literature review of copper-associated hepatitis in different dog breeds

Breed	No. Dogs	Age	Gender	Signs	Liver Enzymes	Copper (ppm dw)	Copper Location	Histology	Therapy and Outcome	Reference
Bedlington terrier	21	8mo–14y	female = male	Partial anorexia, depression, weight loss, vomiting	ALT + ALP elevation	Assessed in wet weight	No assessment in intact lobuli	Chronic hepatitis, cirrhosis, acute hepatocytic necrosis, liver failure	Not assessed	Hardy et al.[48]
	149	1mo–17y	female = male	No signs, family of high copper dog	N/A	N/A	Begin centrolobular, later all zones	Hepatitis	N/A	Thornburg et al.[34]
	68	6mo–15y	female = male	19 dogs: 3 clinical syndromes: 1. acute (6y): anorexia, vomiting, weakness, 2. chronic: (5–12y) 13 dogs: anorexia, weight loss, intermittent vomiting, diarrhea, unthriftiness, 3. Hemolytic/jaundice	ALT increased	850–10,600	Begin centrolobular (stage 1) later all zones	Focal hepatitis – cytologic	d-penicillamine = > improvement	Twedt et al.[31]
	24	1–14y	female = male	No signs	N/A	Numbers not given	N/A	Study compared cytologic versus histologic staining results	N/A	Taske et al.[54]
	18	1.7–11y	female = male	No signs, anorexia, vomiting, weight loss, hemolytic crisis	ALT > AST elevation	2638 (1443–3373)	Periacinar	Necrosis, inflammation, fibrosis, extramedullary hematopoiesis	Preventative feeding of low-copper diet	Hyun et al.[52]

	Age	Sex	Clinical signs	ALT	Value	Histology location	Disease	Treatment	Reference
5	3–10y	female = male	No signs, 1 dog hemolysis	ALT increased	3000–11,000	N/A	Necrosis, chronic hepatitis, cirrhosis	2,3,2-tetramine = > effective chelating drug	Twedt et al.[55]
4	N/A	N/A	N/A	N/A	N/A	N/A	N/A	N/A	Hoff et al.[51]
2	3 + 5y	female = male	anorexia, weight loss > vomiting, PU/PD	ALT × 10, AST × 10	1027 + 10,728	N/A	Chronic hepatitis/cirrhosis	Penicillamine = > died	Kelly et al.[100]
Doberman pinscher									
30	N/A	female >> male	no signs, routine blood screen, ascites, weight loss, jaundice	N/A	650–4700	centrolobular	Chronic hepatitis in zone 3	N/A	Thornburg.[101]
26	1.5–10y	female >> male	Anorexia, weight loss, PU/PD, icterus, ascites, bleeding, seizures vomiting	ALP × 10, ALT × 11, high billirubin	509 (88–722)	N/A	Chronic hepatitis	Prednisolone = > moderate – poor response	Crawford et al.[102]
22	3y	female >> male	No signs	ALT > ALP elevation bile acids elevated	419 ± 414	Centrolobular	Hepatitis	N/A	Mandigers et al.[29]
20	1mo–17y	N/A	no signs, family of high copper dog		140–1500	Begin centro-lobular	Hepatitis	N/A	Thromburg et al.[34]
18	2.5–7y	female >> male	no signs	ALT elevated in 2 dogs	Histology: elevated	Multifocal & portal	Inflammation, necrosis, fibrosis	N/A	Speeti et al.[103]
11	2.5–11y	female >> male	PU/PD, weight loss, decreased activity, poor appetite, vomiting, diarrhea	ALT + ALP > billirubin elevated	404–1700	Centrolobular	Degeneration, inflammation, necrosis, fibrosis, cirrhosis	Diuretics, antibiotics, penicillamine = > 6 dogs died within 9 months	Johnson et al.[104]

(continued on next page)

Table 4
(continued)

Breed	No. Dogs	Age	Gender	Signs	Liver Enzymes	Copper (ppm dw)	Copper Location	Histology	Therapy and Outcome	Reference
	8	2–8y	female	Anorexia, weight loss, apathy, exercise intolerance, vomiting, PD	ALT × 20, AST × 7, ALP × 4.5	Histology: 3 +	Periphery of hyperplastic nodules	Cirrhosis/cholestasis	N/A	van den Ingh et al.[46]
	5	6–8y	female	No signs	ALT × 5, ALP × 2–3	1036 (630–1330)	Centrolobular	Subclinical hepatitis	200 mg d-penicillamine PO q12 h for 4 months = > improvement	Mandigers et al.[59]
	3	N/A	N/A	N/A	N/A	>471	N/A	N/A	N/A	Hoff et al.[51]
	2	3 + 4y	female	N/A	N/A	600 + 804	Juxtaseptal hepatocytes of pseudolobule	Cirrhosis	N/A	Thornburg et al.[105]
	2	3y (f) + 6y (m)	male = female	Partial anorexia, weight loss, vomiting	ALT × 10–20, ALP normal	1465 + 2500	Centrolobular and in macrophages	Focal hepatitis	Died	Thornburg et al.[106]
Dalmatian	10	2–10y	male = female	Inappetence, vomiting	ALT × 6 (2–12x), AST × 7 (2–22x), ALP × 2,7 (07–10x)	3197 (754–8390)	Centrilobular	Necrosis, fibrosis, inflammation	Penicillamine, trientine, zinc = > died/euthanized	Webb et al.[32]
	1	2y	female	Vomiting, PU/PD, diarrhea, seizures	AST, ALT, ALP elevated	1916	N/A	Hepatic necrosis/cirrhosis	Antibiotics, fluid, lactulose, penicillamine = > died	Napier[107]

Breed	n	Age	Sex	Clinical signs	Laboratory	Copper concentration	Distribution	Histology	Treatment/outcome	Reference
	1	1.5y	male	Vomiting, anorexia, weight loss, lethargy	ALT × 10 + AST × 4, ALP × 1.3	2356 up/g wet weight	Centrolobular	Hepatocellular necrosis & inflammation	Manifold = > died	Noaker et al.[108]
	1	2y	female	Lethargy, vomiting, paleness, icterus	ALT × 25, ALP ×3, bili × 15	7940	Centrolobular – midzonal	Hepatocellular necrosis, inflammation & fibrosis	N/A	Cooper et al.[109]
Skye terrier	9	18 mo–15y	male = female	Intermittent anorexia, vomiting, ascites ≫ terminal jaundice	—	358–2257	Centrolobular	Cirrhosis, chronic hepatitis	N/A	Haywood et al.[27]
	1	1y	female	Anorexia, vomiting, melaena, seizures, aggression	Bile acids × 36 fasted, bili × 15 alb (−30%), glop−6% ALP × 1.5, target cells	462	N/A	Micronodular cirrhosis, uneven distribution of inflammation	Antibiotics, lactulose, ursodeoxycholic acid, colchicine, zinc, Waltham hepatic support diet for 12 months, symptom free 2 years post diagnosis	McGrotty et al.[110]
West Highland white terrier	44	3–7y	female> male	N/A	N/A	Normal–3500	24 dogs related	29 dogs: high Cu + normal histology, 15× high copper and hepatitis or cirrhosis	N/A	Thornburg et al.[111]
	395	1mo–17y	female = male	No signs	N/A	20–6800	Begin centrolobular, later all zones	Hepatitis	N/A	Thornburg et al.[34]
	7	N/A	N/A	N/A	N/A	>1100	Copper excretion study	N/A	N/A	Brewer et al.[112]
	2	N/A	N/A	N/A	N/A	>471	N/A	N/A	N/A	Hoff et al.[51]
	2	—	—	—	—					Thornburg et al.[113]
Labrador retriever	23	7y (2–10)	female> male	anorexia> vomiting	ALT × 10, ALP × 4.5	1317 (402–2576)	Centrolobular	Chronic hepatitis, cirrhosis	Penicillamine and prednisolone = > improvement	Hoffmann et al.[28]

(continued on next page)

Table 4
(continued)

Breed	No. Dogs	Age	Gender	Signs	Liver Enzymes	Copper (ppm dw)	Copper Location	Histology	Therapy and Outcome	Reference
	17	9.3y (3.9–14y)	female = male	Decreased appetite, vomiting, lethargy, weight loss diarrhea, PU/PD	mean ALT > ALP	N/A	8 dogs: all 3 zones, 3 dogs: centrolobular, 5 dogs: portal	Inflammation, degeneration (hydropic and necrosis), fibrosis	Ursodeoxycholic acid, prednisone, antibiotics, azathioprin, SAMe	Shih et al.[114]
	1	N/A	N/A	N/A	N/A	>471	N/A	N/A	N/A	Hoff et al.[51]
Other Breeds and Cats:										
German shepherd	3	1.5–3y	male = female	Ascites, icterus	ALP 4× elevated (1–6×), ALT 4× elevated (2–12×)	1441–2921	N/A	Macronodular cirrhosis and high Cu	N/A	Zentek et al.[10]
	3	4mo, 8 + 9y	male = female	N/A	N/A	570, 1352, 2202	Juxtaseptal hepatocytes of pseudolobule	Cirrhosis	N/A	Thornburg et al.[115]
Anatolian shepherd	1	7y	male	Intermittent inappetence, weight loss, decreased endurance, vomiting	ALT × 3, ALP × 1.5	4+	Centrolobular > all zones	Chronic hepatitis	Penicillamine + prednisolone, improvement	Bosje et al.[116]
Keeshond	11	1mo–17y	female = male	No signs, family or high copper dog	N/A	90–2400	Begin centrolobular, later all zones	Hepatitis	N/A	Thornburg et al.[34]
Boxer	1	6y	female	PU/PD	ALT and ALP increased	1101	Centrolobular (zone 3 + 2)	Pigment granulomas, normal architecture	N/A	van den Ingh et al.[117]
European Shorthair cat	1	2y	male	Inappetence, vomiting, fever	—	4170	Centrolobular	Cirrhosis, chronic hepatitis	N/A	Meertens et al.[118]
Siamese cat	1	2y	female	Anorexia, depression	ALT × 15, AST × 6	4074	Centrolobular	Hepatocellular necrosis & inflammation	Died	Heynes et al.[119]

Abbreviations: ALP, alkaline phosphatase; ALT, alanine aminotransferase; AST, aspartate aminotransferase; dw, dry weight liver; N/A, not assessed; PU/PD, polyuria/polydipsia.

a cysteine-rich protein, which acts as an endogenous chelator of metals with high affinity for copper. Metallothionein binds copper from the diet, preventing its transport into the circulation. Most of the bound copper is lost in the feces when intestinal cells are shed from the villi. Zinc might also induce hepatic metallothionein for nontoxic storage of copper. Because the rate of removal of hepatic copper is relatively slow, dogs with severe or fulminant copper-induced hepatitis should not be treated with zinc alone. Theoretically, zinc given orally together with penicillamine may decrease the effectiveness of both drugs.

The type of zinc salt used does not influence efficacy of the drug in people, but may affect tolerability. Acetate and gluconate salts may be more tolerable than sulfate. Theoretically, zinc should be given apart from feeding, because some food constituents (such as phytates) can bind zinc and diminish its efficacy. However, the salts might be an irritant to the gastric mucosa and lead to nausea and vomiting; therefore, mixing of the drug with small amounts of food has been recommended. The plasma zinc concentration of dogs normally ranges from about 90 to 120 μg/dL. As plasma zinc concentration increases above 200 μg/dL, copper uptake may be suppressed. Zinc is a relatively safe drug, but large doses may cause gastrointestinal disturbances. At plasma zinc concentrations above 1000 μg/dL, hemolysis may occur. In a study of three Bedlington terriers and three West Highland white terriers with copper toxicosis, 200 mg of elemental zinc was given daily to each dog to achieve therapeutic plasma concentrations of zinc above 200 μg/dL. The effectiveness of zinc in the prevention of copper uptake from the intestine was assessed by measurement of peak plasma concentrations of radioactive copper after oral application. A minimum of 3 months of zinc treatment was necessary before copper uptake from the intestine was blocked.[61] Although zinc is currently reserved for maintenance treatment, is has been used as first-line therapy in people, most commonly for asymptomatic or presymptomatic patients. For this indication, the drug appears to be equally effective to penicillamine and is much better tolerated.[61,63–65]

TRIENTINE (2-2-2-TETRAMINE TETRAHYDROCHLORIDE)

Recommended dosage: *10 to 15 mg/kg every 12 hours*[28]

Trientine is a chelator, which enhances the urinary excretion of copper. Trientine is poorly absorbed from the gastrointestinal tract. The drug is described for treatment of Wilson's disease in people, where it is used in patients who are intolerant to penicillamine. Symptoms of toxicity in people include bone marrow suppression, proteinuria, and autoimmune disorders, such as systemic lupus erythematosus. In addition trientine has teratogenic effects.[55,61,64–66]

Another tetramine salt, 2,3,2-tetramine (= tetramine) was studied in five Bedlington terriers with copper toxicosis. The drug was very potent and patients remained without adverse effects. Hepatic copper concentrations decreased more than 50% during treatment with tetramine for 6 months, and histologic changes were improved (150 mg trientine salt in capsules twice a day orally per dog, 10 kg average weight, range 6.8 to 13.6 kg). The authors of the study recommended serial copper assessment during long-term treatment with the drug to avoid copper depletion of liver tissue and blood.[55]

TETRATHIOMOLYBDATE

Ammonium tetrathiomolybdate forms a tripartite complex with copper, which is stable. Given with food, tetrathiomolybdate can form complexes between copper and food proteins, and therefore prevents the absorption of copper. When given between meals, tetrathiomolybdate forms complexes with available serum copper (free copper) and albumin, rendering cellular uptake of copper ineffective. The drug is described for intravenous use in sheep with copper toxicosis, as well as a possible emergency approach in patients with acute hemolytic crisis from hepatic copper release. No studies have been performed in dogs. Tetrathiomolybdate is toxic, and copper deficiency can occur with use of this drug, which can lead to anemia because of copper depletion of bone marrow. Tetrathiomolybdate is not commercially available.[15,22,63,64]

REFERENCES

1. Ferenci P, Zollner G, Trauner M. Hepatic transport systems. J Gastroenterol Hepatol 2002;17(Suppl):S105–12.
2. Harris ED. Cellular copper transport and metabolism. Annu Rev Nutr 2000;20: 291–310.
3. Sharp PA. Ctr1 and its role in body copper homeostasis. Int J Biochem Cell Biol 2003;35:288–91.
4. Cox DW. Disorders of copper transport. Br Med Bull 1999;55:544–55.
5. Failla ML, Johnson MA, Prohaska JR. Copper. In: Bowman BA, Russell RM, editors, Present knowledge in nutrition. 8th edition. Washington, DC: ILSI Press; 2001. p. 373–383.
6. Huffman DL, O'Halloran TV. Function, structure, and mechanism of intracellular copper trafficking proteins. Annu Rev Biochem 2001;70:677–701.
7. Huffman DL, O'Halloran TV. Energetics of copper trafficking between the Atx1 metallochaperone and the intracellular copper transporter, Ccc2. J Biol Chem 2000;275:18611–4.
8. Prohaska JR, Gybina AA. Intracellular copper transport in mammals. J Nutr 2004;134:1003–6.
9. Puig S, Thiele DJ. Molecular mechanisms of copper uptake and distribution. Curr Opin Chem Biol 2002;6:171–80.
10. Zentek J, Buhl R, Wolf, et al. [Unusual high frequency of liver cirrhosis with copper storage in German sheperds]. der Praktische Tierarzt 1999;80(3):170–5 [in German].
11. Kastenmayer P, Czarnecki-Maulden GL, King W. Mineral and trace element absorption from dry dog food by dogs, determined using stable isotopes. J Nutr 2002;132:1670S–2S.
12. Prohaska JR, Brokate B. Copper deficiency alters rat dopamine beta-monooxygenase mRNA and activity. J Nutr 1999;129:2147–53.
13. Arnesano F, Banci L, Bertini I, et al. Metallochaperones and metal-transporting ATPases: a comparative analysis of sequences and structures. Genome Res 2002;12:255–71.
14. Handy RD, Eddy FB, Baines H. Sodium-dependent copper uptake across epithelia: a review of rationale with experimental evidence from gill and intestine. Biochim Biophys Acta 2002;1566:104–15.
15. Danks DM. Disorders of copper transport. In: Scriver CR, Beaudet AL, Sly WS, et al, editors. The metabolic and molecular bases of inherited disease. 7th edition. New York: McGraw-Hill; 1995:2211–35.
16. Zakim D, Boyer TD. Hepatology: a textbook of liver disease. Philadelphia: Elsevier Health Sciences; 2002.
17. Dick FD, De Palma G, Ahmadi A, et al. Gene-environment interactions in parkinsonism and Parkinson's disease: the Geoparkinson study. Occup Environ Med 2007;64:673–80.

18. Dong SL, Cadamuro SA, Fiorino F, et al. Copper binding and conformation of the N-terminal octarepeats of the prion protein in the presence of DPC micelles as membrane mimetic. Biopolymers 2007;88(6):840–7.

19. Gaggelli E, Kozlowski H, Valensin D, et al. Copper homeostasis and neurodegenerative disorders (Alzheimer's, prion, and Parkinson's diseases and amyotrophic lateral sclerosis). Chem Rev 2006;106:1995–2044.

20. Klevay LM. Alzheimer's disease as copper deficiency. Med Hypotheses 2007; 70(4):802–7.

21. Leach SP, Salman MD, Hamar D. Trace elements and prion diseases: a review of the interactions of copper, manganese and zinc with the prion protein. Anim Health Res Rev 2006;7:97–105.

22. Haywood S, Simpson DM, Ross G, et al. The greater susceptibility of North Ronaldsay sheep compared with Cambridge sheep to copper-induced oxidative stress, mitochondrial damage and hepatic stellate cell activation. J Comp Pathol 2005;133:114–27.

23. vd Ingh VW, Cullen V, Charles J, et al. Morphological classification of parenchymal disorders of the canine and feline liver. In: Rothuizen J, Bunch S, Charles J, et al, editors. WSAVA standards for clinical and histological diagnosis of canine and feline liver diseases. Philadelphia: Elsevier/Saunders; 2006. p. 85–101.

24. Poffenbarger EM, Hardy RM. Hepatic cirrhosis associated with long-term primidone therapy in a dog. J Am Vet Med Assoc 1985;186:978–80.

25. van de Sluis B, Rothuizen J, Pearson PL, et al. Identification of a new copper metabolism gene by positional cloning in a purebred dog population. Hum Mol Genet 2002;11:165–73.

26. Zudenigo D, Relja M. [Hepatolenticular degeneration]. Neurologija 1990;39: 115–27 [in Croatian].

27. Haywood S, Rutgers HC, Christian MK. Hepatitis and copper accumulation in Skye terriers. Vet Pathol 1988;25:408–14.

28. Hoffmann G, van den Ingh TS, Bode P, et al. Copper-associated chronic hepatitis in Labrador retrievers. J Vet Intern Med 2006;20:856–61.

29. Mandigers PJ, van den Ingh TS, Bode P, et al. Association between liver copper concentration and subclinical hepatitis in Doberman pinschers. J Vet Intern Med 2004;18:647–50.

30. Thornburg LP, Shaw D, Dolan M, et al. Hereditary copper toxicosis in West Highland white terriers. Vet Pathol 1986;23:148–54.

31. Twedt DC, Sternlieb I, Gilbertson SR. Clinical, morphologic, and chemical studies on copper toxicosis of Bedlington Terriers. J Am Vet Med Assoc 1979; 175:269–75.

32. Webb CB, Twedt DC, Meyer DJ. Copper-associated liver disease in Dalmatians: a review of 10 dogs (1998–2001). J Vet Intern Med 2002;16:665–8.

33. Hoffmann G, Mesu S, Jones P, et al. Double blind placebo-controlled treatment with D-penicillamine against hepatic copper in Labrador retrievers. Presented at the American College of Veterinary Internal Medicine forum. Louisville, Kentucky, 2006.

34. Thornburg LP, Rottinghaus G, McGowan M, et al. Hepatic copper concentrations in purebred and mixed-breed dogs. Vet Pathol 1990;27:81–8.

35. Bravo A, Sheth SG, Chopra S. Liver biopsy. N Engl J Med 2001;344:495–500.

36. Cole TL, Center SA, Flood SN, et al. Diagnostic comparison of needle and wedge biopsy specimens of the liver in dogs and cats. J Am Vet Med Assoc 2002;220:1483–90.

37. Rawlings CA, Howerth EW. Obtaining quality biopsies of the liver and kidney. J Am Anim Hosp Assoc 2004;40:352–8.
38. Vasanjee SC, Bubenik LJ, Hosgood G, et al. Evaluation of hemorrhage, sample size, and collateral damage for five hepatic biopsy methods in dogs. Vet Surg 2006;35:86–93.
39. Wang KY, Panciera DL, Al-Rukibat RK, et al. Accuracy of ultrasound-guided fine-needle aspiration of the liver and cytologic findings in dogs and cats: 97 cases (1990–2000). J Am Vet Med Assoc 2004;224:75–8.
40. Mufti AR, Burstein E, Duckett CS. XIAP: cell death regulation meets copper homeostasis. Arch Biochem Biophys 2007;463:168–74.
41. vd Ingh C, Twedt T, van Winkle R, et al. Morphological classification of biliary disorders of the canine and feline liver. In: Rothuizen J, Bunch S, Charles J, et al, editors. WSAVA standards for clinical and histological diagnosis of canine and feline liver diseases. Philadelphia: Saunders/Elsevier; 2006. p. 61–76.
42. Spee B, Arends B, van den Ingh TS, et al. Copper metabolism and oxidative stress in chronic inflammatory and cholestatic liver diseases in dogs. J Vet Intern Med 2006;20(5):1085–92.
43. Shehan H. Theory and practice of histotechnology. In: Sheehan DC, Hrapchak BB, editors. Theory and practice of histotechnology. 2nd edition. St. Louis (MO): CV Mosby Co; 1980. p. 230.
44. Johnson GF, Gilbertson SR, Goldfischer S, et al. Cytochemical detection of inherited copper toxicosis of Bedlington terriers. Vet Pathol 1984;21:57–60.
45. Spee B, Mandigers PJ, Arends B, et al. Differential expression of copper-associated and oxidative stress related proteins in a new variant of copper toxicosis in Doberman pinschers. Comp Hepatol 2005;4:3.
46. van den Ingh TS, Rothuizen J, Cupery R. Chronic active hepatitis with cirrhosis in the Doberman pinscher. Vet Q 1988;10:84–9.
47. Pilloni L, Lecca S, Van Eyken P, et al. Value of histochemical stains for copper in the diagnosis of Wilson's disease. Histopathology 1998;33:28–33.
48. Hardy RM, Stevens JB, Stowe CM. Chronic progressive hepatitis in Bedlington terriers associated with elevated copper concentrations. Minn Vet 1975;15:13–24.
49. Doige SL. Chronic active hepatitis in dogs: a review of 14 cases. J Am Anim Hosp Assoc 1981;17(5):725–30.
50. Fuentealba C, Guest S, Haywood S, et al. Chronic hepatitis: a retrospective study in 34 dogs. Can Vet J 1997;38:365–73.
51. Hoff B, Boermans HJ, Baird JD. Retrospective study of toxic metal analyses requested at a veterinary diagnostic toxicology laboratory in Ontario (1990–1995). Can Vet J 1998;39:39–43.
52. Hyun C, Filippich LJ. Inherited copper toxicosis in Australian Bedlington terriers. J Vet Sci 2004;5:19–28.
53. Owen RA, Haywood S, Kelly DF. Clinical course of renal adenocarcinoma associated with hypercupraemia in a horse. Vet Rec 1986;119:291–4.
54. Teske E, Brinkhuis BG, Bode P, et al. Cytological detection of copper for the diagnosis of inherited copper toxicosis in Bedlington terriers. Vet Rec 1992;131:30–2.
55. Twedt DC, Hunsaker HA, Allen KG. Use of 2,3,2-tetramine as a hepatic copper chelating agent for treatment of copper hepatotoxicosis in Bedlington terriers. J Am Vet Med Assoc 1988;192:52–6.
56. Andersson M, Sevelius E. Breed, sex, and age distribution in dogs with chronic liver disease: a demographic study. J Soc Adm Pharm 1991;32:1–5.

57. Boisclair J, Dore M, Beauchamp G, et al. Characterization of the inflammatory infiltrate in canine chronic hepatitis. Vet Pathol 2001;38:628–35.
58. K Richter. Common canine hepatopathies. Presented at the 15th American College of Veterinary Internal Medicine forum. San Diego, California 1997.
59. Mandigers PJ, van den Ingh TS, Bode P, et al. Improvement in liver pathology after 4 months of D-penicillamine in 5 Doberman pinschers with subclinical hepatitis. J Vet Intern Med 2005;19:40–3.
60. Thornburg LP, Crawford SJ. Liver disease in West Highland white terriers. Vet Rec 1986;118:110.
61. Brewer GJ, Dick RD, Schall W, et al. Use of zinc acetate to treat copper toxicosis in dogs. J Am Vet Med Assoc 1992;201:564–8.
62. Hoffmann G, Rothuizen J. Copper-associated chronic hepatitis. In: Bonagura, editor. Kirk's current veterinary therapy XIV. St. Louis (MO): Elsevier; 2008. p. 557–62.
63. Brewer GJ. Tetrathiomolybdate anticopper therapy for Wilson's disease inhibits angiogenesis, fibrosis and inflammation. J Cell Mol Med 2003;7:11–20.
64. Brewer GJ. Recognition, diagnosis, and management of Wilson's disease. In: Proceedings of the Society for Experimental Biology and Medicine. 2000. p. 39–46.
65. Roberts EA, Schilsky ML. A practice guideline on Wilsons disease. Hepatology 2003;37(6):1475–92.
66. Rolfe D, Twedt DC. Copper-associated hepatopathies in dogs. Vet Clin North Am Small Anim Pract 1995;25:399–417.
67. Klein D, Lichtmannegger J, Heinzmann U. Dissolution of copper-rich granules in hepatic lysosomes by d-penicillamine prevents the development of fulminant hepatitis in Long-Evans cinnamon rats. J Hepatol 2000;32:193–201.
68. Munthe E, Jellum E, Aaseth J. Some aspects of the mechanism of action of penicillamine in rheumatoid arthritis. Scand J Rheumatol Suppl 1979;28:6–12.
69. Jaffe I. Penicillamine: an anti-rheumatoid drug. Am J Med 1983;75:63–8.
70. Stanworth D, Hunneyball IM. Influence of d-penicillamine treatment on the humoral immune system. Scand J Rheumatol 1979;28:37–46.
71. Epstein O, De Villiers D, Jain S. Reduction of immune complexes and immuno-globulins induced by d-penicillamine in primary biliary cirrhosis. N Engl J Med 1979;300:274–8.
72. Harth M, Keown PA, Orange JF. Effects of d-penicillamine on inflammatory and immune reactions. Clin Invest Med 1984;7:45–51.
73. Liu N, Lo LS, Askary SH, et al. Transcuprein is a macroglobulin regulated by copper and iron availability. J Nutr Biochem 2007;18:597–608.
74. Montaser A, Tetreault C, Linder M. Comparison of copper binding components in dog serum with those in other species. Proc Soc Exp Biol Med 1992;200:321–9.
75. Kuo MT, Chen HH, Song IS, et al. The roles of copper transporters in cisplatin resistance. Cancer Metastasis Rev 2007;26:71–83.
76. Fiander H, Schneider H. Compounds that induce isoforms of glutathione S-transferase with properties of a critical enzyme in defense against oxidative stress. Biochem Biophys Res Commun 1999;262:591–5.
77. Mosialou E, Morgenstern R. Activity of rat liver microsomal glutathione trans-ferase toward products of lipid peroxidation and studies of the effect of inhibitors on glutathione-dependent protection against lipid peroxidation. Arch Biochem Biophys 1989;275:289–94.
78. de Bie P, van de Sluis B, Burstein E, et al. Distinct Wilson's disease mutations in ATP7B are associated with enhanced binding to COMMD1 and reduced stability of ATP7B. Gastroenterology 2007;133:1316–26.

79. de Bie P, Muller P, Wijmenga C, et al. Molecular pathogenesis of Wilson and Menkes disease: correlation of mutations with molecular defects and disease phenotypes. J Med Genet 2007;44:673–88.
80. La Fontaine S, Mercer JF. Trafficking of the copper-ATPases, ATP7A and ATP7B: role in copper homeostasis. Arch Biochem Biophys 2007;463:149–67.
81. Puig S, Lee J, Lau M, et al. Biochemical and genetic analyses of yeast and human high affinity copper transporters suggest a conserved mechanism for copper uptake. J Biol Chem 2002;277:26021–30.
82. Dahlman I, Eaves IA, Kosoy R, et al. Parameters for reliable results in genetic association studies in common disease. Nat Genet 2002;30:149–50.
83. Kenney SM, Cox DW. Sequence variation database for the Wilson disease copper transporter, ATP7B. Hum Mutat 2007;28(12):1171–7.
84. Lutsenko S, Petris MJ. Function and regulation of the mammalian copper-transporting ATPases: insights from biochemical and cell biological approaches. J Membr Biol 2003;191:1–12.
85. Lutsenko S, Barnes NL, Bartee MY, et al. Function and regulation of human copper-transporting ATPases. Physiol Rev 2007;87:1011–46.
86. Lutsenko S, LeShane ES, Shinde U. Biochemical basis of regulation of human copper-transporting ATPases. Arch Biochem Biophys 2007;463:134–48.
87. Bertini I, Cavallaro G. Metals in the "omics" world: copper homeostasis and cytochrome c oxidase assembly in a new light. J Biol Inorg Chem 2007;13(1):3–14.
88. Stasser JP, Siluvai GS, Barry AN, et al. A multinuclear copper(I) cluster forms the dimerization interface in copper-loaded human copper chaperone for superoxide dismutase. Biochemistry 2007;46:11845–56.
89. Suazo M, Olivares F, Mendez MA, et al. CCS and SOD1 mRNA are reduced after copper supplementation in peripheral mononuclear cells of individuals with high serum ceruloplasmin concentration. J Nutr Biochem 2007;19(4):269–74.
90. Bertinato J, L'Abbe MR. Maintaining copper homeostasis: regulation of copper-trafficking proteins in response to copper deficiency or overload. J Nutr Biochem 2004;15:316–22.
91. Dolderer B, Echner H, Beck A, et al. Coordination of three and four Cu(I) to the alpha- and beta-domain of vertebrate Zn-metallothionein-1, respectively, induces significant structural changes. FEBS J 2007;274:2349–62.
92. Formigari A, Irato P, Santon A. Zinc, antioxidant systems and metallothionein in metal mediated-apoptosis: biochemical and cytochemical aspects. Comp Biochem Physiol C Toxicol Pharmacol 2007;146:443–59.
93. Burstein E, Hoberg JE, Wilkinson AS, et al. COMMD proteins, a novel family of structural and functional homologs of MURR1. J Biol Chem 2005;280:22222–32.
94. Maine GN, Burstein E. COMMD proteins: COMMing to the scene. Cell Mol Life Sci 2007;64:1997–2005.
95. van de Sluis AJA. Identification of a copper toxicosis gene in Bedlington terriers. Utrecht, Netherlands: University of Utrecht; 2002. p. 9–30.
96. Burstein E, Ganesh L, Dick RD, et al. A novel role for XIAP in copper homeostasis through regulation of MURR1. EMBO J 2004;23:244–54.
97. Tao TY, Liu F, Klomp L, et al. The copper toxicosis gene product Murr1 directly interacts with the Wilson disease protein. J Biol Chem 2003;278:41593–6.
98. Mufti AR, Burstein E, Csomos RA, et al. XIAP is a copper binding protein deregulated in Wilson's disease and other copper toxicosis disorders. Mol Cell 2006;21:775–85.

99. Lim CM, Cater MA, Mercer JF, et al. Copper-dependent interaction of dynactin subunit p62 with the N terminus of ATP7B but not ATP7A. J Biol Chem 2006; 281:14006–14.
100. Kelly, et al. Copet toxicosis in Bedlington terriers in the UK. JSAP 1984;25: 293–8.
101. Thornburg LP. Histomorphical and immunohistochemical studies of chronic active hepatitis in Doberman Pinschers. Vet Pathol 1998;35(5):380–5.
102. Crawford MA, Schall WD, Jensen RK, et al. Chronic active hepatitis in 26 Doberman pinschers. J Am Vet Med 1985;187(12):1343–50.
103. Speeti M, Eriksson J, Saari S, et al. Lesions of subclinical Doberman hepatitis. Vet Pathol 1998;35(5):361–9.
104. Johnson JB, Hagstad HV, Springer WT. Chronic active hepatitis in Doberman pinschers. J Am Vet Med Assoc 1982;180(12):1438–42.
105. Thornburg, Rottinghaus. What is the significance of hepatic copper values in dogs with cirrhosis. Vet Med 1985;50–4.
106. Thornburg, et al. High liver copper levels in Doberman pinschers with subacute hepatitis. JAAHA 1983;20:1003–5.
107. Napier P. Hepatic necrosis with toxic copper levels in a two-year-old Dalmatian. Can Vet J 1996;37(1):45.
108. Noaker LJ, Washabau RJ, Detrisiac CJ, et al. Copper associated acute hepatic failure in a dog. J Am Vet Med Assoc 1999;214(10):1502–6.
109. Cooper, et al. Hepatitis and increased copper levels in a Dalmatian. J Vet Diagn Invest 1997;9(2):201–3.
110. McGrotty YL, Ramsey IK, Knottenbelt CM. Diagnosis and management of hepatic copper accumulation in a Skye terrier. J Small Anim Pract 2003;44(2): 85–9.
111. Thornburg LP, Shaw D, Dolan M, Raisbeck M, et al. Hereditary copper toxicosis in West Highland white terriers. Vet Pathol 1986;23(2):148–54.
112. Brewer GJ, Schall W, Dick R, et al. Use of 64 copper measurements to diagnose canine copper toxicosis. J Vet Intern Med 1992;6(1):41–3.
113. Thornburg LP, Rottinghaus G, Dennis G, et al. The relationship between hepatic copper content and morphologic changes in the liver of West Highland White Terriers. Vet Pathol 1996;33(6):656–61.
114. Shih, et al. Chronic hepatitis in Labrador retrievers: clinical presentation and prognostic factors. J Vet Intern Med 2007;21:33–9.
115. Thornburg, Rottinghaus. What is the significance of hepatic copper values in dogs with cirrhosis. Vet Med 1985;80:50–4.
116. Bosje JT, Van den Ingh TS, Fennema A, et al. Copper-induced hepatitis in an Anatolian shepherd dog. Vet Rec 2003;152(3):84–5.
117. van den Ingh TS, Rothuizen J. Accumulation of copper and iron in the liver of a boxer: a new disease? Tijdschr Diergeneeskd 1992;117(Suppl 1):16S.
118. Meertens NM, Bokhove CA, van den Ingh TS. Copper-associated chronic hepatitis and cirrhosis in a European shorthair cat. Vet Pathol 2005;42(1):97–100.
119. Heynes Wede. Hepatopathy associated with excessive hepatic copper in a Siamese cat. Vet Pathol 1995;32:427–9.

Portosystemic Vascular Anomalies

Allyson C. Berent, DVM[a],*, Karen M. Tobias, DVM, MS[b]

KEYWORDS

• Shunt • Extrahepatic • Intrahepatic
• Malformation • Embolization

Portosystemic shunts (PSS) are vascular anomalies that redirect blood from the portal vein to the systemic circulation, bypassing the hepatic sinusoids and liver parenchyma.[1–5] Normally, blood draining the stomach, intestine, spleen, and pancreas enters the portal vein and perfuses the liver through the sinusoidal network before entering the hepatic veins, and subsequently the caudal vena cava.[3] Portal blood contains nutrients, trophic hormones (intestinal and pancreatic), bacterial products, and intestinal-derived toxins.[1,2,6] The fetal liver has limited function to process these products, and a large shunting vessel (ie, ductus venosus) normally exists to bypass the hepatic circulation as a protective mechanism. This vessel normally closes shortly after birth, establishing hepatic circulation. If the ductus venosus remains patent, intrahepatic portosystemic shunting persists. Persistence of anomalous connections between the fetal cardinal and vitelline systems results in extrahepatic portosystemic shunting.[3,4]

When blood bypasses the liver, delivery of trophic factors (particularly insulin and glucagon) to the liver is decreased, resulting in poor hepatic development, decreased protein production, reticuloendothelial dysfunction, altered fat and protein metabolism, hepatic atrophy, and eventually hepatic failure. The severity of clinical signs is related to the volume and origin of blood bypassing the liver and may include hepatic encephalopathy (HE), chronic gastrointestinal signs, lower urinary tract signs, coagulopathies, and retarded growth.[2,3,5–7] In animals with portosystemic shunting, concentrations of endogenous and exogenous toxins that are normally metabolized or eliminated by the liver (ammonia, gut-associated encephalopathic toxins, hormone metabolism, benzodiazepine-like substances, aromatic amino acids, and so forth; **Table 1**) increase, whereas normal hepatic metabolic function (gluconeogenesis, urea cycle, uric acid cycle, and so forth)[7–10] decreases. This article discusses anomalous macroscopic venous-venous (portocaval or portoazygous shunts, congenital

a Sections of Internal Medicine and Surgery, Veterinary Hospital of the University of Pennsylvania, 3900 Delancey Street, Philadelphia, PA 19104, USA
b Department of Small Animal Clinical Sciences, University of Tennessee, 2407 River Drive, Knoxville, TN 37996, USA
* Corresponding author.
E-mail address: aberent@vet.upenn.edu (A.C. Berent).

Vet Clin Small Anim 39 (2009) 513–541
doi:10.1016/j.cvsm.2009.02.004
0195-5616/09/$ – see front matter © 2009 Published by Elsevier Inc.

Table 1
Toxins implicated in HE

Toxins	Mechanisms Suggested in the Literature
Ammonia	Increased brain tryptophan and glutamine; decreased ATP availability; increased excitability; increased glycolysis; brain edema; decreased microsomal Na,K-ATPase in the brain
Aromatic amino acids	Decreased DOPA neurotransmitter synthesis; altered neuroreceptors; increased production of false neurotransmitters
Bile acids	Membranocytolytic effects alter cell/membrane permeability; blood-brain barrier more permeable to other HE toxins; Impaired cellular metabolism due to cytotoxicity
Decreased a-ketoglutaramate	Diversion from Krebs cycle for ammonia detoxification; decreased ATP availability
Endogenous benzodiazepines	Neural inhibition: hyperpolarize neuronal membrane
False neurotransmitters Tyrosine → octapamine Phenylalanine → phenyethylamine Methionine → mercaptans	Impairs norepinephrine action Impairs norepinephrine action Synergistic with ammonia and short-chain fatty acids Decreases ammonia detoxification in brain urea cycle; derived from the gastrointestinal tract (fetor hepaticus–breath odor in HE); decreased microsomal Na,K-ATPase
GABA	Neural inhibition: hyperpolarize neuronal membrane; increase blood-brain barrier permeability to GABA
Glutamine	Alters blood-brain barrier amino acid transport
Phenol (from phenylalanine and tyrosine)	Syngergistic with other toxins; decreases cellular enzymes; neurotoxic and hepatotoxic
Short-chain fatty acids	Decreased microsomal Na,K-ATPase in brain; uncouples oxidative phosphorylation, impairs oxygen use, displaces tryptophan from albumin, increasing free tryptophan
Tryptophan	Directly neurotoxic; increases serotonin; neuroinhibition

Data from Refs.[2,6,8,9,19,20]

and acquired), venous-arterial (hepatic arteriovenous malformations [HAVM]), and microscopic venous-parenchymal communications (hepatic portal venous hypoplasia [PVH] or microvascular dysplasia [MVD]), involving communications between the portal vein and systemic circulation.

ANATOMY

The portal vein is formed by the convergence of the cranial and caudal mesenteric portal branches within the mesentery. It provides up to 80% of the blood flow (20% through the hepatic artery) and 50% of the oxygen content (50% through the hepatic artery) to the liver.[1-7] Additional tributaries from the spleen, stomach, pancreas, and proximal duodenum join the portal vein before its bifurcation. In dogs the portal vein divides into left and right branches and the left branch divides further to supply the central and left lobes. In the cat the portal vein divides directly into left, central, and right branches.[3,5] The portal vein then branches into smaller venules whereby the blood enters the parenchyma at the portal triads, travels through the hepatic sinusoids, and drains to the central veins, which then confluence to larger hepatic venules and hepatic veins that drain into the caudal vena cava. As it travels through the sinusoids, the portal blood is delivered to the hepatocytes and cleansed by the reticuloendothelial system. If this path is interrupted by an anomalous vessel(s), blood is diverted away from the liver and reaches the systemic circulation before hepatic circulation and cleansing.

PSS can either be congenital or acquired. Congenital PSS most commonly occur as single vessels that provide direct vascular communication between the portal venous supply and the systemic venous circulation (caudal vena cava or azygous vein), bypassing the liver. They commonly occur as a single intra- or extrahepatic communication. Rarely some animals have 2 or more congenital communications. Twenty percent of dogs with PSS have multiple acquired shunts secondary to chronic portal hypertension. Increased portal pressures lead to the opening of fetal, vestigial blood vessels, which reduces the hydrostatic pressure load of the portal veins. Acquired shunts are usually multiple, tortuous, and extrahepatic in nature and are most frequently located near the kidneys. The most common causes for acquired extrahepatic shunts (EHPSS) are hepatic cirrhosis, noncirrhotic portal hypertension (NCPH), HAVM, and congenital PVH.

The types of congenital hepatic vascular malformations found in dogs and cats include single intrahepatic portocaval shunts, single extrahepatic portocaval shunts, portal vein atresia with resultant multiple portal-caval anastomoses, HAVM, and PVH (formally called microvascular dysplasia).[2,11] PVH can be seen with or without portal hypertension. For the purpose of this review, PVH without hypertension is referred to as MVD-PVH and PVH with hypertension as NCPH. Approximately 25% to 33% of congenital PSS are intrahepatic (IHPSS) in dogs and cats. Single EHPSS are noted in 66% to 75% of cats and dogs with congenital PSS, with the most common location being portocaval.[1-3,12] Most IHPSS are found in larger-breed dogs, whereas most EHPSS are seen in smaller breeds.[12] Some EHPSS, such as portoazygous or portophrenic shunts, may be associated with less severe clinical signs, possibly because of intermittent compression by the diaphragm or engorged stomach. Dogs with IHPSS generally have the largest volume of portal blood diverted through their shunt, resulting in more severe clinical signs at an earlier age.[1,2,13]

PVH without a macrovascular shunt is a microscopic pathologic malformation of the hepatic microvasculature, previously called MVD.[11] PVH can occur as an isolated disease or in association with macroscopic PSS. PVH can occur with or without concurrent portal hypertension. It has been suggested that MVD-PVH may represent persistent embryonic vitelline veins, resulting in direct shunting of blood from portal venules to central veins, and finally to the systemic circulation, resulting in microvascular shunting.[11,14] Clinical signs in dogs with MVD-PVH can be similar to PSS, although they are often less severe, present later in life, and have a better long-term prognosis with medical management alone. Breeds overrepresented are the Cairn terrier and Yorkshire terrier.[11,15] Animals with PSS or MVD-PVH have the same histologic changes and preoperative clinical signs, therefore the 2 conditions cannot be distinguished.

HAVM is a rare condition comprised of single or multiple high-pressure arterial and low-pressure venous communications. The condition, previously termed hepatic arteriovenous fistulae (HAVF), is more appropriately named a malformation because most affected animals have numerous communications rather than a single fistula. The condition is usually congenital and has been described in dogs and cats.[16,17] Typically a branch of the hepatic artery communicates directly with the portal vein by multiple (tens to hundreds) aberrant shunting vessels within the liver. This creates a high pressure system, resulting in hepatofugal blood flow and arterialization of the portal vein. Because of excessive portal hypertension, multiple EHPSS open to decompress the portal system.[2,3,16]

PATHOPHYSIOLOGY

Most of the clinical signs associated with PSS result from HE, the pathogenesis of which is complex and largely unknown in our veterinary patients. HE is a neuropsychiatric syndrome involving a gamut of neurologic abnormalities that manifest if more than 70% of hepatic function is lost.[8,10,18–20] The healthy liver serves a filtration function against a multitude of neurotoxic substances that are absorbed across the gastrointestinal barrier. If liver function is altered or shunting occurs, the liver cannot appropriately perform its role in either metabolism or substance clearance. Toxic substances subsequently accumulate in the systemic circulation and alter multiple aspects of central nervous system (CNS) function. More than 20 different compounds can be found in increased concentrations in the circulation if liver function is impaired (**Table 1**).[8–10,18,19] Ammonia may be considered the most important because increased concentrations trigger a sequence of metabolic events that have been implicated in HE in rats, humans, and dogs.[9,10,18,19] Ammonia is the easiest substance measured in veterinary patients and treatments to decrease ammonia concentration reduce the signs of HE. The degree of encephalopathy is not well associated with the blood ammonia levels,[21] however, suggesting that other suspected neurotoxins are also important in the pathophysiology.

DIAGNOSTIC EVALUATION
Signalment

Congenital EHPSS are most commonly seen in the small- and toy-breed dogs. In a study of more than 2,400 dogs in North America, odds ratios for development of PSS were near 20 or greater for breeds such as the Yorkshire terrier, Havanese, Maltese, Dandie Dinmont terrier, pug and miniature Schnauzer.[5,12,22] In cats, EHPSS are more common,[3,23] although IHPSS have been reported.[24,25] PSS seem to be most commonly reported in domestic short hair, Persian, Siamese, Himalayan, and Burmese cats.[4,26–28] Intrahepatic shunts are overrepresented in larger-breed dogs with an increased prevalence in the Irish wolfhound, retriever (Labrador, golden), Australian cattle dog, and Australian shepherd.[3,4,26,29–31] Left divisional IHPSS have been considered heritable in the Irish wolfhound,[32,33] and right divisional IHPSS have been overrepresented in males and Australian cattle dogs in Australia.[31] Inheritance has been documented in the Maltese dog and is also believed to occur in the Yorkshire terrier.[3,4,34] The Cairn terrier has been documented to have hereditary MVD-PVH, which is believed to be an autosomal inherited trait; Yorkshire terriers are also overrepresented with this condition.[11,15]

History

Most dogs and cats evaluated for congenital PSS present with signs of chronic or acute illness at less than 1 to 2 years of age, although some animals have presented at greater than 10 years of age.[12,35] This condition is far more common in dogs than cats. Median age of animals with multiple acquired EHPSS was 3 years (range 7 months to 7 years), and the median age of dogs diagnosed with MVD-PVH was 3.25 years (range up to 10 years).[2,11] There is no clear gender predisposition in dogs; however, male cats may be overrepresented.[1,2] The history typically suggests the patient has shown failure to thrive since birth, is small in stature (or the runt of the litter), has weight loss (11%) or failure to gain weight, has anesthetic intolerance, is dull or lethargic at times, and displays bizarre behavior (41%–90%; star-gazing, head-pressing, staring into walls or corners, random barking, intermittent blindness, pacing, or aggression).[1,2,5,12,36] Some animals present with a history of hematuria, stranguria, pollakiuria, or urinary obstruction (20%–53%). Polyuria and polydipsia (PUPD) are common complaints in dogs, and the cause has been associated with various theories, including increased secretion of ACTH and associated hypercortisolism, poor medullary concentration gradient because of a low blood urea nitrogen (BUN) level, increased renal blood flow, and psychogenic polydipsia from HE.[3,5,6] Correlation of the onset of signs with meal ingestion has been reported in only 30% to 50% of patients.[5] Gastrointestinal signs of vomiting, pica, anorexia, or diarrhea are also common.[2]

Abdominal effusion is seen in 75% of dogs with HAVM[16] and has been reported in dogs with congenital PSS and severe hypoalbuminemia. Abdominal effusion is most common if the animal has a concurrent protein-losing enteropathy, which can be associated with GI ulceration/bleeding or inflammatory bowel disease with or without lymphangiectasia. The author has found abdominal effusion to be common in dogs with IHPSS.

Clinical Signs

The 3 most common systems affected are the CNS, the gastrointestinal tract, and the urinary tract. Nonspecific signs have been described earlier. Signs of HE can be either obvious or subtle, and are typically associated with bizarre behaviors (as discussed earlier). More obvious CNS signs include ataxia, unresponsiveness, pacing, circling, blindness, seizures, and coma.[3,7,13,36] Gastrointestinal signs, such as vomiting, diarrhea, anorexia, or gastrointestinal bleeding/melena/hematemesis, occur in approximately 30% of dogs but are less frequent in cats.[5,12,13,24] Ptyalism is extremely common in cats (75%) and is believed to be a manifestation of HE or gastrointestinal upset.[5,6,24,36]

Signs of lower urinary tract disease (stranguria, pollakiuria, hematuria, dysuria) are common in dogs with PSS. Because of decreased urea production, increased ammonia excretion, and decreased uric acid metabolism, ammonium urate stones may develop. These were documented in 30% of patients with PSS in 1 study and can result in secondary bacterial urinary tract infections.[12]

Other congenital defects reported in animals with PSS include cryptorchidism (up to 30% of cats and 50% of dogs in some studies) and heart murmurs.[3,5,37,38] Copper-colored irises inappropriate for the breed have also been documented, particularly in cats.[39] Animals with MVD-PVH have a similar signalment and clinical signs to those described earlier, although these animals are typically older and their signs are milder.[5,11]

Intrahepatic PVH with associated portal hypertension has been described in a variety of breeds of dogs.[40,41] This condition has recently been termed idiopathic NCPH. Other names for this similar condition include hepatoportal fibrosis,[42] idiopathic hepatic fibrosis,[43] veno-occlusive disease,[44] and nonfibrosing liver disease.[45] Diagnosis is based on the presence of portal hypertension with a patent portal vein and lack of cirrhosis on liver biopsy. Affected animals are often purebred dogs; Doberman pinchers (27% of dogs) are overrepresented. Dogs most affected are less than 4 years of age and weigh more than 10 kg.[40] Signs are similar to those of PSS or cirrhosis; concurrent portal hypertension results in ascites (in 60%), PUPD, gastro-intestinal upset, HE, weight loss and multiple EHPSS. The underlying cause of this condition is unknown but speculation includes severe, diffuse intrahepatic vascular malformations without concurrent cirrhosis, resulting in portal hypertension.

Clinical signs associated with HAVM result from PSS and portal hypertension. The condition has been reported in dogs of all sizes and in a small number of cats.[5,16] Gastrointestinal signs are common, and many dogs present with stunted growth and lethargy.[16] Ascites was documented in 75% of dogs, and heart murmurs were documented in 20%.[16] Signs of HE are reported less frequently with HAVM. In some animals, the sound of turbulent blood flow (bruit) can be heard over the fistula when the liver is auscultated.

CLINICAL DIAGNOSIS
Clinicopathologic Findings

In animals with PSS, the most common hematological changes include mild to moderate, microcytic, normochromic nonregenerative anemia (60%–72% of dogs, 30% of cats).[3,46,47] The cause of the microcytic anemia is not fully known, although studies suggest a defective iron-transport mechanism, decreased serum iron concentrations, decreased total iron-binding capacity, and increased hepatic iron stores in Kupffer cells. This suggests that iron sequestration may be the cause.[3,46,47] Typically, microcytosis resolves after shunt fixation. Microcytosis is not reported in dogs with MVD-PVH.[5,11] Erythrocyte target cells are commonly seen on morphology evaluation in dogs and poikilocytes in cats.[48] Leukocytosis can occur and is suspected to be secondary to stress or inadequate hepatic endotoxin and bacterial clearance.[1,2,12,29,49]

Serum biochemical abnormalities are extremely common in animals with PSS. In dogs the most common deficiencies include hypoalbuminemia (50%), decreased BUN (70%), hypocholesterolemia, and hypoglycemia, which result from decreased hepatic synthesis. In cats hypoalbuminemia is uncommon, but decreased BUN concentrations are typical.[24,50] Mild to modest increases (2- to 3-fold) in alkaline phosphatase (ALP) and alanine aminotransferase (ALT) are also reported. These abnormalities are typical of any hepatic vascular anomaly and levels of biochemical changes are not a hallmark for any 1 of these particular conditions. The ALP is typically higher than the ALT with PSS and likely secondary to increased bone isoenzyme in growing animals.[5]

Abnormalities on urinalysis include decreased urine specific gravity (>50% are hyposthenuric or isosthenuric) and ammonium biurate crystalluria.[3,5,36,51] Decreased urine specific gravity most likely results from polydipsia and poor medullary concentration gradient.[6,51] Hyperammonuria from a deficient hepatic urea cycle, along with inappropriate uric acid metabolism, results in excessive ammonia and urate excretion in the kidneys and ultimately ammonium biurate crystalluria (26%–57% of dogs and 16%–42% of cats)[38,52,53] or stone formation (30% of dogs in 1 study).[12,39,51] Proteinuria can be seen and this is suspected to be secondary to glomerular sclerosis or another glomerulopathy. In 1 study of 12 dogs, 100% had evidence of a moderate to severe glomerulofibrosis or membranoproliferative glomerulonephritis.[54] This link between severe liver disease and glomerulonephritis has been seen in humans for many years and has been speculated to be secondary to the accumulation of antigens bypassing hepatic clearance.[55]

Liver function testing

Fasting (12 hours) and 2-hour postprandial serum bile acids (SBA) are the most widely used tests for evaluating liver function in animals with PSS. Bile acids, which are synthesized in the liver from cholesterol, conjugated, secreted into the bile canaliculi, and stored in the gallbladder, are then released into the duodenum after a meal, aiding in fat emulsification, metabolism and lipid absorption. Bile acids are reabsorbed from the ileum, transported into the portal venous system, and extracted by hepatocytes for recirculation.[56,57] By measuring these levels this entire circuit is evaluated. Bile acid concentrations are affected by the timing of the gallbladder contraction, the rate of intestinal transport, the degree of bile acid deconjugation in the small intestine, the rate and efficiency of bile acid absorption in the ileum, the portal blood flow, and the function of the hepatocyte uptake and canalicular transport. Although increases in postprandial bile acids have been found to be 100% sensitive for detection of a PSS in dogs and cats in some studies,[56,58] others have found that paired samples are 100% sensitive, but not individual measurements. There is a small subset of animals that have normal postprandial bile acids with elevated fasting samples, and an even larger number that have normal fasting and elevated postprandial bile acids.[12,56] It has also been found that normal Maltese dogs have elevated serum bile acids without evidence of hepatocellular dysfunction. Increases in bile acids are not specific to PSS and have been reported with other hepatobiliary diseases, cholestasis, glucocorticoid or anticonvulsant therapy, tracheal collapse, seizures, and gastrointestinal disease.[48,59]

If a false-negative bile acid test is suspected, measurement of plasma ammonia can be performed. Basal ammonia in fasting animals is close to 100% sensitive[60] so that an ammonia tolerance test is rarely necessary to detect PSS. Bile acid concentrations have been shown to be somewhat less sensitive but also considerably less specific than ammonia to detect portosystemic shunting.[60,61] An ammonia tolerance test (ATT) is always abnormal in dogs with PSS[62,63] but should be avoided in animals in which the basal value is already highly increased.[62,63] The ATT gives semiquantitative values of the degree of portosystemic shunting and can therefore be used to evaluate the postoperative course after surgical attenuation of the shunt. The ATT can be performed by administration of ammonium chloride orally or rectally. The rectal route is much better tolerated and easy to perform, and is therefore the best way for routine use. Samples are evaluated before and 30 minutes after (or 20 and 40 minutes for semiquantitative analysis[62]) ammonium chloride administration (100 mg/kg [not to exceed 3 g]; 2 mL/kg of a 5% solution in water) with a deep rectal catheter. Plasma separation and laboratory analysis need to be done within 20 minutes of sample collection, making this test difficult to perform in many practices. However, nowadays a reliable and affordable desktop analyzer brings this sensitive and specific test for portosystemic shunting within reach for routine use.[61] Prolonged fasting, a low-protein diet, and administration of lactulose may decrease the basal ammonia concentration, but they do not affect the ATT.[12,38,64,65] False-positive tests in Irish wolfhound puppies[66] have been documented due to an inborn error of ammonia metabolism in this breed.[12]

Coagulation profiles

Prolonged coagulation times are found in most dogs with PSS before fixation; however, spontaneous bleeding is rare and does not usually occur until surgical intervention is attempted.[67,68] In 1 study, postoperative mortality increased in those dogs that had a dramatic worsening of their coagulopathy after surgical fixation.[69] Because the liver parenchymal cells synthesize most of the clotting factors (I, II, V, IX, X, XI, and XIII [and VIII by way of the liver vascular endothelium]), animals in liver failure, as seen in PSS, would be expected to have deficiencies in some of these factors. Approximately 65% to 80% of factor loss must occur before prothrombin time (PT) or activated partial thromboplastin time (PTT) becomes prolonged.[10,67] The liver is also involved in the regulation of coagulation by aiding in the clearance of the activated factors so that regeneration of inactivated factors and fibrinolytic factors can occur.[67–71] Dogs with PSS may have prolonged PTT, without prolonged PT, potentially because of impaired hepatic synthesis, qualitative abnormalities, and clearance of coagulation factors.[67–71] The factors that were evaluated to be deficient involved the common (factors II, V, and X) and the extrinisic pathway (factor VII), which suggests that the PT should be prolonged as well. The exact reason for this has not been clarified.[67] Platelet counts in dogs with PSS were also lower preoperatively than in normal dogs and even more so after surgery (a 27% decrease from baseline).[67] This may be supportive of a postoperative consumptive coagulopathy.

Abdominal effusion
Ascites is rarely seen in dogs with single congenital PSS unless there is severe hypoproteinemia, severe GI bleeding, or portal hypertension (HAVM, NCPH, or acquired multiple EHPSS). Typically, the fluid for any of these conditions would be a clear pure transudate.[48]

Histopathology
Most dogs with congenital PSS have microscopic changes in liver biopsy samples, including ductular proliferation, hypoplasia of intrahepatic portal tributaries, hepatocellular atrophy (lobular), arteriolar proliferation or duplication, lipidosis and cystoplasmic vacuolar changes (lipogranulomas), smooth muscle hypertrophy, increased lymphatics around central veins, and Ito cell and Kupffer cell hypertrophy.[6,51,72–75] Some animals have evidence of mild fibrosis around the central veins, and some have signs of necrosis or inflammation.[5,6,72] One recent article evaluating histopathologic data and prognosis in dogs with congenital macroscopic EHPSS or IHPSS did not find any statistical association between histologic features and survival times.[72] Another recent article investigated the presence of lipogranulomas in liver biopsy samples of dogs with PSS (55.4% of cases).[75] Lipogranulomas were defined as focal lesions consisting of cells (Kupffer cells or macrophages) with cytoplasmic brown pigments (ceroid and hemosiderin) and lipid vacuoles.[75] Although some investigators have suggested an association between lipogranulomas and a poor prognosis, no evidence of this has been documented.[72]

Histologic changes in dogs with PVH-MVD and NCPH are similar to those with macroscopic congenital shunts.[11,40–45] Dogs with NCPH often have more significant fibrosis extending along the portal tracts or bridging to other portal areas and central veins.[40] Biopsies from unaffected liver lobes in dogs with HAVM also show similar findings to those with venovenous PSS. The liver tissue in close proximity to the malformation often has largely dilated portal venules, marked arteriolar hyperplasia and muscular proliferation, and sinusoidal capillarization. Some portal veins have evidence of thrombus formation and recanalization.[5,16]

Diagnostic Imaging

PSS are easily diagnosed with various imaging modalities. Survey abdominal radiographs often show microhepatica (60%–100% of dogs and 50% of cats)[3,5] and bilateral renomegaly. In dogs with PVH the liver and kidneys are often normal in size.[5,11,15] Marginally radiopaque calculi can be seen in the bladder, ureters, or kidneys. To diagnose a macroscopic shunt definitively, imaging such as abdominal ultrasonography

(AUS), angiography (portal or arterial), computed tomographic angiography (CTA) or magnetic resonance angiography (MRA) is needed.

Abdominal ultrasonography
Ultrasound is the most widely used diagnostic tool for PSS in many practices. It is noninvasive, does not require general anesthesia like angiography (although sedation makes finding EHPSS more reliable in many circumstances), and does not require special licensing/handling (like scintigraphy). Decreased numbers of hepatic and portal veins, a subjectively small liver, and an anomalous vessel are readily seen with ultrasound in PSS. Extrahepatic shunts are typically more difficult to diagnosis due to the small patient and vessel size, and the presence of gas in the bowel and lungs obscuring the image. Multiple EHPSS are often harder to find, and are typically located near the kidney. There is considerable variation in the reported accuracy of ultrasonography for detection of shunts (sensitivity 74%–95% and specificity 67%–100%).[76–78] Overall sensitivity is higher for IHPSS (95%–100%).[5,76] The results of ultrasound are dependent of the equipment, operator, and experience. Using a well-evaluated protocol for ultrasonographic examination, it is possible to reach high sensitivity and specificity.[79] Color-flow and pulse-wave Doppler imaging are useful to look for changes in flow direction; classically, HAVM have hepatofugal flow, and venous-venous shunts have hepatopedal flow in the portal vein. Ultrasound is also useful for detecting uroliths in dogs and cats with vascular anomalies.[76,80]

Scintigraphy
Transcolonic scintigraphy is a useful, noninvasive method for detecting PSS. Technetium pertechnetate (^{99m}Tc pertechnetate) is the radioisotope most commonly used.[81] A bolus of the isotope is infused high into the colon, per rectum, and the animal is imaged using a gamma camera. In animals, the isotope is taken up by the colonic veins, which drain to the caudal mesenteric vein and then the portal vein. In a patient with a PSS, the isotope is delivered from the portal vein to the heart, bypassing the liver, and then returning to the liver through the arterial circulation. In a normal patient, it should take approximately 8 to 14 seconds before it reaches the heart, reaching the liver first.[81] If a shunt is present, a shunt fraction can be calculated, giving an estimate of the percentage of portal blood bypassing the liver. A fraction <15% is considered normal, with most dogs with shunt having fractions >60%. Some cats (52% in 1 study) have lower fractions than dogs.[82] There is considerable variation in shunt fraction calculations so comparisons at different time points are difficult and should not be used to assess changes reliably.[83] The half-life of technetium pertechnetate is 6 hours, so animals must be isolated for at least 24 hours after the procedure. Transcolonic scintigraphy does not give morphologic information on the type and location of the shunt, cannot differentiate IHPSS from EHPSS, and cannot differentiate between a single or multiple shunts. The information obtained with transcolonic scintigraphy is therefore comparable with that of the ammonia tolerance test. Scintigraphy is typically normal in dogs with MVD-PVH if there is no macrovascular PSS.[16] Another group evaluated the use of trans-splenic portal scintigraphy for the diagnosis of PSS, using ^{99M}TCO$_4$$^{-}$.[84] Trans-splenic scintigraphy was useful for differentiating portoazygous from portocaval shunts, MVD-PVH from PSS, and, in some patients, single congenital from multiple acquired shunts. Clearance times are faster with trans-splenic scintigraphy and a smaller amount of radionuclide is used, reducing exposure to personnel.

Computed tomographic angiography (CTA)
Computed tomographic angiography is the gold standard for the evaluation of the portal venous system in human medicine.[85] It is noninvasive, fast, and provides

images of all portal tributaries and branches from a single peripheral venous injection of contrast. CTA can be performed with accuracy in dogs and cats of any size, and images can be reconstructed and manipulated for further evaluation after the study is complete. Dual-phase CTA provides a complete evaluation of portal and hepatic vasculature and is considered superior to single-phase CT.[86] This study is most valuable in animals with suspected IHPSS or HAVM or in animals in which ultrasound is not clear and more invasive imaging is not desired. CTA is helpful in planning surgical or interventional radiologic (IR) approaches to IHPSS or HAVM, which can eliminate excessive liver dissection or manipulation, and minimizing contrast load during IR procedures.

Magnetic resonance angiography

MRA also provides a three-dimensional preoperative image of the shunt(s), aiding in preprocedural planning. Magnetic resonance imaging without the use of gadolinium-enhanced angiography was less promising with sensitivities ranging from 63% to 79%, although the specificity was 97%.[5]

Portovenography

Portography is less commonly performed in many large facilities than previously because of availability of less invasive imaging modalities (ultrasound, scintigraphy, CT angiography). Surgical mesenteric portography is the most commonly performed angiographic diagnostic test for documenting PSS in dogs and cats. This procedure requires a laparotomy, portable fluoroscopy (C-arm; or closing an abdomen after jejunal or splenic vein catheterization to transport the patient to a standing fluoroscopy unit, and then returning to the operating room for shunt repair), and intravenous contrast material. Sensitivity of intraoperative portography has been reported to be between 85% and 100% and is dependent on patient positioning.[3–5] An alternative to surgical portal venography is percutaneous ultrasound-guided splenic venography, performed with simultaneous ultrasound access and fluoroscopic evaluation of contrast material. Caudal EHPSS can be missed with this technique if the portal branch communicates with the caudal vena cava in a more caudal location than the splenic vein and retrograde flow is absent. Injection of contrast material into the mesenteric artery (cranial mesenteric arteriography) with access through the femoral artery has also been performed, but is less in favor than other modalities due to its more invasive nature and the difficult interpretation of portal flow after venous dilution of contrast occurs (**Table 2**).[1–3,5,6,8]

TREATMENT
Medical Management

Medical management of animals with portovascular anomalies is required in patients with MVD-PVH or NCPH, or for macrovascular shunts for which surgery is not possible or declined, and is recommended before surgical or IR treatment. Medical management controls the clinical signs associated with shunting but does not treat the underlying diminished hepatic perfusion from the portal vein.

When a patient presents with signs of HE, abrupt stabilization is required and aggressive efforts to decrease the ammonia levels to near normal should be implemented. Intravenous fluid therapy to replace and maintain hydration is necessary if an animal presents recumbent and unable to drink, or dehydrated from gastrointestinal fluid losses. Potassium supplementation is often needed due to potassium depletion from chronic diarrhea; hypokalemia may also contribute to HE.[8,36] Metabolic acidosis may also contribute to HE and should be corrected slowly with fluid therapy.

Table 2
Medical managements of portal vascular anomalies

Symptom	Therapy
Bacterial translocation/decreasing bacterial byproduct absorption (ammonia)	Cleansing enemas with warm water or 30% lactulose solution at 5–10 mL/kg Oral lactulose: 0.5–1.0 mL/kg by mouth every 6–8 h to effect 2–3 soft stools/d Antibiotics Metronidazole 7.5 mg/kg intravenously or by mouth every 12 h Ampicillin 22 mg/kg intravenously every 6 h Neomycin 10–22 mg/kg PO q8h (avoid if any evidence of intestinal bleeding, ulcerations or renal failure)
Coagulopathy (symptomatic; postoperative)	Fresh frozen plasma 10–15 mL/kg over 2–3 h Vitamin K_1 1.5–2 mg/kg subcutaneously or intramuscularly every 12 h for 3 doses then every 24 h
Gastrointestinal ulceration (common with IHPSS, treat before intervention) (common with HAVM due to portal hypertension)	Antacid Famotidine 0.5–1 mg/kg/d intravenously or by mouth Omeprazole 0.5–1 mg/kg/d by mouth Esomeprazole 0.5 mg/kg intravenously every 12–24 h Misoprostol 2–3 μg/kg by mouth every 12 h Protectant Sucralfate 1 g/25 kg by mouth every 8 h Correct coagulopathy
Seizure control	Benzodiazepines (controversial) Phenobarbital (16 mg/kg intravenously, divided into 4 doses for loading over 12–24 h) Potassium bromide (should be avoided in cats because of bronchospasm) Loading 400–600 mg/kg/d divided over 1–5 d by mouth with food; can be given per rectum if needed Maintenance 20–30 mg/kg/d by mouth Sodium bromide can be used if an intravenous form is necessary Propofol 0.5–1.0 mg/kg intravenous bolus, CRI at 0.05–0.1 mg/kg/min (controversial)
Decrease cerebral edema	Mannitol 0.5–1.0 g/kg bolus over 20–30 min
Nutritional support	Moderate protein restriction 18%–22% for dogs and 30%–35% for cats (on dry matter basis); dairy or vegetable proteins preferred Vitamin B complex supplementation (1 mL/L intravenous fluid therapy) Multivitamin supplementation
Hepatoprotective therapy (for chronic conditions that are unable to be fixed MVD, NCPH, MEHPSS, and so forth)	S-Adenosylmethionine (SAMe) 17–22 mg/kg/d by mouth Ursodeoxycholic acid 10–15 mg/kg/d Vitamin E 15 IU/kg/d Milk thistle (silymarin) 8–20 mg/kg divided every 8 h L-Carnitine 250–500 mg/d (cats)

Glucose should be supplemented in the intravenous fluids, particularly in young puppies with PSS in which glycogen stores and gluconeogenesis are minimal. Therapy for HE includes cleansing enemas with warm water or lactulose, oral lactulose therapy, antibiotic therapy (metronidazole, ampicillin, or neomycin), and anticonvulsant therapy if necessary. Using a benzodiazepine antagonist, such as flumazenil, has been shown to be of benefit in humans with HE-induced coma, because GABA and its receptors have been implicated in HE.[8] Mannitol is often considered in patients with severe HE, or after significant seizure activity. In humans there is an association between HE and cerebral edema.[2,8]

Seizure control is often initiated with low-dose midazolam (a benzodiazepine that is preferred to diazepam due to the lack of propylene glycol as a carrying agent, which requires liver metabolism). Once the seizure is controlled, loading with either phenobarbital, potassium bromide, or sodium bromide can be considered (doses are given in **Table 2**).

Lactulose, a disaccharide that is metabolized by colonic bacteria to organic acids, can be administered either by enema or orally. It promotes the acidification of colonic contents, trapping ammonia in the form of ammonium, while decreasing bacterial numbers and eliminating ammonium and bacteria in the feces. The osmotic effect will result in catharsis, reducing fecal transit time and exposure to bacteria for proliferation and ammonia production. Antibiotics will decrease GI bacterial numbers, allowing for a decrease in ammonia production, and will help to decrease the risk of associated bacterial translocation and systemic bacterial infections. In patients that have signs of bleeding, or are significantly anemic or coagulopathic, packed red blood cells, whole blood, or fresh frozen plasma may be of benefit. If there is evidence of HE, fresh whole blood should be used, because stored blood has high ammonia levels.

Nutritional management is important in patients, particularly young animals, that have extremely poor body conditions. The diet should be readily digestible, contain a protein source of high biologic value (enough to meet the animal's needs, but not enough to encourage HE), supply enough essential fatty acids and maintain palatability, and meet the minimum requirements for vitamins and minerals. Low-protein diets should not be used routinely unless HE is noted. Milk and vegetable proteins are lower in aromatic amino acids (tyrosine and phenylanaline) and higher in branched-chain amino acids (BCAA), such as valine, leucine, isoleucine, than animal proteins. These sources are less likely to precipitate HE.[2,8]

Gastric bleeding/ulceration should be treated with acid receptor blockade, such as famotidine or omeprazole, along with sucralfate. Animals with IHPSS and HAVM have a predisposition to the development of gastrointestinal ulcerations.[83,84] Since the authors started life-long antacid therapy in dogs with IHPSS, the morbidity associated with GI bleeding has decreased dramatically (see section on Interventional Radiologic Management). For the same reason, nonsteroidal antiinflammatory drugs (NSAIDs) should be avoided in any dog with IHPSS or HAVM.

Ascites and fibrosis may be seen in patients with HAVM and NCPH, as discussed earlier. It is rarely seen in animals with PSS unless there is severe hypoalbuminemia. If ascites results from decreased oncotic pressure, colloidal therapy should be considered. If the ascites is secondary to portal hypertension, administration of diuretics and a low-sodium diet should be considered. Spironolactone is the initial diuretic of choice because of its potassium-sparing effects. Furosemide may be necessary as well but should be used with caution, because it potentiates further hypokalemia. There are several drugs that theoretically decrease connective tissue formation and may be helpful in patients with hepatic fibrosis. Prednisone (1 mg/kg/d), D-penicillamine (10–15 mg/kg twice a day), and colchicine (0.03 mg/kg/d) have been recommended.

Supportive nutraceutical therapy has been recommended for a variety of liver diseases and is usually unnecessary in portovascular anomalies that can be fixed either surgically or interventionally. Nutraceuticals that may be useful for animals that do not have a correctable condition (MVD, NCPH, multiple EHPSS) include S-adenosyol-L-methionine (SAMe), ursodeoxycholic acid, vitamin E, and milk thistle (silymarin).

Progonsis with Medical Management Alone

Prospective studies on the medical management of dogs or cats with portosystemic vascular anomalies have not been reported. In 1 retrospective study of 27 dogs with congenital PSS evaluated after long-term medical management alone, 52% were euthanized with a median survival time (MST) of 9.9 months and 15% were lost to follow-up. One third of the animals survived long term (MST of 56.9 months; range 5 months to >7 years), with many of those still alive at the time of evaluation.[29] Of the 27 dogs, 9 had EHPSS and 17 had IHPSS. Dogs with IHPSS on medical management alone often had persistent neurologic signs with treatment compared with dogs with EHPSS whose clinical signs were either similar or occurred less often once medicated.[29] Of dogs with IHPSS, 65% were euthanized, mostly due to uncontrolled signs of HE. One third of dogs with EHPSS were euthanized because of persistent clinical signs. There were no correlations between levels of bile acid, serum protein, albumin, ALP, ALT, and MCV and survival times.[29]

Presurgical Considerations

Patients that are cachectic, encephalopathic, or unstable should be managed medically until they can tolerate the stress of anesthesia and surgery (as discussed earlier). Patients in poor body condition or young animals should be managed medically with a strong effort to put on weight before shunt fixation. One study of IHPSS found a worse outcome in dogs <10 kg at the time of shunt fixation.[87] Cats with preoperative, uncontrolled, generalized seizures should be given phenobarbital (2–4 mg/kg every 8 to 24 hours) 2 to 4 weeks before surgery, with the final dosage ultimately based on blood levels and response to therapy. In dogs with preoperative generalized seizures, potassium bromide is preferred because of limited hepatic effects. Prophylactic use of anticonvulsants is not recommended in patients that are not seizing before surgery.

Anesthetic agents that are metabolized by the liver, highly protein-bound, or hepatotoxic should be used with caution because of poor hepatic function and hypoalbuminemia. Anesthesia can be induced with opioids, propofol, or mask delivery of isoflurane or sevoflurane in oxygen, and maintained with isoflurane or sevoflurane. Intraoperative treatment with hetastarch or dextrose (2.5%–5%) is recommended in patients with hypoalbuminemia or hypoglycemia, respectively.

Exploratory Laparotomy

A definitive diagnosis of extrahepatic PSS can usually be made during exploratory laparotomy if the veterinarian is familiar with the anatomy of the abdomen.[83] Most extrahepatic portocaval shunts terminate on the caudal venal cava cranial to the renal veins at the level of the epiploic foramen. Occasionally, they may travel along the lesser curvature of the stomach and terminate on the phrenic or left hepatic vein cranial to the liver. Portoazygous shunts usually traverse the diaphragm at the level of the crura or aortic hiatus. Thorough exploration is warranted in all dogs with single congenital PSS because of the possibility, although rare, of a second shunt.[12,88] In addition, the bladder should be palpated for calculi if preoperative ultrasonography was not performed. IHPSS are more difficult to detect during exploratory surgery. If not readily visible, they may be located intraoperatively by palpation, portography, ultrasound, catheterization by way of the portal vein, or measurement of portal pressure changes during digital vascular occlusion or portal or hepatic vein branches.[3]

Many surgeons obtain liver biopsies to provide a basis for future comparison. Unfortunately, preligation liver biopsies cannot be used to differentiate or prognosticate animals.[72] Because PSS are considered hereditary in many breeds, castration or ovariohysterectomy of affected animals is recommended.[89,90]

Surgical Options for Shunt Occlusion

Congenital PSS can be completely or partially ligated with nonabsorbable sutures or gradually attenuated with an ameroid constrictor, cellophane band, or hydraulic occluder.[69,91–96] Gradual attenuation is preferred to reduce the risk of postoperative complications. Extrahepatic shunts are occluded as close to their terminus as possible to reduce blood flow from shunt tributaries. Blood flow through intrahepatic shunts is usually reduced by attenuating the portal vein branch supplying the shunt or the hepatic vein draining the shunt.[97] Rarely, intrahepatic shunts are approached through a venotomy during inflow occlusion.[98,99]

Suture ligation

Shunt ligation in dogs is often performed with silk because of its superior handling characteristics. Nonabsorbable synthetic monofilament is recommended in cats because of the risk of shunt recanalization.[27] Nonencephalopathic dogs can often tolerate complete shunt ligation; however, up to 80% of animals undergoing acute shunt occlusion require partial attenuation.[69,100] Degree of attenuation is based on visual inspection for evidence of portal hypertension, such as pallor or cyanosis of the intestines, increased intestinal peristalsis, cyanosis or edema of the pancreas, and increased mesenteric vascular pulsations.[101] In addition, the surgeon can measure portal and central venous pressures. Recommendations for postligation pressures include a maximum portal pressure to 17 to 24 cmH_2O, maximal change in portal pressure of 9 to10 cmH_2O, and maximal decrease in central venous pressure of 1 cmH_2O.[3] Objective pressure measurements should not be used as the sole criterion for degree of shunt attenuation, because blood pressures can vary with depth of anesthesia, hydration status, phase of respiration, degree of splanchnic compliance, and other systemic factors.

Pre- and postligation, intraoperative mesenteric portograms have been used to evaluate portohepatic blood supply in animals undergoing suture attenuation of congenital PSS. Absence of arborizing intrahepatic vasculature on preligation portograms has been correlated with greater occurrence of postoperative complications.[74,97]

Long-term outcome, however, is not correlated with portogram findings before or after temporary shunt occlusion.[102] Results of intraoperative mesenteric portography cannot be used to determine the degree of shunt attenuation.[103]

Some investigators recommend second surgery for animals undergoing partial suture ligation of congenital PSS.[96,102,104] Partially attenuated shunts can be completely ligated during a subsequent surgery in 75% of animals.[96] Liver function returns to normal in up to 70% of dogs undergoing a single partial ligation, however, indicating that many shunts continue to narrow after the initial attenuation.[69,95,105]

Ameroid constrictors

Ameroid constrictors (Research Instruments N.W., Inc, Lebanon, OR 97355; researchinstrumentsnw.com) have an inner ring of casein that is surrounded by a stainless steel sheath. Casein is a hygroscopic substance that swells as it slowly absorbs body fluid, reducing the ring's internal diameter by 32%.[95] It also stimulates a fibrous tissue reaction that results in gradual shunt occlusion over 2 or more weeks. In some animals, thrombus formation could result in more rapid obstruction of partially attenuated shunts. The choice of ameroid constrictor size for PSS occlusion is based on shunt diameter; preferably, the constrictor should have an internal diameter larger than the shunt. Extrahepatic PSS are most commonly attenuated with ring of 5 mm inner diameter; intrahepatic shunt attenuation may require rings of 5 to 9 mm inner diameter.

Before placement of an ameroid constrictor, the perivascular fascia is gently dissected away from the shunt. Dissection should be minimized to prevent postoperative movement of the ring and subsequent acute shunt occlusion. The ameroid constrictor is slipped over the flattened vessel, and the slot in the constrictor ring is obstructed with a stainless steel key. Measurement of portal or central venous pressures is unnecessary with ameroid constrictor placement as long as the shunt is not attenuated at the time of surgery.

Cellophane bands

Cellophane bands can be constructed from clear, nonmedical-grade cellophane like that used to wrap flowers and candy baskets. The cellophane is cut into 1 by 10 cm strips and gas sterilized. During surgery, a strip is folded longitudinally into thirds to make a thick, flexible band. The shunt is dissected with right-angle forceps, which are then used to gently thread the band around the shunt. The band is held in place by securing the ends together with surgical clips; excess cellophane is removed 1 to 2 cm beyond the clips. Like ameroid constrictors, cellophane bands cause fibrous tissue reaction and gradual shunt occlusion.[95] Initially, attenuation of the shunt to less than 3 mm in diameter was performed to encourage complete shunt closure.[26] In more recent studies, complete occlusion was demonstrated in dogs and cats that underwent cellophane banding without intraoperative attenuation.[92,106]

Hydraulic occluders

Hydraulic occluders has been used for gradual attenuation of IHPSS.[91] A hydraulic occluder consists of a silicone and polyester cuff (DOCXS Biomedical Products and Accessories, Ukiah, CA) connected by tubing to a vascular access port (Access Technologies, Skokie, IL).[91,95] The cuff is secured around the shunt with suture and the attached access port is inserted under the skin. After surgery, a small amount of sterile saline is injected through the port every 2 weeks to gradually inflate the cuff. Shunt closure usually occurs in 6 to 8 weeks and is not dependent on fibrous tissue formation.[91] In most animals, the vascular access port is left in place permanently.

Complications of Portosystemic Shunts Attenuation

Acute complications of shunt attenuation include refractory hypoglycemia, prolonged anesthetic recovery, hemorrhage, seizures, intraoperative hemorrhage, and portal hypertension. Hypoglycemia occurs in 44% of dogs after EHPSS attenuation and is refractory to dextrose administration in 29% of affected dogs.[107] Dogs that have refractory hypoglycemia or delayed anesthetic recovery may respond to glucocorticoid administration (eg, dexamethasone, 0.1–0.2 mg/kg intravenously). In dogs that have undergone acute shunt ligation, packed cell volume, platelet count, and coagulation times should be monitored because platelet count and coagulation factor activity significantly decrease after surgery, as discussed earlier.[67]

Clinical signs of portal hypertension include pain, abdominal distension from ileus or ascites, decreased central venous pressure, prolonged capillary refill time, pale mucous membranes, poor peripheral pulses, and gastrointestinal hemorrhage.[3,89]

Acute portal hypertension is most commonly seen in animals undergoing suture liga-tion. Mild portal hypertension may result in ascites and wound drainage and is usually self-limiting. Ascites may improve with administration of hetastarch. Animals with severe ascites may require diuretics or abdominal drainage if respiration is compro-mised. Moderate portal hypertension is treated with intravenous crystalloids, hetas-tarch, gastrointestinal protectants (eg, omeprazole and sucralfate) and systemic antibiotics. Affected animals are evaluated for hypotension and evidence of dissemi-nated coagulopathy (DIC). Ligature removal should be performed immediately in animals with severe clinical signs, such as DIC, or hypotension that does not respond to fluid therapy. Multiple EHPSS have been reported to occur after ameroid placement in dogs and cats for single congenital EHPSS in nearly 10% to 20% of cases.[5]

Postoperative seizures develop in 3% to 7% of dogs and 8% to 22% of cats after shunt attenuation.[12,35,50,69,88,92–94,96,102,105,108] Seizures may occur up to 80 hours after surgery and are not associated with hypoglycemia, hyperammonemia, or atten-uation technique. Initial treatment includes intravenous boluses of midazolam or pro-pofol. If seizures persist or reoccur, the animal is anesthetized with an intravenous bolus of propofol (5–8 mg/kg) and maintained under anesthesia on a propofol contin-uous-rate infusion (CRI; 0.1–0.2 mg/kg/minute). There is a suggestion that propofol may not eliminate cerebral seizure activity when monitored on EEG, and other inject-able anticonvulsants should be considered, although in the authors' experience pro-pofol has been effective in seizure management of PSS patients. Mannitol is administered intravenously every 6 hours to reduce intracranial swelling. Electrolyte and glucose abnormalities are corrected, and supportive care is provided. Propofol is discontinued after 12 hours. Some patients may benefit from a low dose of acepro-mazine before propofol is discontinued, because anxiety during anesthetic recovery may be difficult to differentiate from early seizure activity. If seizures reoccur with anesthetic recovery, the animal is reanesthetized with a propofol bolus and CRI, and treatment with intravenous barbiturates is instituted. Some animals may require 72 hours of anesthesia to resolve seizure activity. Once the animal has recovered from anesthesia, oral anticonvulsant therapy (phenobarbital in cats; potassium bromide or phenobarbital in dogs) is initiated. Prognosis is poor for animals with post-operative seizures; mortality rates are high and those that survive often continue to have neurologic problems.[88,94,96,109,110]

The most common chronic complication of PSS attenuation is persistence or recur-rence of clinical signs. Differentials include continued flow through the original shunt, the presence of a second shunt, development of multiple acquired shunts, or the pres-ence of congenital PVH. In animals with cellophane bands or ameroid constrictors, high-dose steroids can interfere with fibrous tissue formation and shunt closure. Animals with clinical signs or biochemical changes that indicate liver dysfunction should be evaluated with ultrasonography, scintigraphy, portography, computed tomography, or magnetic resonance imaging for evidence of shunting. Surgical inter-vention is recommended for patients with a second shunt or clinical signs related to persistent flow through the original shunt. If shunting is not detected, the most common cause is congenital PVH (MVD-PVH), which can be confirmed by histologic evaluation of liver biopsy samples. Animals that have focal or generalized seizures, have minimal hepatic dysfunction, and do not respond to medical management for encephalopathy should be evaluated for central neurologic disorders.

Prognosis for Congenital Portosystemic Shunts Treated Surgically

In dogs with congenital EHPSS, mortality rates were 2% to 32% after ligation, 7% after ameroid constrictor placement, and 6% to 9% after cellophane banding.[12,69,92–94,102,105] In dogs with IHPSS, mortality rates were 6% to 23% after ligation, 0% to 9% after ameroid constrictor placement, and 27% after cellophane banding with intraoperative attenuation.[12,26,69,98,111,112] The most common cause of death after PSS attenuation is severe persistent neurologic signs. Other causes include intraoperative hemorrhage, postoperative coagulopathy, portal hypertension, and hemorrhagic gastroenteritis.[69,94] Age is not correlated with mortality or long-term complications; however, degree of shunt closure during ligation is correlated with postoperative mortality.[12,35,69,104,113]

In surviving dogs available for follow-up, good to excellent outcomes were noted in 84% to 94% of animals undergoing ligation, cellophane banding, or ameroid constrictor placement for EHPSS.[26,69,94] Most dogs continued to have mildly increased bile acids.[12,69,102]

Clinical outcome was more variable in surviving dogs after IHPSS attenuation. Good to excellent outcomes were noted in 70% to 89% of dogs with IHPSS that underwent ameroid constrictor placement,[94,111] 76% to 100% of dogs that underwent ligation,[94,98] and 50% of dogs that underwent cellophane banding with intraoperative attenuation[93] In many dogs, clinical signs resolved despite persistent shunting.[94,105,114] Immediate survival was 100% for 10 dogs undergoing hydraulic occluder attenuation of intrahepatic shunts, but long-term survival was only documented in 8/10 dogs, with 2 lost to follow-up.[91] Clinical signs resolved in all dogs, although 1 dog required reinflation of the cuff 9 months after surgery and a second developed sinus tracts that resolved with port removal.[91] In dogs undergoing ameroid constrictor placement, preoperative hypoalbuminemia was associated with persistent postoperative shunting.[94] Preoperative hypoalbuminemia or leukocytosis, occurrence of seizures after surgery, and persistent shunting at 6 to 10 weeks after surgery were predictive of poor long-term outcome.

In cats, perioperative mortality rates are 0% to 4% after ligation or ameroid constrictor placement, and 0% to 23% after cellophane banding.[50,96,106,108] Up to 75% of cats have postoperative complications.[108] The most common complication is neurologic dysfunction, including generalized seizures in 8% to 22% and central blindness in up to 44%.[50,96,108] Blindness usually resolves within 2 months after surgery.[108] Of surviving cats available for follow-up, good or excellent long-term outcome was reported in 66% to 75% undergoing ligation, 33% to 75% undergoing ameroid constrictor placement, and 80% undergoing cellophane banding.[50,96,106,108,115] Excellent outcome has been reported in 25% of cats with persistent shunting, and continued or recurrent neurologic abnormalities have been reported in 57% of cats with normal scintigraphy or hepatic function tests.[50,108]

Surgical Treatment of Hepatic Arteriovenous Malformations

Treatments for HAVM include liver lobectomy, ligation of the nutrient artery, or fluoroscopically guided glue embolization of abnormal arterial vessels.[16,116] Most HAVM are located in the right or central liver lobes, and 25% involved 2 lobes. Lobectomy may be challenging because of proximity to the gall bladder and caudal vena cava and extensive vascularity. Temporary occlusion of the portal vein and celiac artery is recommended during partial lobectomy to reduce intraoperative hemorrhage.[116] Complications of surgery include hemorrhage, portal hypertension, systemic hypotension, bradycardia, and portal or mesenteric vein thrombus formation.[16] Perioperative survival of dogs undergoing surgery alone was 75% to 91%.[16] Long-term outcome of dogs treated with surgery alone was fair or good for 38% to 57%. Overall, 75% of dogs continue to require dietary or medical management of clinical signs.[16]

Interventional Radiologic Management

Interventional radiology (IR) uses contemporary imaging modalities, such as fluoroscopy, to gain access to various parts of the body through a small incision (jugular vein for the treatment of IHPSS or femoral artery for the treatment of HAVM). Devices can be introduced percutaneously through these small holes and deployed once inside the vessel in the proper position. With the use of contrast, catheters, wires, and embolization devices (coils, vascular occluders, cyanoacrylate glue, stents, and so forth), shunts can be attenuated either abruptly (cyanoacrylate, coils, vascular occluders) or slowly (coils). Because of the technical difficulty of surgery for these 2 conditions, along with the high perioperative complication rates reported (0%–77%),[87,91,93,98,108,111,117] these minimally invasive alternatives are currently being investigated and performed in a small number of facilities around the world.[2,25,118–125] In the author's practice, IR procedures involving portovascular anomalies are mainly reserved for IHPSS and HAVM; EHPSS are routinely fixed surgically.

Percutaneous Transjugular Coil Embolization

Transvenous coil embolization has been described from various institutions in the past decade,[2,25,118,120–125] for repair of IHPSS and EHPSS[124,125] in dogs and cats.[118] The most common complication of this technique has been coil migration, which has been diminished with the addition of caval stent placement before coil deployment. Portal hypertension, which is 1 of the most common complications reported with surgical fixation, was not commonly seen in the patients treated with PTCE.

Percutaneous venous access to the jugular vein is obtained. Under fluoroscopic guidance, a guidewire is passed down the jugular vein into the cranial vena cava, through the right atrium, and into the caudal vena cava (CdVC) (**Fig. 1**A). The shunting vessel is then selected (hepatic vein to portal vein) (**Fig. 1**A). Next, a catheter is advanced over the guidewire and the guidewire is subsequently removed (**Fig. 1**B). An angiogram is performed, using contrast material under fluoroscopic guidance, and visualized with digital subtraction (DSA), confirming shunt location and anatomy (**Fig. 1**B). Next, in a similar fashion as above, a catheter is placed into the caudal vena cava, caudal to the shunting tributary, and another angiogram is performed marking the communication of the shunt to the caudal vena cava (**Fig. 1**B). With a measuring catheter, the maximal diameter of the vena cava is determined facilitating sizing for stent placement (**Fig. 1**B). Once the location of the shunt entry point into the CdVC is identified and the size of the cava is determined, a wire is advanced back into the CdVC and the catheters are removed. Next, an ensheathed, laser-cut, self-expanding nitinol stent is advanced over the guidewire into the CdVC (**Fig. 1**C), ensuring that the entire mouth of the shunting vessel is covered. Then, the sheath of the stent is removed as the stent is deployed in the chosen location (**Fig. 1**D). Finally, using the guidewire and catheter, the shunt is again selected through the interstices of the stent (**Fig. 1**E) and an angiogram is performed as above, to confirm that the shunt is completely covered by the stent (**Fig. 1**F). Through the catheter, thrombogenic coils are placed into the shunt to monitor portal pressures. Coils are added until the mouth of the shunt is covered or the portal pressures increase to >10 CmH$_2$O over baseline or to a maximum of 20 cmH$_2$O (**Fig. 1**G, H). The stent is used as a cage to prevent coil migration cranially. The procedure allows an abrupt (presence of the coils) and a slow attenuation of the shunting vessel; the thrombogenic coils allow a clot to form, organize, and occlude the blood flow. If necessary additional coils can be easily added at a future date if clinical signs persist, liver functional parameters do not improve, or medications cannot be weaned. The addition of coils has been necessary

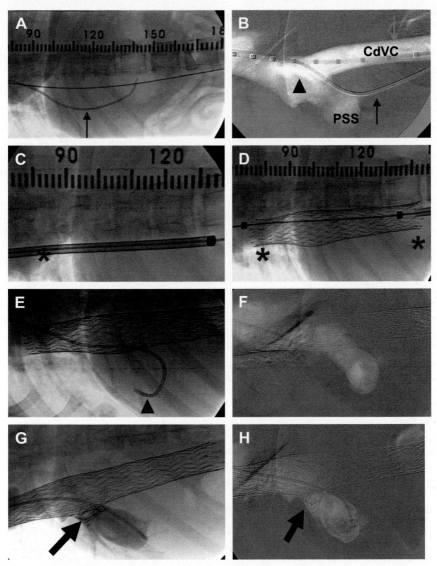

Fig. 1. A study of a dog with a right divisional IHPSS, during a PTCE. The animal is placed in dorsal recumbency with the head to the left and the tail to the right of the image. (*A*) A guidewire (*yellow arrow*) is placed from the jugular vein, through the cranial vena cava and the CdVC and extending down the CdVC. A catheter ends in the portal vein (*red arrow*), extending from the jugular vein, through the cranial and CdVC, transversing the right hepatic vein, the portosystemic shunt (PSS) and extending to the portal vein. (*B*) An angiogram being performed under DSA fluoroscopy. Contrast material is in the CdVC and portosystemic shunting vessel (PSS). The mouth of the shunt is identified (*black triangle*). Using a marker catheter (*yellow arrow*), the magnification is adjusted for, and the vena cava can be accurately measured for appropriate selection of stent size. (*C*) Over a guidewire, the ensheathed stent (*red asterisk*) is advanced to cover the mouth of the shunt that was previously determined in (*B*). (*D*) The stent is then deployed in the selected location with each end confirmed to cover the shunt (*red asterisk*). (*E*) The mouth of the shunt is again selected with a catheter (*blue triangle*) and (*F*) another angiogram is done using contrast, to confirm that the stent is covering the entire mouth of the shunt. This image is under DSA. (*G*) Through the catheter, thrombogenic coils are placed in the shunting vessel (*black arrow*). (*H*) Once completed the catheter is removed and the stent and coils remain in place until a final angiogram is performed under DSA and final portal pressures are obtained.

in <10% of cases. In the rare cases in which portal perfusion is excellent, the shunt can be occluded abruptly. This has been performed in approximately 5% of cases.

Complications

Of 70 patients undergoing this procedure, fewer than 5% had perioperative complications in our experience,[87] (Weisse and Berent, direct communications, Philadelphia, PA, July 2008). Complications included coil migration, excessive bleeding at the site of the jugular catheter postprocedure, and aspiration at the time of induction before the procedure. Of 40 dogs reported in abstract form,[118] the long-term mortality rate was 30% and more than 50% of the deaths were secondary to severe GI ulcerations and bleeding. More than 30% of dogs have (or had) evidence of GI ulcerations either before or after PTCE. Since initiating life-long antacid therapy at the time of diagnosis, the overall long-term mortality rate (6 months to >7 years follow-up) has decreased dramatically, with fewer than 3% of deaths secondary to GI ulcerations.

Because GI bleeding has become so apparent, nearly all dogs with IHPSS undergo upper GI endoscopy with gastrointestinal biopsies before PSS correction. Evidence of petechiation and active or healing ulcerations are commonly seen. More than 85% of dogs with IHPSS have evidence of moderate to severe lymphoplasmacytic with or without eosinophilic mucosal and submucosal inflammation. Hypergastrinemia, which is currently being evaluated in a large group of dogs, does not seem to be associated with or prognostic to the development of GI ulceration in dogs with IHPSS, EHPSS, or normal age-matched dogs. Visual endoscopy scores, gastrointestinal histopathology, and gastrin levels seem to have minimal statistical correlation with overall outcome in the author's preliminary data. Morbidity and mortality have significantly improved since the start of life-long antacid use. The only prognostic factor appreciated as a marker for GI bleeding and postprocedural gastrointestinal symptoms (severe vomiting, diarrhea, and inappetance) is albumin; concentrations ≤1.8 g/dL increase the odds of bleeding by more than 5 times and the odds of chronic vomiting and diarrhea by 4.7 times. Treatment of dogs, particularly those with IHPSS, with life-long antacid therapy (particularly, omeprazole) has improved the morbidity and mortality rates.

Hepatic Arteriovenous Malformations Cyanoacrylate Glue Embolization

Hepatic arteriovenous fistula/malformations (HAVM) are rare vascular anomalies involving multiple arterial communications to the portal vein. Because they usually involve multiple, rather than a single communication, the term malformation is more appropriate than fistula. These communications are usually from the hepatic artery, but have been seen to involve other arteries, such as the gastroduodenal artery and left gastric artery. Angiography helps to determine the origin of these numerous vessels. Due to high-pressure arterial blood shunting to the portal vein, there is severe portal hypertension and this most commonly results in multiple EHPSS to help decompress the portal vein. Cyanoacrylate glue embolization has been performed in 11 cases to date at the author's institution (University of Pennsylvania).

Access to the femoral artery is obtained and, under fluoroscopic guidance, a wire is advanced retrograde into the aorta, and the hepatic artery is selected by way of the celiac artery. A catheter is advanced over the wire and an angiogram is done using contrast material and digital subtraction (DSA). The communication can be appreciated (Fig. 2A), and centrifugal blood flow is seen as the contrast material enters the portal vein traveling caudally until it reaches the multiple EHPSS, whereby it travels through the caudal vena cava cranially. Then, the small vessels feeding the malformation are selected with a microcatheter, and cyanoacrylate (a glue) is infused. The glue polymerizes and occludes the small communications of the malformation.

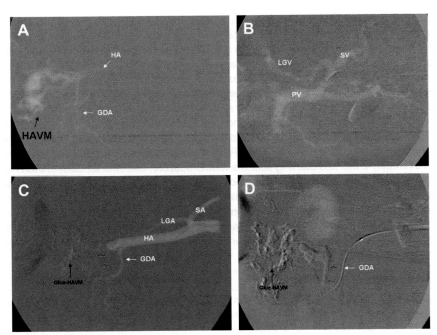

Fig. 2. Fluoroscopic images of a glue embolization in a 4-month-old female intact boxer with an HAVM. Left is cranial and right is caudal. (*A*) Angiogram from the hepatic artery (HA) showing the contrast filling the gastroduodenal artery (GDA) and the malformation (HAVM). (*B*) Hepatofugal portal flow after the malformation is filled is traveling in the wrong direction caudally down the portal vein (PV) resulting in retrograde filling of the left gastric vein (LGV) and splenic vein (SV). (*C*) After glue is injected into the hepatic artery the malformation is filled. The contrast is seen to stop at the hepatic arterial branch but there is still filling of the malformation from a branch of the GDA (*yellow arrows*). (*D*) A microcatheter in the branch off the GDA filling with glue (*yellow arrows*).

Cyanoacrylate infusion is continued until the flow into the portal vein from the artery is eliminated, or dramatically decreased (**Fig. 2**).

Complications with this procedure include nontarget embolization of glue entering the portal system to the extrahepatic shunts, or elsewhere, on catheter removal. These events have not been clinically significant and have not resulted in any long-term complications. After this procedure, most dogs require life-long medical management due to continued shunting from their multiple EHPSS. Recurrence of arteriovenous communications can occur and recurrence of clinical signs has been seen requiring serial embolizations. Long-term survival is considered good with this technique.

POSTOPERATIVE CARE

After surgery or IR treatment, patients are maintained on intravenous fluids until they are eating and drinking. Dextrose is added to the fluids if the blood glucose level is less than 80 mg/dL. Patients are monitored for hypoglycemia, hypothermia, delayed anesthetic recovery, hemorrhage, seizures, and signs of portal hypertension. Animals usually require opioid analgesics such as buprenorphine for 1 to 3 days. Sedation with a low dose (0.01–0.02 mg/kg intravenously) of acepromazine may be necessary if dogs are vocalizing or abdominal pressing, because these activities will increase

22. Tobias KM, Rohrbach BW. Association of breed with the diagnosis of congenital portosystemic shunts in dogs: 2,400 cases (1980–2002). J Am Vet Med Assoc 2003;223(11):1636–9.
23. Birchard SJ, Sherding RG. Feline portosystemic shunts. Compend Contin Educ Vet 1992;14:1295–300.
24. Schunk CM. Feline portosystemic shunts. Semin Vet Med Surg (Small Anim) 1997;12:45–50.
25. Weisse C, Schwartz K, Stronger R, et al. Transjuglar coil embolization of an intra-hepatic portosystemic shunt in a cat. J Am Vet Med Assoc 2002;221(9): 1287–91.
26. Hunt GB. Effect of breed on anatomy of portosystemic shunts resulting from congenital diseases in dogs and cats: a review of 242 cases. Aust Vet J 2004;82(12):746–9.
27. Blaxter AC, Holt PE, Pearson GR, et al. Congenital portosystemic shunts in the cat: a report of nine cases. J Small Anim Pract 1988;29:631–45.
28. Tillson DM, Winkler JT. Diagnosis and treatment of portosystemic shunts in the cat. Vet Clin North Am Small Anim Pract 2002;32:881–99.
29. Watson PJ, Herrtage ME. Medical management of congenital portosystemic shunts in 27 dogs – a retrospective study. J Small Anim Pract 1998;39:62–8.
30. Wolschrijn CF, Mahapokai W, Rothuizen J, et al. Gauged attenuation of congen-ital portosystemic shunts: results in 160 dogs and 15 cats. Vet Q 2000;22:94–8.
31. Krotscheck U, Adin CA, Hunt GB, et al. Epidemiologic factors associated with the anatomic location of intrahepatic portosytemic shunts in dogs. Vet Surg 2007;36:31–6.
32. Kerr MG, van Doorn T. Mass screening of Irish wolfhound puppies for portosys-temic shunts by the dynamic bile acid test. Vet Rec 1999;144(25):693–6.
33. Meyer HP, Rothuizen J, Ubbink GJ, et al. Increasing incidence of hereditary in-trahepatic portosystemic shunts in Irish wolfhounds in the Netherlands (1984–1992). Vet Rec 1995;136:13–6.
34. Tobias KM. Determination of inheritance of single congenital portosystemic shunts in Yorkshire terriers. J Am Anim Hosp Assoc 2003;39:385–9.
35. Worley DR, Holt DE. Clinical outcome of congenital extrahepatic portosystemic shunt attenuation in dogs aged five years and older: 17 cases (1992–2005). J Am Vet Med Assoc 2008;232:722–7.
36. Broome CJ, Walsh VP, Braddock JA. Congenital portosystemic shunts in dogs and cats. N Z Vet J 2004;52(4):154–62.
37. Forster-Van Hijfte MA, McEvoy FJ, White RN, et al. Per rectal portal scintigraphy in the diagnosis and management of feline congenital portosystemic shunts. J Small Anim Pract 1996;37(1):7–11.
38. Johnson CA, Armstrong PJ, Hauptman JG. Congenital portosystemic shunts in dogs: 46 cases (1979–1986). J Am Vet Med Assoc 1987;191:1478–83.
39. Center SA, Magne ML. Historical, physical examination, and clinicopathologic features of portosystemic vascular anomalies in the dog sand cat. Semin Vet Med Surg (Small Anim) 1990;5:83–93.
40. Bunch SE, Johnson SE, Cullen JM. Idiopathic noncirrhotic portal hypertension in dogs: 33 cases (1982–1998). J Am Vet Med Assoc 2001;218(3):392–9.
41. DeMarco J, Center SA, Dykes N, et al. A syndrome resembling idiopathic non-cirrhotic portal hypertension in 4 young Doberman pinschers. J Vet Intern Med 1998;12(3):147–56.
42. Van den Ingh TS, Rothuizen J. Hepatoportal fibrosis in three young dogs. Vet Rec 1982;110:575–7.

43. Rutgers HC, Haywood S, Kelly DF. Idiopathic hepatic fibrosis in 15 dogs. Vet Rec 1993;133:115–8.
44. Rand JS, Best SJ, Mathews KA. Portosystemic vascular shunts in a family of American cockers spaniels. J Am Anim Hosp Assoc 1988;24:265–72.
45. Hunt GB, Malik R, Chapman BL, et al. Ascites and portal hypertension in three young dogs with non-fibrosing liver disease. J Small Anim Pract 1993;34: 428–33.
46. Simpson KW, Meyer DJ, Boswood A, et al. Iron status and erythrocyte volume in dogs with congenital portosystemic vascular anomalies. J Vet Intern Med 1997; 11:14–9.
47. Bunch SE, Jordan HL, Sellon RK, et al. Characterization of iron status in young dogs with portosystemic shunt. Am J Vet Res 1995;56:853–8.
48. Willard MD, Twedt DC. Gastrointestinal, pancreatic, and hepatic disorders. In: Willard MD, Tvedten H, Turnwald GH, editors. Small animal clinical diagnosis by laboratory methods. 3rd edition. Philadelphia: WB Saunders Company; 1999. p. 172–207.
49. Tobias KM, Besser TE. Evaluation of leukocytosis, bacteremia, and portal vein partial oxygen tension in normal dogs and dogs with portosystemic shunt in a dog. J Am Vet Med Assoc 1997;211:715–8.
50. Havig M, Tobias KM. Outcome of ameroid constrictor occlusion of single congenital extrahepatic portosystemic shunts in cats: 12 cases (1993–2000). J Am Vet Med Assoc 2002;220:337–41.
51. Swalec KM. Portosystemic shunts. In: Bojrab MJ, editor. Disease mechanisms in small animal surgery. Philadelphia: Lea & Febiger; 1993. p. 298–305.
52. VanGundy TE, Boothe HW, Wolf A. Results of surgical management of feline portosystemic shunts. J Am Anim Hosp Assoc 1990;26:55–62.
53. Cornelius LM, Thrall DE, Halliwell WH, et al. Anomalous portosystemic anastomoses associated with chronic hepatic insufficiency in 6 young dogs. J Am Vet Med Assoc 1975;167:220–8.
54. Tisdall PC, Tothwell TW, Hunt GB, et al. Glomerulopathy in dogs with congenital portosystemic shunts. Aust Vet J 1997;73:52–4.
55. Bloodworth JB, Sommers SC. "Cirrhotic glomerulosclerosis," a renal lesion associated with hepatic cirrhosis. Lab Invest 1959;8:962–78.
56. Center SA, ManWarren T, Slater MR, et al. Evaluation of twelve-hour preprandial and two-hour postprandial serum bile acid concentrations for diagnosis of hepatobiliary disease in dogs. J Am Vet Med Assoc 1991;199:217–26.
57. Center SA. Serum bile acids in companion animal medicine. Vet Clin North Am Small Anim Pract 1993;23:625–57.
58. Center SA, Erb HN, Joseph SA. Measurement of serum bile acids concentrations for diagnosis of hepatobiliary disease in cats. J Am Vet Med Assoc 1995;207:1048–54.
59. Center SA, Baldwin BH, Erb HN, et al. Bile acid concentrations in the diagnosis of hepatobiliary disease in the dog. J Am Vet Med Assoc 1985;187(9):935–40.
60. Sterczer A, Meyer HP, Boswijk HC, et al. Evaluation of ammonia measurements in dogs with two analysers for use in veterinary practice. Vet Rec 1999;144: 23–6.
61. Gerritzen-Bruning MJ, van den Ingh TS, Rothuizen J. Diagnostic value of fasting plasma ammonia and bile acid concentrations in the identification of portosystemic shunting in dogs. J Vet Intern Med 2006;20:13–9.
62. Rothuizen J, Ingh TSG. Rectal ammonia tolerance test in the evaluation of portal circulation in dogs with liver disease. Res Vet Sci 1982;33:22–5.

63. Meyer DJ, Strombeck DR, Stone EA, et al. Ammonia tolerance test in clinically normal dogs and dogs with portosystemic shunts. J Am Vet Med Assoc 1978; 173:377–9.
64. Tisdall PLC, Hunt GB, Bellenger CR, et al. Congenital portosystemic shunts in Maltese and Australian cattle dogs. Aust Vet J 1994;71:174–8.
65. Walker MC, Hill RC, Guilford WG, et al. Postprandial venous ammonia concentrations in the diagnosis of hepatobiliary disease in dogs. J Vet Intern Med 2001;15:463–6.
66. Meyer HP, Rothuizen J, Tiemessen I, et al. Transient metabolic hyperammonemia in young Irish wolfhounds. Vet Rec 1996;138:105–7.
67. Kummeling A, Teske E, Rothuizen J, et al. Coagulation profiles in dogs with congenital portosystemic shunts before and after surgical attenuation. J Vet Intern Med 2006;20:1319–26.
68. Niles JD, Williams JM, Cripps PJ. Hemostatic profiles in 39 dogs with congenital portosystemic shunts. Vet Surg 2001;30:97–104.
69. Kummeling A, van Sluijs FJ, Rothuizen J. Prognostic implications of the degree of shunt narrowing and of the portal vein diameter in dogs with congenital portosystemic shunts. Vet Surg 2004;33:17–24.
70. Prater MR. Acquired coagulopathy II: liver disease. In: Feldman BF, Zinkl JG, Jain NC, editors. Schalm's veterinary hematology. Philadelphia: Lippincott Williams & Wilkins; 2000. p. 560–4.
71. Badylak SF, Dodds WJ, Van Vleet JF. Plasma coagulation factor abnormalities in dogs with naturally occurring hepatic disease. Am J Vet Res 1983;44:2336–40.
72. Parker JS, Monnet E, Posers BE, et al. Histologic examination of hepatic biopsy samples as a prognostic indicator in dogs undergoing surgical correction of congenital portosystemic shunts: 64 cases (1997–2005). J Am Vet Med Assoc 2008;232:1511–4.
73. Baade S, Aupperle H, Grevel V, et al. Histopathologic and immunohistochemical investigations of hepatic lesions associated with congenital portosystemic shunts in dogs. J Comp Pathol 2006;134:80–90.
74. Swalec KM, Smeak DD. Partial versus complete attenuation of single portosystemic shunts. Vet Surg 1990;19:406–11.
75. Isobe K, Matsunage S, Nakayama H. Histopathological characteristics of hepatic lipogranulomas with portosystemic shunt in dogs. J Vet Med Sci 2008; 70(2):133–8.
76. Lamb CR. Ultrasonographic diagnosis of congenital portosystemic shunts in dogs: results of a prospective study. Vet Radiol Ultrasound 1996;37:281–8.
77. Holt DE, Schelling CG, Saunders HM, et al. Correlation of ultrasonographic findings with surgical, portographic, and necropsy findings in dogs and cats with portosystemic shunts: 63 cases (1987–1993). J Am Vet Med Assoc 1995;207: 1190–3.
78. Tiemessen I, Rothuizen J, Voorhout G. Ultrasonograpthy in the diagnosis of congenital portosystemic shunts in dogs. Vet Q 1995;17:50–3.
79. Szatmári V, Rothuizen J, Voorhout G. Standard planes for ultrasonographic examination of the portal system in dogs. J Am Vet Med Assoc 2004;224: 713–6, 698–9.
80. Lamb CR, Forster-van Hijfte MA, White RN, et al. Ultrasonographic diagnosis of congenital portosystemic shunt in 14 cats. J Small Anim Pract 1996;37:205–9.
81. Lamb CR, Daniel GB. Diagnostic imaging of dogs with suspected portosystemic shunting. Compend Contin Educ Vet 2002;24:626–35.
82. Daniel GB, Bright R, Monnet E, et al. Comparison of per-rectal portal scintigraphy using 99m technetium pertechnetate to mesenteric injection of radioactive

microspheres for quantification of portosystemic shunts in an experimental dog model. Vet Radiol Ultrasound 1990;31:175–81.

83. Samii VF, Kyles AE, Long CD, et al. Evaluation of interoperator variance in shunt fraction calculation after transcolonic scintigraphy for diagnosis of portosystemic shunts in dogs and cats. J Am Vet Med Assoc 2001;218:1116–9.

84. Morandi F, Cole RC, Tobias KM, et al. Use of 99MTCO4(-) trans-splenic portal scintigraphy for diagnosis of portosystemic shunts in 28 dogs. Vet Radiol Ultrasound 2005;46(2):153–61.

85. Henseler KP, Pozniak MA, Lee FT, et al. Three-dimensional CT angiography of spontaneous portosystemic shunts. Radiographics 2001;21:691–704.

86. Zwingenberger A, Schwarz T, Saunders HM. Helical computed tomographic angiography of canine portosystemic shunts. Vet Radiol Ultrasound 2005; 46(1):27–32.

87. Papazoglou LG, Monnet E, Seim HB. Survival and prognostic indicators for dogs with intrahepatic portosystemic shunts: 32 cases (1990–2000). Vet Surg 2002; 31:561–70.

88. Yool DA, Kirby BM. Neurologic dysfunction in three dogs and one cat following attenuation of intrahepatic portosystemic shunts. J Small Anim Pract 2002;43:171–6.

89. Tobias KM, Rohrbach BW. Proportional diagnosis of congenital portosystemic shunts in dogs accessed by veterinary teaching hospitals: 1980–2002. J Am Vet Med Assoc 2003;223:1636–9.

90. van Straten G, Leegwater PAJ, de Vries M, et al. Inherited congenital extrahepatic portosystemic shunts in Cairn terriers. J Vet Intern Med 2005;19:321–4.

91. Adin CA, Sereda CW, Thompson MS, et al. Outcome associated with use of a percutaneously controlled hydraulic occluder for treatment of dogs with intrahepatic portosystemic shunts. J Am Vet Med Assoc 2006;229:1749–55.

92. Frankel D, Seim H, MacPhail C, et al. Evaluation of cellophane banding with and without intraoperative attenuation for treatment of congenital extrahepatic portosystemic shunts in dogs. J Am Vet Med Assoc 2006;228:1355–60.

93. Hunt GB, Kummeling A, Tisdall PLC, et al. Outcomes of cellophane banding for congenital portosystemic shunts in 106 dogs and 5 cats. Vet Surg 2004;33:25–31.

94. Mehl ML, Kyles AE, Hardie EM, et al. Evaluation of ameroid ring constrictors for treatment for single extrahepatic portosystemic shunts in dogs: 168 cases (1995–2001). J Am Vet Med Assoc 2005;226:2020–30.

95. Sereda CW, Adin CA. Methods of gradual vascular occlusion and their applications in treatment of congenital portosystemic shunts in dogs: a review. Vet Surg 2005;34:83–91.

96. Lipscomb VL, Jones HJ, Brockman DJ. Complications and long term outcomes of the ligation of congenital portosystemic shunts in 49 cats. Vet Rec 2007;160: 465–70.

97. Tobias KMS, Rawlings CA. Surgical techniques for extravascular occlusion of intrahepatic shunts. Compend Contin Educ Vet 1996;18:745–55.

98. White RN, Burton CA, McEvoy FJ. Surgical treatment of intrahepatic portosystemic shunts in 45 dogs. Vet Rec 1998;142:358–65.

99. Hunt GB, Bellenger CR, Pearson MRB. Transportal approach for attenuating intrahepatic portosystemic shunts in dogs. Vet Surg 1996;25:300–8.

100. Harvey J, Erb HN. Complete ligation of extrahepatic congenital portosystemic shunts in nonencephalopathic dogs. Vet Surg 1998;27:413–6.

101. Mathew K, Grofton N. Congenital extrahepatic portosystemic shunt occlusion in the dog: gross observation during surgical correction. J Am Anim Hosp Assoc 1988;24:387–94.

102. Lee KCL, Lipscomb VJ, Lamb CR, et al. Association of portovenographic findings with outcome in dogs receiving surgical treatment for single congenital portosystemic shunts: 45 cases (2000–2004). J Am Vet Med Assoc 2006;229:1122–9.

103. White RN, MacDonald NJ, Burton CA, et al. Use of intraoperative mesenteric portovenography in congenital portosystemic shunt surgery. Vet Radiol Ultrasound 2003;44:514–21.

104. Hottinger HA, Walshaw R, Hauptman JG. Long term results of complete and partial ligation of congenital portosystemic shunts in dogs. Vet Surg 1995;24: 331–6.

105. Hunt GB, Hughes J. Outcomes after extrahepatic portosystemic shunt ligation in 49 dogs. Aust Vet J 1999;77:303–7.

106. Cabassu J, Seim H, MacPhail C, et al. Outcome of surgical attenuation of congenital extrahepatic portosystemic shunts using ameroid ring constrictors or cellophane banding in 13 cats. Proceedings of the 7th Annual Scientific Meeting of the Society of Veterinary Soft Tissue Surgery. Sante Fe (NM), June 19-21, 2008 (or personal communication E Monnet June 2008).

107. Holford AL, Tobias KM, Bartges JW, et al. Adrenal response to adrenocorticotropic hormone in dogs before and after surgical attenuation of a single congenital portosystemic shunt. J Vet Intern Med 2008;22:832–8.

108. Kyles AE, Hardie EM, Mehl M, et al. Evaluation of ameroid ring constrictors for the management of single extrahepatic portosystemic shunts in cats: 23 cases (1996–2001). J Am Vet Med Assoc 2002;220:1341–7.

109. Hardie EM, Kornegay JN, Cullen JM. Status epilepticus after ligation of portosystemic shunts. Vet Surg 1990;19:412–7.

110. Matushek KJ, Bjorling D, Mathews K. Generalized motor seizures after portosystemic shunt ligation in dogs: five cases (1981–1988). J Am Vet Med Assoc 1990; 196:2014–7.

111. Bright SR, Williams JM, Niles JD. Outcomes of intrahepatic portosystemic shunts occluded with ameroid constrictors in nine dogs and one cat. Vet Surg 2006;35:300–9.

112. Mehl ML, Kyles AE, Case JB, et al. Surgical management of left-divisional intrahepatic portosystemic shunts: outcome after partial ligation of, or ameroid constrictor placement on, the left hepatic vein in twenty-eight dogs (1995–2005). Vet Surg 2007;36:21–30.

113. Windsor RC, Olby NJ. Congenital portosystemic shunts in five mature dogs with neurological signs. J Am Anim Hosp Assoc 2007;43:322–31.

114. Landon BP, Abraham LA, Charles JA. Use of transcolonic portal scintigraphy to evaluate efficacy of cellophane banding of congenital extrahepatic portosystemic shunts in 16 dogs. Aust Vet J 2008;86:169–79.

115. White RN, Forster van Hijfte MA, Petrie G, et al. Surgical treatment of intrahepatic portosystemic shunts in six cats. Vet Rec 1996;139:314–7.

116. Whiting PG, Breznock EM, Moore P, et al. Partial hepatectomy with temporary hepatic vascular occlusion in dogs with hepatic arteriovenous fistulas. Vet Surg 1986;15:171–80.

117. Komtebedde J, Forsyth SF, Breznock EM, et al. Intrahepatic portosystemic venous anomaly in the dog. Perioperative management and complications. Vet Surg 1991;20:37–42.

118. Weisse C, Berent A, Todd K, et al. Percutaneous transjugular coil embolization for intrahepatic portosystemic shunts in 40 dogs [abstract]. In: Programs and abstracts of the American College of Veterinary Internal Medicine Conference. Louisville (KY): 2006.

119. Leveille-Webster CR, Center SA. Chronic hepatitis: therapeutic considerations. In: Bonagura JD, Kirk RW, editors. Kirks current veterinary therapy. Philadelphia: WB Saunders Company; 1995. p. 749–56.
120. Weisse C, Mondschein JI, Itkin M, et al. Use of a percutaneous atrial septal occluder device for complete acute occlusion of an intrahepatic portosystemic shunt in a dog. J Am Vet Med Assoc 2005;227(2):249–52.
121. Bussadori R, Bussadori C, Millan L, et al. Transvenous coil embolisation for the treatment of single congenital portosystemic shunts in six dogs. Vet J 2008;176: 221–6.
122. Gonzalo-Orden JM, Altonaga JR, Costillla S, et al. Transvenous coil embolization of an intrahepatic portosystemic shunt in a dog. Vet Radiol Ultrasound 2000; 41(6):516–8.
123. Asano K, Watari T, Kuwabara M, et al. Successful treatment by percutaneous transvenous coil embolization in a small-breed dog with intrahepatic portosystemic shunt. J Vet Med Sci 2003;65(11):1269–72.
124. Leveille R, Johnson S, Birchard S. Transvenous coil embolization of portosystemic shunt in dogs. Vet Radiol Ultrasound 2003;44(1):32–6.
125. Schneider M, Plassmann M, Rabuer K. Coil embolization of portosystemic shunts in comparison with conventional therapies. Proc 15th European College of Internal Medicine, 2005.
126. Boothe HW, Howe LM, Edwards JF, et al. Multiple extrahepatic shunts in dogs: 30 cases (1981–1993). J Am Vet Med Assoc 1996;208:1849–54.
127. Butler-Howe LM, Boothe HW Jr, Boothe DM, et al. Effects of vena caval banding in experimentally induced multiple portosystemic shunts in dogs. Am J Vet Res 1993;54:1774–83.

Diseases of the Gallbladder and Biliary Tree

Sharon A. Center, DVM

KEYWORDS

- Bile ducts • Canalilculi
- Gall bladder • Biliary mucocele
- Cholangiohepatitis • Choledochitis
- Extrahepatic bile duct obstruction
- Feline polycystic liver disease

ANATOMY OF THE BILIARY SYSTEM

The biliary system consists of the gallbladder (GB), cystic duct, common bile duct (CBD), hepatic ducts, interlobular ducts, intralobular ducts, bile ductules (first biliary component lined by cuboidal epithelium), and hepatic canaliculi (**Fig. 1**). Hepatocytes have basolateral (sinusoidal membranes containing microvilli) and apical-polar (canalicular) plasma membranes that contain transporters involved with bile formation. Basolateral membranes abut the space of Disse and are bathed in sinusoidal ultrafiltrate. The canalicular membranes represent a specialized component of the hepatocyte cell membrane anatomically delimited by tight junctions that segregate bile from sinusoidal blood and ultrafiltrate. Canaliculi (1-mm diameter) are the site of initial bile formation. While histologic or cytologic observation of canalicular cholestasis (microscopic bile plugs within canaliculi) is common (**Fig. 2**), this finding has no diagnostic or prognostic significance because it occurs with diverse disorders that may or may not directly involve liver disease.

The GB, located and attached to the liver to the right of midline within a fossa between the right medial and quadrate liver lobes, units with the CBD by means of the cystic duct. The cystic duct extends from the neck of the GB to its junction with the first hepatic duct (see **Fig. 1**).

The communication of the CBD and duodenum is anatomically distinct in the dog and cat. In a medium-sized dog, the CBD is 5-cm long and 2.5 mm in diameter and empties into the duodenum 1.5 cm to 6.0 cm distal to the pylorus at the major duodenal papilla. At the junction with the intestine, the CBD courses intramurally for 2 cm.[1] The CBD of the dog opens near the smaller of two pancreatic ducts (minor pancreatic duct) at the major duodenal papilla; the larger pancreatic duct (accessory

Department of Clinical Sciences, Cornell University, College of Veterinary Medicine, Vet Box 33, Ithaca, NY, USA
E-mail address: sac6@cornell.edu

Vet Clin Small Anim 39 (2009) 543–598
doi:10.1016/j.cvsm.2009.01.004
0195-5616/09/$ – see front matter © 2009 Elsevier Inc. All rights reserved.

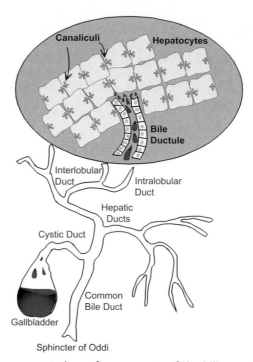

Fig. 1. Diagrammatic representations of components of the biliary system. (*Adapted from* Johns Hopkins Pathology. Anatomy and physiology of the gallbladder and bile ducts. Available at: http://pathology2.jhu.edu/gbbd/images/hepatocyte2.gif. Accessed April 23, 2009; with permission.)

pancreatic duct) opens a few centimeters distally. The bile duct of the cat is long and sinuous compared with the dog. In the cat, the CBD fuses in an ampulla with the pancreatic duct just before entering the duodenal papilla 3-cm caudal to the pylorus.[2] In some cats the major pancreatic duct opens separately but immediately adjacent to the CBD. Approximately 2-cm caudal to the major duodenal papilla, the accessory pancreatic duct enters the duodenum (minor duodenal papilla) in 20% of cats.[2] While the pancreas in each species is nearly always drained by two ducts, a great deal of variation exists. Because of the close proximity of the pancreas and CBD, pancreatitis commonly influences bile flow through the major bile duct, causing obstruction to flow

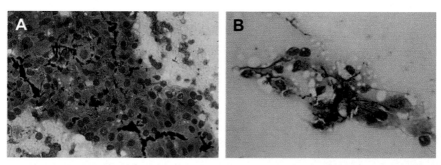

Fig. 2. Photomicrograph of aspiration cytology from a cat (*A*) and dog (*B*) showing canalicular bile stasis (canalicular cholestasis) (*modified* Wright Giemsa, original magnification x600 [*A*] and ×900 [*B*]).

and jaundice. In the cat, inflammatory, neoplastic, or obstructive disorders involving the distal CBD can affect both the biliary tree and pancreas. In fact it is possible that microlithiasis or sludged bile transiently obstructing the distal CBD causes intermittent bile duct occlusion and idiopathic pancreatitis in the cat. Blood supply to the intrahepatic bile ducts is provided by the hepatic arterial and portal venous circulations. Consequently, hematogenously disseminated infectious agents may involve the intrahepatic biliary tree.

Nestled deep within its fossa, an empty GB may not be readily apparent on gross inspection during surgical exploration or laparoscopy. Embryologically derived from the foregut, the structure of the GB resembles the intestines. Its luminal surface is covered with mucosa containing fine microvilli that expand the surface area for resorptive and exchange processes. Similar to the intestine, the GB also has a lamina propria with a resident lymphoplasmacytic population, a muscularis, a layer of connective tissue, and an outermost serosa. Mucus glands within the GB provide mucin that protects the luminal epithelium from the cytolytic effects of bile acids. Mucin production is stimulated by inflammatory cytokines, endotoxins, and prostaglandins and excessive GB mucin production in the dog seemingly contributes to biliary mucocele formation. Having fewer mucus glands in their GB may explain why mucoceles do not develop in the cat.[3] Numerous lymphatics in the GB may be grossly visible during portal hypertension, chronic passive congestion, or hepatobiliary inflammation. Fluid leaked from these lymphatics contributes to GB wall thickening observed ultrasonographically. Innervation of the GB and CBD is provided by the vagal nerve. Arterial perfusion is solely derived from the left branch of the proper hepatic artery (cystic artery). Having only a single source of perfusion makes the GB and CBD uniquely susceptible to ischemic necrosis following blunt abdominal trauma (ie, vascular shearing trauma). Compromised perfusion can lead to biliary tree rupture and bile peritonitis. The GB functions as a storage reservoir where bile is concentrated, acidified, and modified. However, its function is not essential such that cholecystectomy is usually well tolerated.

Bile enters the GB continuously in a low-flow low-pressure system. Pressure within the system is generated by hepatic bile secretion and the tonic contraction of the sphincter of Oddi, the one-way sphincter at the duodenal papilla. The sphincter of Oddi provides protection against retrograde passage of enteric contents up the biliary tree. After food ingestion, the GB mucosa produces a mucinous, bicarbonate-rich fluid that mixes with stored hepatic bile. This action is facilitated by several gastrointestinal peptides, including secretin and vasoactive intestinal peptide.

GALLBLADDER

Hepatic canalicular bile is continuously delivered to the intrahepatic ductal system, with the majority being diverted into a relaxed GB. Bile is markedly concentrated and modified by the GB (**Table 1**). After a prolonged fast, most of the bile salt pool is stored in the GB, where it is concentrated up to 10-fold. Isotonicity with plasma is maintained by formation of mixed-micelles (bile salt anions and cations [Na^+ and Ca^{2++}] aggregated with phospholipids, lecithin, and cholesterol). GB bile is acidified by absorption of Na^+ in exchange for H^+, while K^+ and Ca^{2++} are passively equilibrated with plasma. Most biliary HCO_3^- is lost by neutralization with H^+ and diffusion of liberated CO_2 into the circulatory system. Small amounts of bilirubin glucuronides are hydrolyzed to unconjugated bilirubin, and some of this is resorbed into the systemic circulation. The GB is a dynamic organ responsive to myoelectric motor complexes similar to the intestines. During the interdigestive interval, "bellows-like" gallbladder contractions divert bile directly into the CBD and intestines. Motilin is

Table 1
Characteristics of hepatic and GB bile

Characteristic	Hepatic Bile	Gallbladder Bile
Color	Golden yellow to orange	Dark brown to greenish brown
Water	95%–97%	85%–90%
Bile salts	35 mM	310 mM
Cholesterol	2 mM–5 mM 3 mM	10 mM–30 mM 25 mM
Bilirubin (total)[a]	0.3 mM–0.8 mM 0.8 mM	1.5 mM–7.0 mM 3.2 mM
Lecithin	1.0 mM	8.0 mM
Proteins	250 mg/dL	700 mg/dL
Fatty acids	250 mg/dL	350 mg/dL
pH	7.0–7.8	6.0–7.0
HCO_3-	20 mM–30 mM 45 mM	≤ 1 mM 8 mM
Ca^{++}/Ca_{Total}	0.8 mM–1.2 mM/2 mM–3 mM	2 mM–3 mM/10 mM–18 mM
Na^+	165	280
K^+	5	10
Cl-	90	15
Osmolality	Similar to plasma	Similar to plasma

Abbreviation: mM = millimole.
[a] Less than 2% of bilirubin in normal bile is unconjugated.

associated with this activity and can be induced pharmacologically with certain drugs (eg, erythromycin). Rhythmic or phasic contractions of the sphincter of Oddi regulate duodenal bile release in spurts. GB motility is initiated through interplay of neuroendocrine signals that coordinate contraction with meal ingestion. Free fatty acids and amino acids in food and gastric distention initiate vagal stimulation (parasympathetic), and cholecystokinin (CCK) and motilin released from the duodenum signal GB contraction and relaxation of the sphincter of Oddi (enhanced by secretin). This coordinated activity allows postprandial release of bile in the duodenum. CCK also stimulates intestinal peristalsis, facilitating meal digestion and propulsion of bile salts to the ileum, where they are actively recycled in the enterohepatic circulation. Negative feedback signals from bile acids returning to the liver inhibit further CCK release. After meal-initiated GB contraction, the GB relaxes and the sphincter of Oddi tone returns, diverting hepatic bile into a relaxed GB. Dysmotility of the GB may be an emerging clinical syndrome in the dog associated with GB mucocele and cholelith formation (see sections on GB mucocele and cholelith formation later in this article).

Hepato-Biliary-Enteric Bacterial Circulation

An hepato-biliary-enteric bacterial circulation is acknowledged, whereby transmural passage of enteric organisms into the portal vein navigate canaliculi and transcend the biliary tree into bile. Consequently, disorders impairing bile flow within the ductal systems or GB are permissive to bacterial opportunists.

Bile Formation

To understand the rational of choleretic therapy, it is essential to consider basic mechanisms of bile formation. Bile primarily functions as a digestive vehicle for bile acids and elimination of lipophilic metabolic products and xenobiotics. Initial canalicular bile is modified by diverse hepatic and ductular mechanisms during transport through the biliary tree.[4]

Hepatic bile formation

Hepatic bile formation is classically defined as either bile acid-dependent or independent. Independent mechanisms involve active transport of glutathione (GSH) at the canaliculus and modification of bile in the ductal system.

Canalicular bile formation

Canalicular bile formation is a continuous osmotic process predominantly driven by active pumps excreting organic solutes (eg, GSH, bile acids) followed passively by water, electrolytes, and nonelectrolytes (eg, glucose, amino acids). In parallel with transport of water-soluble bile constituents, lipid vesicles are detached from the apical membrane of the canaliculus, forming micelles composed of phospholipid, phosphatidylcholine (also called lecithin), free cholesterol, and bile salts. Vesicles and mixed micelles attenuate the osmotic effect of free bile salts and their toxicity to biliary epithelium. Delivery of mixed micelles to the alimentary canal augments the intermingling of bile salts and lipid, thereby facilitating fat digestion. The cholesterol composition of bile influences risk for bile lithogenicity. High cholesterol saturation in bile increases risk for cholesterol choleliths (common to human beings). Neither the dog nor cat have similar cholesterol bile saturation and thus do not form primary cholesterol choleliths. It is important to consider this difference when deciding on the propriety of ursodeoxycholate (UDCA) as a choleretic in dogs and cats when medical management of choleliths is considered. The cholelith dissolution response, well reported in human beings, likely does not occur in these species because of a different cholelith composition.

The role of bile acids

Amphipathic organic anions synthesized in the liver, bile acids are conjugated exclusively to taurine in the cat and to either taurine or glycine in the dog. Maintained largely in conjugated form in mixed micelles, bile acids circulate efficiently in an enterohepatic circulation. Active transport uptake in the ileum and active transporters on the surface of the liver provide for high system efficiency ($\leq$ 5% fecal loss per day). Bile salt-dependent bile flow has a powerful influence at the canaliculus (direct linear relationship), with nonmicelle-forming bile salts (eg, dehydrocholate) bestowing the greatest effect. Thus, dehydrocholate imparts prominent choleresis. Transcellular transport of bile salts along with micelle formation maintains a marked concentration gradient between bile and blood; biliary concentrations exceed plasma bile acid concentration by 100- to 1,000-fold.

The role of Glutathione

GSH is the only endogenous anion known to promote bile salt-independent canalicular bile formation under physiologic conditions.[5] Similar to the secretion of bile acids, the rate of GSH secretion is quantitatively related to bile flow. Its strong osmotic influence derives from its hydrophilic nature, active membrane exportation at the canaliculus, and its hydrolysis by membrane-affiliated gamma glutamyl transferase (GGT) into its three constituent amino acids (cysteine, glutamate, glycine). This triples its osmolar impact and draws water and electrolytes into bile through paracellular pathways. Consequently, thiol donors may impart a choleretic influence, particularly in animals with cholestatic liver disease who are at risk for low hepatic GSH concentrations.[6] A choleretic influence of s-adenosylmethionine (SAMe, a GSH donor) was shown in

GB bile in clinically healthy cats treated with 40–60 mg/kg SAMe (Denosyl [Nutramax Laboratories, Edgewood, MD] by mouth daily).[7]

Modification of hepatic bile

Primary hepatic bile is modified during transport in the biliary system by secretion and reabsorption of fluid and inorganic electrolytes. Cholangiocytes also uptake bile salts (Na^+-dependent transporter) as the initial step in a cholehepatic shunt pathway that permits intrahepatic cycling of bile salts through a periductular capillary plexus. Under normal conditions, the high luminal concentration of bile salts (millimolar range) negates the impact of this process on bile. However, cholehepatic shunting is physiologically important for signaling ductular mucin and bicarbonate secretion in bile and contributes to the very high serum-bile acid concentrations in animals with cholestatic liver disease. Bile ducts substantially contribute to bile formation and flow through bicarbonate production, primarily influenced by secretin (derived from duodenal and jejunal mucosa). Ductal secretions account for 10% to 40% of basal bile flow, depending on the species. In human beings, 40% of bile volume is of ductular origin.

Bile flow

Variables influencing bile flow mediate canalicular or ductal processes involved with bile formation and modification. Vagal stimulation, CCK, and gastrin weakly stimulate hepatic bile production, secretin potently stimulates ductule bile flow (increasing bicarbonate secretion), glucagon modestly stimulates canalicular bile formation and ductule bicarbonate secretion, and somatostatin potently inhibits bile secretion (canalicular and ductular sites). While the entire spectrum of effects of drugs on bile flow remains largely unexplored, certain drugs have been shown to modulate bile formation at the canalicular level by inducing transport pump activity (ie, multidrug resistance-associated protein-2 or MRP-2). MRP-2 levels are modified by certain glucocorticoids (and steroid hormones) and structurally unrelated xenobiotics, such as rifampicin, phenobarbital, oltipraz, and cisplatin.[8,9] The MRP-2 activity is down-regulated during cholestasis.

Furosemide has been shown to stimulate bile flow in the dog, but can impose a detrimental effect if the patient becomes dehydrated. UDCA and dehydrocholic acid induce choleresis and have been specifically studied in the dog.[10] Oral UDCA (50 mg/kg) increased bile flow by 70% within 1 hour, as well as the concentration of phospholipid, cholesterol, bile acids, and bilirubin in bile. Oral dehydrocholic acid (50 mg/kg) produced a considerable increase in bile flow (270%) by increasing secretion of electrolytes and water. In human beings, UDCA reduces biliary cholesterol and increases HCO_3^- secretion in bile; these changes remarkably enhance solubility of cholesterol gallstones but not pigment gallstones.

Pathologic Changes In Bile

White bile syndrome, inspissated bile syndrome, bile acid deconjugation

In animals with bile stasis, nonabsorbable bile constituents (bile salts, phospholipids, and cholesterol) are subject to concentration or dilution when water and inorganic electrolytes (sodium, chloride, bicarbonate) are resorbed or added to bile by biliary epithelium. Major bile-duct obstruction can produce a "white bile" syndrome (white reflecting the absence of bilirubin pigments) when bile containing pigment is segregated from bile in the large ducts or GB (eg, obstructed hepatic ducts, cystic duct, chronic extrahepatic bile duct obstruction [EHBDO]). Stasis of bile flow and dehydration promote pathologic thickening of bile and formation of inspissated dark green/black biliary material. Formation of a GB mucocele involves the entrapment, retention, or local over-production of mucin that profoundly increases bile viscosity. Choleresis (enhanced bile flow) produces thin, watery dilute bile and is a therapeutic goal in disorders involving stasis of bile flow in large bile ducts. Disease states causing bile ductule proliferation (inflammation) may modify bile composition and alter bile flow by increasing ductular secretions of bicarbonate and mucin. Increased mucin production can be identified histologically within intrahepatic bile ducts in certain disorders (cholangitis, EHBDO). Although virtually all bile acids derived from the biliary tree are conjugated, a bacterial infection or low pH in the biliary system can result in bile acid deconjugation. Unconjugated bile acids are cytotoxic, alter permeability of vascular structures, and induce tissue inflammation. These likely contribute to inflammatory changes and epithelial edema in septic cholecystitis and choledochitis.

EVALUATION OF THE PATIENT WITH BILIARY TRACT DISEASE

A general diagnostic approach for disorders of the biliary tract is presented in **Fig. 3**; differential diagnosis of these disorders requires skilled abdominal ultrasonography. Initial assessments are usually pursued upon recognition of increased enzyme activities (especially alkaline phosphatase [ALP] or GGT) or hyperbilirubinemia. If a septic process is involved, fever and a neutrophilic leukocytosis with a left shift are often apparent. Animals with complete EHBDO, necrotizing cholecystitis or choledochitis, pain producing cholelithiasis, or septic bile peritonitis are most symptomatic. Cats with severe cholangiohepatitis may fail to disclose signs of illness. Clinical signs and clinicopathologic features for separate disease entities are discussed separately in this article.

Sequential assessments of enzyme activity, bilirubin, and cholesterol concentrations are important to gain a perspective of disease continuation or progression. Finding acholic stools in an overtly jaundiced patient indicates high likelihood of EHBDO or feline diffuse sclerosing cholangitis. Abdominal pain associated with peritoneal

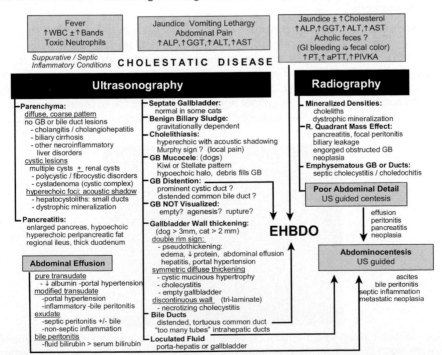

Fig. 3. Diagnostic algorithm for diagnosis of disorders of the gallbladder and biliary tree.

effusion containing a disproportionately high bilirubin concentration suggests a ruptured biliary tree, often attributable to cholecystitis, choledochitis, neoplasia, or blunt abdominal trauma. An abdominal effusion should be sampled as close to the biliary structures as safely possible and fluid examined for particulate bile. In febrile animals with suspected biliary disease, early submission of cultures of blood, urine, hepatic or bile aspirates for aerobic and anaerobic bacteria can expedite identification of involved organisms and appropriate treatment.

IMAGING
Radiography

Abdominal radiographs have limited utility in diagnosis of biliary system disorders. Mineralized densities involving the biliary tree can reflect stasis of bile flow or dystrophic mineralization associated with congenital malformations, acquired duct "sacculation," chronic duct inflammation, or choleliths (**Fig. 4**). Some choleliths contain enough calcium bilirubinate to be radiographically visible. A mass effect in the right cranial quadrant in suspected EHBDO may represent an engorged GB, pancreatitis, neoplasia, or focal bile peritonitis. Radiographic suspicion of abdominal effusion (poor abdominal detail) may prompt early diagnosis of bile peritonitis. Gas within biliary structures or liver indicates an emphysematous process (eg, cholecystitis, choledochitis, infected biliary cyst, hepatic abscess, necrotic tumor mass) and warrants prompt antimicrobial therapy and either surgical intervention or percutaneous ultrasound-guided aspiration or lavage. Thoracic radiography is used to survey for systemic disease (ie, metastatic lesions, pleural fluid). Sternal lymphadenopathy is common in cats with the cholangitis/cholangiohepatitis syndrome (CCHS), as this lymph node functions as a sentinel for the cranial abdomen (**Fig. 5**).

Cholecystography

Contrast radiographic imaging of the biliary system is rarely pursued in veterinary medicine. Rather, abdominal ultrasound (US) takes important first priority as a diagnostic modality. However, a number of radiographic contrast agents pertinent to the biliary tree have been studied in dogs and cats (**Table 2**).[1] Cholecystography can be accomplished with iodinated contrast given by oral or intravenous routes. Distribution and concentration of such contrast agents for interrogation of biliary structures is influenced by numerous variables, including hyperbilirubinemia and major duct

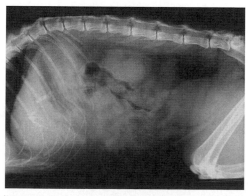

Fig. 4. Abdominal radiograph from a cat with mineralized hepatocystoliths and dystrophic mineralization of small bile ducts secondary to chronic cholangitis. (*Courtesy of* the Section of Diagnostic Imaging, College of Veterinary Medicine, Cornell University, Ithaca, NY.)

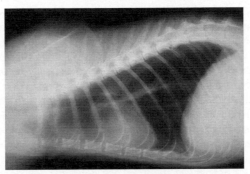

Fig. 5. Thoracic radiograph from a cat with the CCHS demonstrating a prominent sternal lymph node, reflecting inflammatory response in the abdominal cavity. (*Courtesy of* the Section of Diagnostic Imaging, College of Veterinary Medicine, Cornell University, Ithaca, NY.)

occlusion. At best, these agents may disclose choleliths, polyps, or sludged bile, but are insufficient for confirming bile peritonitis or for localizing the site of leakage.

Ultrasonography

Abdominal US has become an essential diagnostic tool for assessment of the liver and biliary system. However, overconfidence in its ability to predict histologic diagnoses can lead to grave prognosis and treatment errors. Findings must always be reconciled with a patient's history, physical examination findings, and clinicopathologic data by the veterinarian with case responsibility. A rigorous criterion-referenced investigation of the diagnostic utility of US to predict parenchymal liver disorders recently confirmed its insufficiency in discriminating among diffuse canine and feline liver disease.[11] A further complication is that in clinically ill inappetent cats, hepatic lipidosis can complicate assessment of hepatic parenchyma because of the hyperechogenicity imparted by triglyceride stores.

Abdominal US can be used to subjectively estimate liver size, to identify changes in parenchymal echogenicity, mass lesions, distension and wall thickness of components of the biliary system, size and echogenicity of the pancreas and perihepatic lymph nodes, and the presence of abdominal effusion. Investigation for abdominal lymphadenopathy and other organ system abnormalities should be undertaken concurrent with investigation of the liver. In healthy dogs and cats, the wall of the GB is often poorly

Table 2
Radiographic contrast agents pertinent to the biliary tree studied in dogs and cats

Agent	Species	Dose (mg/kg)	Route	Exposure Time Interval
Iodipamide	Dog	0.5	IV	1 hr
Iobenzamic acid	Dog	2 g–3 g/10 kg–15 kg 5 mg/kg–150 mg/kg	PO	12 hrs
Meglumine iotrixanate	Dog	0.5 mg/kg–1.0 mg/kg	IV slow	30 min
Ipodate calcium	Dog	150 mg/kg–450 mg/kg	PO	12 hrs
	Cat	150 mg/kg–500 mg/kg	PO	12 hrs
Ipodate sodium	Cat	150 mg/kg–500 mg/kg	PO	12 hrs
Iodipamide meglumine	Cat	0.5 mL/kg–1.5 mL/kg	IV slow	3 hrs–5 hrs

visualized (**Fig. 6**). Occasionally a septate or bilobed GB is identified in cats reflecting a benign developmental anomaly (**Fig. 7**). Thickness of the GB wall in healthy dogs is 2 mm to 3 mm and in healthy cats is less than or equal to 1 mm, measured in longitudinal or cross-sectional dimension.[12,13] However, wall thickness varies according to the degree of GB distension. Care must be taken to rule out imaging artifacts when determining GB wall thickness (eg, pseudo-thickening may be caused by reverberation or refraction).[13] Pseudo-thickening of the GB wall may occur with peritoneal effusion as a result of the acoustic interface between fluid and the GB wall (**Fig. 8**). A double-rim pattern may reflect edema associated with hepatitis, passive congestion, severe hypo-albuminemia, or disease involving the GB (**Fig. 9**).[14] A diffusely thick GB wall usually represents cholecystitis (**Fig. 10**A). A discontinuous or tri-laminar appearance of the GB wall (**Fig. 10**B,C) is definitively abnormal and suggests wall necrosis. Diffuse hyper-echogenicity of the GB wall may be observed with mineralization secondary to chole-cystitis (**Fig. 11**). Gravitational dependency of biliary sediment (moving with positional change) confirms the liquid nature of bile and is typical for nonpathologic bile sludge (see **Figs. 6** and **8**). Finding sludged bile is common in inappetent or fasted animals and this typically is not associated with a postacoustic shadow. Echogenic material in bile represents conglomerates (1 mm–3 mm) of calcium bilirubinate and cholesterol suspended in the viscous mucin-rich phase of bile. Lipid droplets may also contribute echogenic particulates. The inability to image a GB may be because of technical difficulties, agenesis of the GB, or GB rupture.

During examination of the biliary structures, the cystic duct often can be traced into the CBD and the union between the CBD and duodenal papilla identified. In cats, the duodenal papilla ranges from 2.9 mm to 5.5 mm in width and has a maximum height of 4.0 mm (transverse section).[2] In dogs, size is more variable because of the wide range of body mass among breeds.

Assessment of Gallbladder Motility

Impaired gallbladder motility has been associated with a number of conditions in human beings and may be antecedent to choleliths or GB mucocele formation in dogs. Compromised integration between GB motor function, the intestinal migrating motor complex, and motilin is hypothesized. Detection of diminished GB contractility in the presence of choleliths or a developing mucocele is now used in the author's hospital to recommend prophylactic cholecystectomy. We have adopted this approach because of the complications and high mortality associate with cholecystectomy for necrotic or septic cholecystitis. Functional US and biliary scintigraphy have

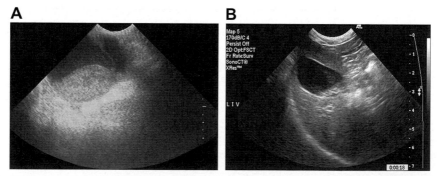

Fig. 6. Ultrasonographic image of a gallbladder from a (*A*) healthy dog and (*B*) healthy cat. In (*A*) the wall is not evident (<1 mm thick); in (*B*) the wall is less than 2 mm. (*Courtesy of* the Section of Diagnostic Imaging, College of Veterinary Medicine, Cornell University, Ithaca, NY.)

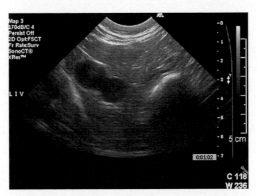

Fig. 7. Ultrasonographic image of a bipartate (septate or bilobed) GB in a healthy cat; a corresponding gross image is shown in **Fig. 23**. (*Courtesy of* the Section of Diagnostic Imaging, College of Veterinary Medicine, Cornell University, Ithaca, NY.)

been used to study GB motility in vivo. Because scintigraphy is expensive, not widely available, and exposes the patient to radiation, functional US is preferable. A practical clinical protocol for real-time assessment of GB contractility in dogs has been established.[15] Time-related changes in GB volume are determined after an overnight fast and sequentially after administration of a test meal plus or minus low-dose oral erythromycin (motilin stimulus); the protocol is described in **Fig. 12**. If on initial abdominal US, a GB is of less than or equal to 1 mL/kg body weight, there is no need for motility assessment. An example of data from a dog with GB hypomotility is shown in **Fig. 13**.

Ultrasonographic Features of Specific Disorders

Extrahepatic bile duct obstruction
Engorgement of the GB and dilated cystic duct are evident within 24 hours of acute complete EHBDO; distention of intrahepatic bile ducts is evident within 5 to 7 days (**Fig. 14**).[1,16,17] Ducts are differentiated from portal vasculature by their irregular branching patterns, tortuosity, and absence of blood flow on Doppler interrogation.[17] Bile duct diameter is variable among dogs and cannot be used to determine the chronicity of obstruction, although profound duct dilation develops after 4 to 6 weeks of complete EHBDO. Obstruction of hepatic ducts (one or more) within a single liver lobe can be difficult to image. Affected animals are not hyperbilirubinemic but have

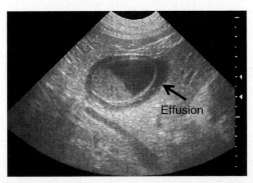

Fig. 8. Ultrasonographic image from a dog with abdominal effusion and "pseudo" thickening of the GB wall. Abdominal effusion can be observed adjacent to the GB wall. (*Courtesy of* the Section of Diagnostic Imaging, College of Veterinary Medicine, Cornell University, Ithaca, NY.)

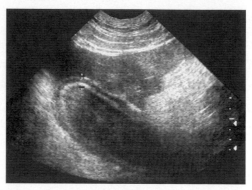

Fig. 9. Ultrasonographic image from a dog with hepatitis demonstrating a double-rim sign attributable to GB wall edema. Note the irregular hepatic contour ("nodular"). (*Courtesy of* the Section of Diagnostic Imaging, College of Veterinary Medicine, Cornell University, Ithaca, NY.)

increased liver enzyme activity. Once distended by obstructive phenomenon, intra- and extra-hepatic bile ducts may remain larger than normal.

Feline cholangitis/cholangiohepatitis syndrome

Ultrasonographic assessment may fail to detect abnormalities or may detect diffuse hepatic parenchymal echogenicity attributable to hepatic lipidosis (confirmed by

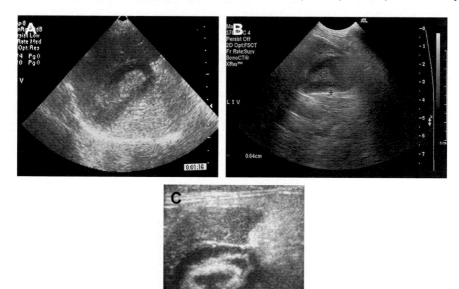

Fig. 10. Ultrasonographic image of the gallbladder from two dogs with cholecystitis. (*A*) The GB wall is difficult to distinguish and is adjacent to hyperechoic tissue that corresponded to adhesions and apparent focal bile peritonitis. (*B*) The GB wall is discontinuous, associated with necrosis. (*C*) The wall demonstrates a tri-laminar appearance at the location of necrosis. (*Courtesy of* the Section of Diagnostic Imaging, College of Veterinary Medicine, Cornell University, Ithaca, NY.)

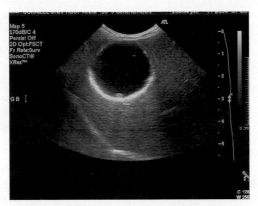

Fig. 11. Ultrasonographic image of a GB with a hyperechoic wall caused by mineralization and a small cholecystolith (small acoustic shadow) in a dog with hyperadrenocorticism. (*Courtesy of* the Section of Diagnostic Imaging, College of Veterinary Medicine, Cornell University, Ithaca, NY.)

hepatic aspirate cytology) (**Fig. 15**A). Some cats with CCHS have choleliths, cholecystitis, and large duct choledochitis associated with heteroechoic parenchymal foci reflecting inflammation and fibrosis (**Fig. 15**B and C). In febrile cats with a left-shifted leukogram, liver aspirates and cholecystocentesis (in the absence of suspected EHBDO) provide samples for bacterial culture and cytologic confirmation of sepsis that augment prompt treatment recommendations.

Cholelithiasis
Both radiodense and radiopaque choleliths are identified with US. Cholecystoliths are most easily imaged and produce strong acoustic shadows when of sufficient size and density (**Figs. 16–19**). Choleliths can be identified within intrahepatic bile ducts (hepatolithiasis), large hepatic ducts, the cystic duct, the CBD, the sphincter of Oddi, or in

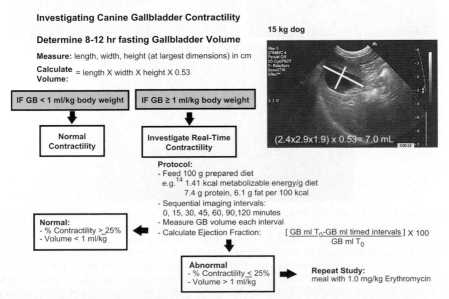

Fig. 12. Investigating canine GB contractility.

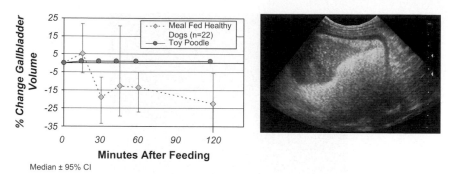

Median ± 95% CI

Fig. 13. Ultrasonographic assessment of GB motility in a 3.2-kg Toy Poodle. GB volume was 11.3 mL (3.5 mL/kg body weight) and did not change after feeding with 1.0 mg/kg erythromycin. Elective cholecystectomy and liver biopsies were performed because of progressive increases in ALP activity. (*Data from* Ramstedt KL, Center SA, Randolph JF, et al. Changes in gallbladder volume in healthy dogs after food was withheld for 12 hours followed by ingestion of a meal or a meal containing erythromycin. Am J Vet Res 2008;69:647–51.)

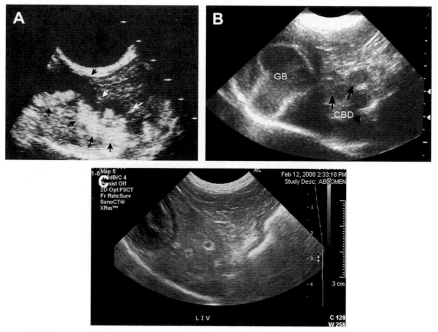

Fig. 14. (*A*) Ultrasonographic images from a cat with major bile duct obstruction that corresponds to **Fig. 28**; a dilated common bile duct is filled with dense sludge (*ventral black arrows*) and liquid bile (black anechoic material marked by *dorsal black and white arrows*). (*B*) Ultrasonographic image of chronic bile duct occlusion in a dog showing GB and CBD that is tortuous and dilated, indicated by black arrows. (*C*) Intrahepatic bile ducts are distended and have hyperechoic walls; these bile ducts were differentiated from blood vessels using color-flow Doppler. (*Courtesy of* the Section of Diagnostic Imaging, College of Veterinary Medicine, Cornell University, Ithaca, NY.)

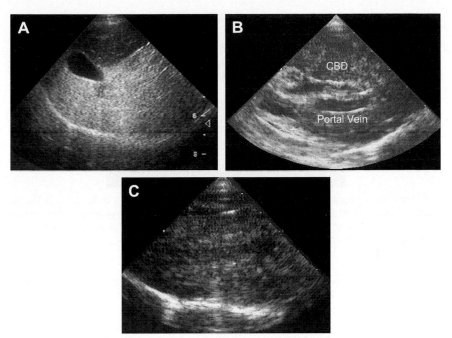

Fig. 15. (A) Ultrasonographic image of a cat with cholangiohepatitis complicated by the hepatic lipidosis syndrome associated with a diffuse hyperechogenic parenchymal pattern. (B) Ultrasonographic image of a cat with CCHS associated with involvement of the CBD; note the increased echogenicity and thickness of the duct. (C) Ultrasonographic image of the liver of a cat with the CCHS showing a coarse echogenic pattern associated with inflammatory infiltrates and fibrosis. (*Courtesy of* the Section of Diagnostic Imaging, College of Veterinary Medicine, Cornell University, Ithaca, NY.)

the GB. However, the most common cholelith location is within the GB. Stones within the common or cystic ducts may be challenging to identify because adjacent visceral structures and bowel gas may obscure their detection, and because they are not surrounded by anechoic bile. Calculi are differentiated from mural lesions by demonstrating gravitational mobility. Finding a dilated CBD associated with high liver enzyme activity (especially ALP and GGT) and hyperbilirubinemia is consistent with symptomatic cholelithiasis.

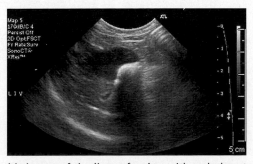

Fig. 16. Ultrasonographic image of the liver of a dog with a cholecystolith; note the prominent acoustic shadow. (*Courtesy of* the Section of Diagnostic Imaging, College of Veterinary Medicine, Cornell University, Ithaca, NY.)

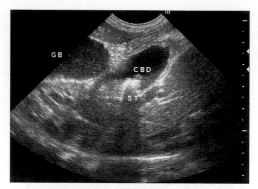

Fig. 17. The ultrasonographic image of a dog showing the GB with a distended CBD caused by obstruction with a calcium bilirubinate stone (ST) that is casting an acoustic shadow. (*Courtesy of* the Section of Diagnostic Imaging, College of Veterinary Medicine, Cornell University, Ithaca, NY.)

Gallbladder masses

Sessile or polypoid lesions in the gallbladder may be identified in dogs with GB cystic mucosal hyperplasia. Adenomas or adenocarcinomas are less common and usually produce an irregular and focal wall involvement or appear to compress the GB lumen (**Fig. 20**). Sometimes a large pedunculated mass can cause GB obstruction.

Cystic biliary syndromes

Cats with an hepatic polycystic disorder may not have cystic malformations easily identified on US because of small cyst size (< 2 mm in diameter) (**Fig. 21**A). Larger cysts are easily detected (**Fig. 21**B). Complex cystic structures in the porta hepatitis may be associated with the hepatic polycystic syndrome or an isolated cystadenoma (**Fig. 21**C).

Gallbladder mucocele

An exclusive diagnosis in the dog, GB mucoceles are easily detected. The US image is diagnostic and is characterized by finding a large GB filled with hyperechoic nongravitationally dependent contents and a hypoechoic "rim sign" (an immobile star-like or kiwi fruit-like appearance) (**Fig. 22**). This pattern reflects a dense central biliary conglomerate comprised of thick sludge containing tenacious mucin that is tightly

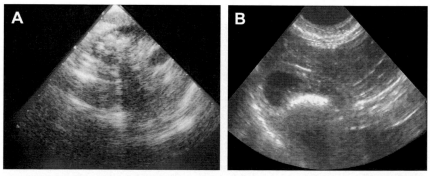

Fig. 18. (*A*) A GB from a 10-year-old cat is filled with numerous choleliths. (*B*) Choleliths are observed within a thick walled GB caused by biopsy-confirmed cholecystitis. (*Courtesy of* the Section of Diagnostic Imaging, College of Veterinary Medicine, Cornell University, Ithaca, NY.)

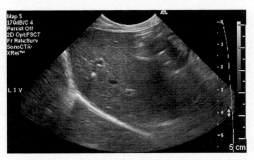

Fig. 19. Ultrasonographic image of the liver of a dog with hepatocholeliths in small bile ducts; small stones with mineral produce an acoustic shadow. (*Courtesy of* the Section of Diagnostic Imaging, College of Veterinary Medicine, Cornell University, Ithaca, NY.)

adhered to the GB mucosa (hypoechoic rim sign). In some cases, a mixed echogenic, mosaic-like appearance characterizes the GB image. In either case, luminal contents are not gravitationally dependent and the GB is distended. The hepatic parenchyma is often hyperechoic because of coexistent vacuolar hepatopathy.[18–21] Progressive GB distention may lead to necrotizing cholecystitis. US may disclose a GB wall within normal limits that appears hyperechoic or thickened, or a wall that is discontinuous, suggesting rupture. In the circumstance of rupture, pericholecystic fat will appear bright and the GB may be surrounded by a mantle of fluid that imparts a hypoechoic "halo." Abdominal fluid also may be identified and suggests GB rupture. A ruptured GB can be difficult to identify; in addition, the associated abdominal pain is inconsistent and the omentum appears hyperechoic and may shroud the region of interest. The diagnostic utility of US for detecting GB rupture in dogs with biliary mucoceles is good but imperfect (sensitivity, 86%; specificity, 100%).[21]

Cholecystitis
Symmetric or asymmetric thickening of the GB wall is often associated with cholecystitis (**Figs. 10** and **18B**). Necrotizing cholecystitis involves devitalization of the GB wall and often appears as an asymmetric focal lamination or discontinuation of the GB wall, and often is associated with an adjacent small volume of fluid and hyperechoic fat (omental adhesions, chemical peritonitis). Untreated necrotizing cholecystitis culminates in GB rupture and bile peritonitis (see **Fig. 10**).

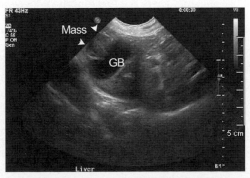

Fig. 20. Ultrasonographic image of the GB of a dog with an attached neoplasm (*arrowheads*) pushing on the wall; the mass was an adenocarcinoma. (*Courtesy of* the Section of Diagnostic Imaging, College of Veterinary Medicine, Cornell University, Ithaca, NY.)

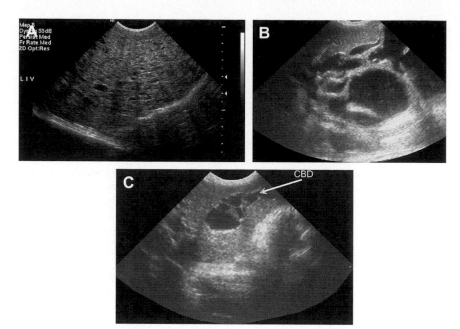

Fig. 21. (*A*) Ultrasonographic image of the liver from a cat with fibrocystic liver disease; this 5-year-old female spayed (FS) domestic longhaired cat had too numerous to count small cysts throughout the liver. (*B*) Ultrasonographic image of the liver from a cat with fibrocystic liver disease; this 10-year-old FS Persian-cross had many small and large biliary cysts. (*C*) Ultrasonographic image of a biliary cystadenoma in the porta hepatis of a geriatric cat, adjacent to the CBD. Note the complex nature of the cystic structure. (*Courtesy of* the Section of Diagnostic Imaging, College of Veterinary Medicine, Cornell University, Ithaca, NY.)

Hepatobiliary Scintigraphy

Alternative methods for imaging the biliary tree are available at some referral practices, involving short-lived radioisotopes (eg, technicium 99mTC) as labels on a new class of organic anions, the iminodiacetic analogs. In human beings, these agents are used to achieve early diagnosis of CBD occlusion, acute and chronic cholecystitis, segmental biliary tree obstruction, and problems associated with GB or sphincter of Oddi function. Studies also have shown that these imaging agents may assist in the identification of small-volume bile leakage. There are few reports of these analogs in veterinary

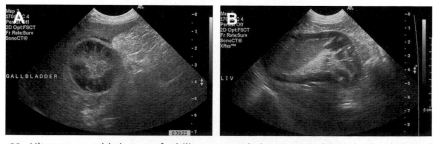

Fig. 22. Ultrasonographic image of a biliary mucocele in a 9-year-old FS Shetland Sheepdog (*A*) and an 8-year-old FS Cocker Spaniel (*B*); note the kiwi or stellate pattern of biliary-mucin conglomerate within each gallbladder. (*Courtesy of* the Section of Diagnostic Imaging, College of Veterinary Medicine, Cornell University, Ithaca, NY.)

patients relevant to clinical practice. Two studies document their utility in dogs with spontaneous cholestatic disease.[22,23]

At the present time, hepatobiliary scintigraphy is not a practical means of patient assessment.

Cholecystocentesis

Cholecystocentesis, the aspirate sampling of GB bile, can be completed using a percutaneous US-guided method, by laparoscopic-assistance, or during exploratory abdominal surgery.[24–27] Samples of bile are collected for cytologic investigation and bacterial culture. A transhepatic approach or a direct fundic approach can be used; the author prefers a transhepatic approach using an US guide and the patient under deep sedation or anesthesia. Adherence of the GB to liver in its fossa limits leakage from the puncture site with a transhepatic approach. If a direct fundic approach is used, it is useful to empty the GB of bile to avoid spillage into the abdominal cavity. Re-evaluation of cats undergoing laparoscopic cholecystocentesis 4 months after initial bile aspiration demonstrated local omental adhesions to areas of asymptomatic bile leakage (Sharon A. Center, DVM, unpublished data, 2004). With either approach, a 22-gauge spinal needle is usually sufficient. However, animals with suspected thick or inspissated bile may require a larger bore needle (eg, 18-gauge, used only via transhepatic aspiration). Lavage of the GB with saline is not routinely advised.[24] Complications of cholecystocentesis include intraperitoneal bile leakage, hemorrhage, hemobilia, bacteremia, and vasovagal reaction that may result in ventilatory arrest, severe bradycardia, and death.[28] Lethal vasovagal responses should be anticipated any time this procedure is completed and the clinician should be prepared to provide anticholinergics and ventilatory assistance. Blunt pressure on the GB should be avoided during this procedure, as this provokes high vagal tone.

SPECIFIC DISORDERS
Disorders of the Gallbladder

Gallbladder agenesis
Congenital absence of the GB is occasionally encountered. In the absence of congenital malformations of the intrahepatic biliary structures this is an inconsequential abnormality.

Biliary atresia
Congenital maldevelopment of intrahepatic biliary structures is uncommon but has been observed in dogs. This developmental anomaly is associated with jaundice and progressive liver injury in young animals.

Bilobed gallbladder
Bilobed GB is occasionally identified in cats but is uncommon. While this may cause confusion during US imaging, it is an inconsequential abnormality (**Figs. 7** and **23**).

Cystic mucosal hyperplasia of the gallbladder
This syndrome is cited in the veterinary literature as cystic mucinous hypertrophy, cystic mucinous hyperplasia, and mucinous cholecystitis. It has long been recognized as an incidental finding in elderly dogs and was described in dogs treated with progestational compounds more than 40 years ago. That study also first described GB mucocele formation.[29] The role of steroid hormones in lesion induction remains unclear. Affected GB mucosa is usually riddled with cystic sessile or polypoid hyperplastic lesions that trap mucin within cystic structures and between polypoid villi (**Fig. 24**). Usually there is no inflammation and the serosal surface remains intact. This lesion

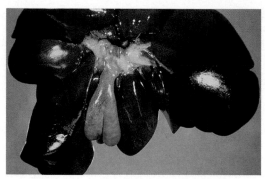

Fig. 23. Gross appearance of aseptate or bilobed GB in a cat corresponding to the US image shown in **Fig. 7**.

is routinely found in dogs with GB mucoceles, where it may play a causal role in the trapping of mucin or disturbing mechanical evacuation of bile. In some cases, mucosal "fronds" have been visible on US examination. An affected GB has a thickened proliferative surface and the lumen is typically filled with thick green, viscous mucoid debris.

Gallbladder dysmotility

GB dysmotility may be an emerging syndrome in the dog. Reduced GB contractility has been identified in a small number of dogs in the author's hospital before development of a mature GB mucocele.[19] A syndrome of GB dysmotility is recognized in human beings who are at risk for asymptomatic cholelithiasis. The asymptomatic nature of this cholelith syndrome relates to the underlying cause of pain: duct obstruction and biliary tree pressure. A dysmotile GB has limited influence on the driving force of bile flow within the cystic and common bile duct. Asynchronous function of the sphincter of Oddi also has been described in these patients. It is possible that GB dysmotility is linked with exposure to steroid hormones in dogs, considering initial studies with progestational compounds and recent in vitro work confirming that both progesterone and testosterone impair GB smooth muscle contractility.[30,31] A circumstantial link between adrenal steroid production or glucocorticoid administration, antecedent to mature GB mucocele formation, has been reported.[19] Diagnosis of GB dysmotility requires investigation of real time GB contractility, as previously described (see **Figs. 12** and **13**).[15]

Cholecystitis

Non-necrotizing cholecystitis

Inflammation of the GB may involve nonsuppurative or suppurative processes, may associate with infectious agents, systemic disease, or neoplasia, and may reflect blunt abdominal trauma or GB obstruction by occlusion of the cystic duct (eg, cholelithiasis, neoplasia, or choledochitis). Cystic duct occlusion incites GB inflammation secondary to bile stasis; this process can be augmented by a mechanical irritant, such as a cholelith. After cystic duct occlusion, the GB wall thickens and its volume decreases. Thereafter, a hydrops develops as the GB distends with a white-viscid mucin-laden bile. If GB distention imposes wall ischemia, necrotizing cholecystitis follows. If infection occurs during the process, acute septic cholecystitis emerges.

Necrotizing cholecystitis is a severe syndrome requiring prompt surgical intervention (cholecystectomy and potential biliary diversion, see below). Clinical signs include abdominal pain, fever, and increased liver enzymes. However, signs may remain vague and episodic and hyperbilirubinemia is inconsistent. US detection of a thickened GB wall or CBD, and sometimes a tenderness noted during the imaging procedure or

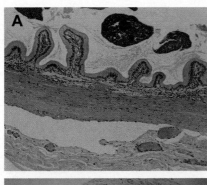

Mucosa

Lamina propria

Muscularis

(nerves, lymphatics
microvasculature)

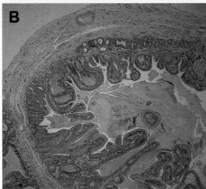

Fig. 24. Photomicrograph of normal gallbladder (*A*) and of a gallbladder from dog with a biliary mucocele and cystic mucosal hyperplasia (*B*). In (*B*), note the cystic epithelium and entrapped mucin. Elongated villi "fronds" and cyst formation impair gallbladder "cleansing" on contraction. Cystic hyperplasia also may be associated with gallbladder dysmotility (hematoxylin and eosin, original magnification ×40).

on deep abdominal palpation (positive Murphy sign), may be the only evidence of illness. Imaging may disclose focal free-peritoneal fluid adjacent to the GB, reflecting transmural bile leakage, focal inflammation, or wall rupture. Confusion with other causes of GB wall thickening (see secton on "Imaging") necessitates that a diagnosis of cholecystitis be carefully considered.

A common cause of GB rupture in the dog, necrotizing cholecystitis is associated with interrupted perfusion from the cystic artery by thromboembolism, a shearing tear delivered from blunt abdominal trauma, bacterial infection, cystic duct obstruction (choleliths, neoplasia), or a mature GB mucocele imposing wall ischemia.[1,32] Extension of an inflammatory or neoplastic process from adjacent hepatic tissue also may be an underlying cause. Necrotizing cholecystitis can present with or without GB rupture, or as a chronic syndrome associated with adhesions between the GB, omentum, and adjacent viscera. One study in dogs (*n* = 23)[33] reported a mean age of 9.5 years and that clinical signs preceded case presentation for only 3 days. Histologic GB lesions resembled those associated with EHBDO, suggesting that chronic GB obstruction was an underlying causal factor. Gallbladder rupture was confirmed surgically in 78% of dogs and 81% of these had bacteria cultured from their GB wall. Another study of dogs indentified GB wall infarction in the absence of inflammation as the acute causal factor of necrotizing cholecystitis.[34] A diagnosis of necrotizing cholecystitis is based on reconciliation of clinical signs (severe cholecystitis), clinicopathologic features, and US imaging. The GB wall may appear trilaminate, discontinuous, or markedly thickened (see **Fig. 10**). Finding focal-fluid accumulation should prompt a presumptive diagnosis of necrotizing cholecystitis and GB rupture, and triage for exploratory laparotomy and cholecystectomy. Because necrotizing cholecystitis is often associated with a mature GB mucocele (see the section on GB mucocele in dogs, below), early intervention by prophylactic cholecystectomy has seemingly reduced the incidence in the author's hospital.

Emphysematous cholecystitis/choledochitis
Emphysematous cholecystitis is an uncommon condition (gas within the wall or lumen of the GB or segments of the biliary tree) in the dog that has been associated with diabetes mellitus, acute cholecystitis with or without cholecystolithiasis, traumatic ischemia, mature GB mucocele formation, and neoplasia. Gas within biliary structures implicates serious septic inflammation likely associated with *Escherichia coli* or *Clostridial* sp. Treatment requires cholecystectomy and antimicrobial therapy based on culture and sensitivity of bile and involved biliary tissues.

Clinical signs of cholecystitis
Clinical signs of acute cholecystitis include abdominal pain, fever, vomiting, ileus, and mild to moderate jaundice. A mass effect may be detected in the right cranial abdominal quadrant and some animals present in endotoxic shock. The hemogram discloses variable leukocytosis, with or without toxic neutrophils, with or without a left shift. Hyperbilirubinemia may be mild or associated with jaundice; development of jaundice depends on chronicity, involvement of extrahepatic biliary structures, presence or extent of biliary tree occlusion, or bile peritonitis. Liver enzyme activity is variable but cholestatic enzymes (ALP, GGT) are moderately to markedly increased. Gallbladder rupture leads to pericholecystic abscess formation (localized by the omentum) or generalized bile peritonitis. Abdominal radiography may disclose indistinct detail in the cranial abdomen consistent with focal peritonitis; a sentinel loop may implicate a focal ileus. Rarely, the GB wall may become radiodense because of dystrophic mineralization. In some animals, choleliths are found on US imaging (**Fig. 18**B). Detection of gas within the biliary tree or GB heralds an emphysematous process associated with sepsis and should prompt antibiotic administration and emergency cholecystectomy. Pericholecystic fluid should be sampled using US guidance to confirm bile leakage and infection. Comparison of total bilirubin concentration in any effusion to serum will help confirm bile leakage.

Treatment of cholecystitis
Medical and surgical management focuses on restoration of fluid and electrolyte status, provision of broad-spectrum antibiotics effective against enteric opportunists, and prompt surgical intervention. In some cases, colloids and plasma transfusion are necessary to restore and preserve normal blood pressure and oncotic pressure. For jaundice, notable for several weeks, EHBDO must be a considered differential and vitamin K_1 administered (intramuscularly or subcutaneously, 0.5 mg/kg–1.5 mg/kg, three doses at 12-hour intervals) before surgery to avoid hemorrhagic complications. If emergency surgery is necessary, fresh frozen plasma should be given judiciously. Considering potential causal factors, careful exploration of all biliary structures is warranted. Patency of the cystic and CBD must be determined and viability of the GB ascertained. A cholecystectomy is the treatment of choice for most patients. However, some animals benefit from a cholecystoenterostomy or choledochoenterostomy to circumvent a permanently occluded distal CBD. Placement of a temporary biliary stent (see section on EHBDO) may be appropriate in some of these patients. Cultures of bile, GB wall, choleliths, and liver tissue should be submitted for aerobic and anerobic

bacteria. Cytologic evaluations of tissue imprints and bile assist in initial antimicrobial selection. Combination of metronidazole, ampicillin clavulinate, and enrofloxacin provides broad protection against commonly encountered enteric opportunists. If only the GB is involved, simple cholecystectomy may be curative. If the CBD, cystic, or hepatic ducts are involved, a more guarded prognosis is warranted and long-term antibiotic therapy necessary.

Consequences of cholecystectomy
There are few side effects of cholecystectomy, although episodic abdominal pain and diarrhea associated with fat malabsorption have been described in human beings.[35,36] Cholecystectomy results in loss of the absorptive and pressure-regulating function of the GB and the fasting reservoir where bile is concentrated.[37,38] After cholecystectomy, the volume of bile increases because of reduced Na^+ resorption in the GB, the size of the bile-acid pool diminishes, and the enterohepatic circulation of bile becomes a continuous process.[37–40] Six to 8 weeks after cholecystectomy in cats, the size of the bile-acid pool diminished by 80%.[35] A shift in the composition of the bile-acid pool also occurs commensurate with an increase in the dihydroxy forms. This reflects increased exposure of bile acids to enteric flora causing increased bacterial dehydroxylation of primary bile acids (trihydroxy forms to the dihydroxy forms: eg, cholic acid $\rightarrow$ dehydrocholate).[35,41,42] In the dog, early work reported that the CBD may enlarge after cholecystectomy, but this remains controversial.

Consequences of biliary enteric-anastomosis
Animals undergoing biliary tree decompression by biliary enteric-anastomoses are susceptible to retrograde septic cholangitis and choledochitis (**Fig. 25**). Dogs seem to tolerate this procedure with fewer clinical signs than cats. Owners should monitor these patients for fever, inappetence, and vomiting, and seek veterinary assistance if cyclic illness is suspected. A complete blood count and serum biochemistry profile (liver enzymes) should be monitored quarterly. Chronic or pulsitile (intermittent) antimicrobial administration may be needed to control ascending infection of biliary structures. Usually, illness is antibiotic-responsive and transient.

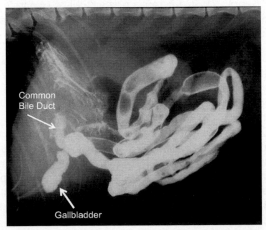

Fig. 25. Radiograph from a dog with a cholecystoduodenostomy after administration of gastrointestinal contrast as a diagnostic test investigating the cause of chronic vomiting. Note contrast refluxing through the biliary-enteric anastomosis, detailing a collapsed GB and a dilated CBD. Residual contrast remains within gastric rugal folds. (*Courtesy of* the Section of Diagnostic Imaging, College of Veterinary Medicine, Cornell University, Ithaca, NY.)

Gallbladder mucocele
With the routine integration of abdominal ultrasonography in clinical practice, an increase in the diagnosis of canine GB mucoceles has emerged.[19–21] This disorder is characterized by progressive accumulation of tenacious mucin-laden GB bile, which may extend into the cystic, hepatic, and common bile ducts, resulting in variable degrees of EHBDO. Progressive expansion of a biliary mucocele leads to GB ischemic necrosis, bile peritonitis, and sometimes opportunistic infection. Serious attention to consideration of a GB mucocele is warranted when sequential US examinations fail to indicate a reduction in GB size or content after feeding, and confirms lack of gravitational movement of sludge. Gallbladder stasis, perhaps reflecting dysmotility, and distention predispose to cholecystitis.[43,44]

Diagnostic features Three recent retrospective studies described the clinical scenario and surgical outcome in dogs with biliary mucocele, reviewing 70 cases.[19–21] A median age of 10 years (dogs as young as 3 years) without apparent gender predisposition, and an increased incidence in Shetland Sheepdogs were confirmed. There also seemingly is an increased incidence in Cocker Spaniels and Miniature Schnauzers. Clinical illness averages 5 days, although some dogs have vague episodic signs for months (ie, inappetance, vomiting, vague abdominal pain). In decreasing order and frequency, clinical signs have included: vomiting (87%), abdominal pain (87%), anorexia (78%), jaundice (57%), tachypnea (65%), tachycardia (44%), polyuria and polydipsia (30%), fever (26%), diarrhea (26%), and abdominal distension (13%). Dogs progressing to GB rupture demonstrate abdominal pain (93%), jaundice (64%), tachycardia and tachypnea (36%), and fever (29%). Clinicopathologic indicators include leukocytosis (50%, mature neutrophilia: 40%, monocytosis: 27%), high liver enzymes including ALP (100%), GGT (86%), alanine aminotransferase (ALT) (77%), and aspartate aminotransferase (AST) (60%), and hyperbilirubinemia (63%). Dogs with GB rupture that died generally had higher liver enzyme activity, bilirubin concentrations, and total white blood cell counts than survivors. Aerobic bacteria have been cultured from bile or GB wall, with a number of enteric organisms identified (ie, *E. coli, Enterobacter* spp, *Enterococcus* spp, *Staphylococcus* spp, *Micrococcus* spp, *Streptococcus* spp).[19–21] In different studies 6 out of 14 and 2 out of 23 bacterial cultures were positive; discordance between studies likely reflects antibiotic administration before collection of diagnostic samples.

Gallbladder and liver histologic lesions Histologically, cystic mucosal hyperplasia is common in the GB wall. All dogs have had abnormally thick biliary debris: some is viscous and mucin laden, some is more liquid, some is dark green-black, some with a white bile component, some with gritty black material, and some with a firm gelatinous matrix. Cysts in the GB mucosa are common (single layer of epithelial cells surrounding mucus-filled lumen) and mucus-secreting glands are widely distended with mucus resembling GB debris (see **Fig. 24**). Transmural ischemic necrosis may develop, leading to necrotizing cholecystitis and GB rupture. The most common site of rupture is the fundus.[21] Liver biopsies may disclose a vacuolar hepatopathy (consistent with a steroidogenic hormone link) or mild to moderate portal hepatitis/fibrosis associated with bile ductule proliferation.[45] The latter lesion reflects biliary tree obstruction. Some dogs lack concurrent hepatic lesions.

Predisposing factors Factors predisposing to GB mucocele formation include middle to geriatric age, hyperlipidemia/hypercholesterolemia (idiopathic, associated with pancreatitis or nephrotic syndrome or endocrinopathies, including typical and atypical hyperadrenocorticism and hypothyroidism), GB dysmotility, and cystic hyperplasia of the GB mucosa that entraps mucinous debris and compromises mechanical GB cleansing. The inciting cause of mucus hypersecretion is unknown and may be multifactorial. Decreased GB motility (geriatric or possibly steroidal influence) leads to luminal bile stasis and enhanced absorption, promoting formation of biliary sludge. An apparent risk factor is hyperlipidemia/hypercholesterolemia (breed predisposition: hyperlipidemic Shetland Sheepdogs and Miniature Schnauzers). We also have witnessed dogs (with sequential US monitoring) with antecedent risk factors to rapidly developing a mature GB mucocele after initiating glucocorticoid therapy. Because a vacuolar hepatopathy is a common coexistent problem, investigation for underlying disorders associated with this syndrome is advised.[45] Vacuolar hepatopathy develops in dogs with and without exposure to steroidogenic hormones (approximately 1:1). It is intriguing to consider a potential link between steroidogenic hormones, GB cystic mucinous hyperplasia, and GB dysmotility, as previously discussed.[30,31,46] Clearly, risk factors described, including adrenal hyperplasia, need to be explored in affected dogs.

Ultrasonographic imaging (See "Imaging" section above.) In the event of loculated pericholecystic fluid, aspiration should be done as close to the GB as safely possible. Samples collected near the GB are more likely to disclose bacteria or bilirubin crystals important for diagnosis of septic or bile peritonitis. Measurement of total bilirubin in collected fluid and comparison to the serum bilirubin concentration helps clarify the likelihood of bile peritonitis (eg, fluid bilirubin $\geq$ 10-fold the serum concentration). GB rupture should be suspected if the wall is discontinuous, trilaminated, or the GB is surrounded by hyperechoic pericholecystic fat or a hypoechoic fluid ring; these patterns warrant recommendation for emergency surgery. However, the author has observed bile staining of adjacent visceral surfaces and omental adhesions at surgery in some dogs lacking an apparent bile leakage; transmural passage of bile pigments across the GB wall is suspected. US-guided cholecystocentesis should not be performed if a GB mucocele is probable. Ultrasonography also may detect hepatomegaly and either a heterogenous or hyperechoic hepatic parenchymal pattern. In some dogs, hypoechoic "nodules" correspond to a severe vacuolar hepatopathy. After GB removal, sequential hepatic US evaluations are necessary to see if parenchymal lesions resolve. Persistent abnormalities likely reflect underlying medical disorders that need investigation. Rarely, a ruptured GB will release a well-organized mucocele into the peritoneal cavity, where it may cause pain and effusion; these are sometimes discovered during US examination.

Medical treatment Dogs lacking clinical signs of mucocele leakage or biliary tree obstruction at the time of initial diagnosis may benefit from administration of UDCA, SAMe (Denosyl, Nutramax Laboratory, Edgewood, Maryland) as a GSH donor providing both a choleretic and antioxidant benefit, and antimicrobials, providing that sequential biochemical and US evaluations are used to monitor syndrome progression (every 6 weeks). At the author's institution, we have observed two dogs resolve an apparent GB mucocele with medical treatment only. The UDCA is dosed at 15 mg/kg to 25 mg/kg by mouth per day (tablet form providing improved bioavailability), given twice daily with food (to increase bioavailability). The Denosyl (Nutramax Laboratory, Edgewood, Maryland) must be given on an empty stomach to optimize bioavailability (overnight fast, abstain from feeding 2 hours after dosing), at a dose of 20 mg/kg to 40 mg/kg by mouth per day (20-mg/kg dose provided antioxidant and metabolic benefits, choleretic influence in cats was achieved with 40 mg/kg).[7,47] In addition to the beneficial effects of UDCA on the bile-acid profile, it protects hepatocytes and biliary epithelium against injurious effects of cholestasis (along with other benefits), with recent work suggesting that it reduces lipid peroxidation and mucin secretagogue activity of GB bile (in human beings with cholelithiasis) and that it may improve GB motility.[48-52] The ideal course of therapy must be tailored to each patient. Improved clinical, clinicopathologic, and US features indicate control of causal factors. However, progression in any parameter indicates poor control and recommends surgical intervention.

Surgical treatment Cholecystectomy is the best course of treatment for GB mucocele and is essential for dogs with clinical signs and clinicopathologic findings consistent with biliary tree inflammation. At surgery, it is important that the CBD is cleansed of obstructing debris and that the distal duct is canulated and flushed to ascertain patency through the duodenal papilla. Opening the bowel to identify the duct stoma has been necessary in some cases. Because bile stasis predisposes to infection, broad-spectrum antimicrobials are initially recommended (aerobic and anaerobic bacteria), while cultures of bile, GB wall, and liver are pending. Antibiotics should be started before or during the cholecystectomy. Evidence of bacteria in cytologic samples or the presence of suppurative cholecystitis affirm a need for chronic antimicrobial administration.

The resected GB should be submitted for histologic characterization, and a liver biopsy should be collected distant to the site of surgery to survey for concurrent liver disease. A portion of the liver biopsy should be submitted for tissue copper, iron, and zinc concentrations, as these may help guide future treatment recommendations. While cholecystectomy is an effective treatment for GB mucocele, perioperative mortality is high for symptomatic dogs with a ruptured GB complicated by sepsis. If bile peritonitis is present, the peritoneal cavity must be extensively cleansed with sterile warm polyionic fluids to remove debris, bacteria, and injurious bile salts. Abdominal drains may be necessary in the case of septic peritonitis. Antibiotics should be administered for 4 to 6 weeks; presurgical antibiotic therapy can compromise reliable culture of complicating infection.

Cholecystotomy for removal of GB contents without cholecystectomy is not advised because mucoceles have recurred in several dogs so treated (Center SA, unpublished observation). Furthermore, microscopic mural necrosis may exist at the time of surgery that is not grossly evident, leading to postoperative GB rupture. For dogs with a firm US diagnosis of GB mucocele, elective cholecystectomy as a prophylactic procedure is now recommended in the author's hospital. This averts mucocele maturation and subsequent GB ischemic necrosis. Dynamic US studies are used to confirm GB dysmotility/amotility, as this will confirm a need for GB resection as an early surgical intervention. After GB resection, chronic choleretic therapy is recommended, as described above. Underlying causes of hyperlipidemia or endocrine disorders (as described above) should be identified and managed appropriately. Clinicopathologic abnormalities normalize after GB removal in most dogs, except those with associated suppurative cholangiohepatitis or unresolved endocrinopathies. There is no evidence that affected dogs need dietary protein restriction; rather, it may be detrimental to feed a protein-restricted high-fat diet to some of these patients (see hyperlipidemia under "Predisposing factors," above).

DISORDERS OF BILE DUCTS
Benign Biliary Cysts

Benign biliary cysts are occasionally encountered in dogs and cats. These are limited to a single liver lobe and usually cause no substantial compressive injury. Enlarging cysts may be removed in their entirety or managed with periodic cystocentesis.

Hepatic Fibropolycystic Disorders

Fibropolycystic liver diseases have been identified in most of the companion animals and often involve the biliary structures and renal tubules.[53-56] This unique group of entities reflect deranged embryonic ductal plate development, at various stages forming cystic lesions involving intrahepatic or extrahepatic bile ducts.[54] Embryologic development of the ductal plate is schematically presented in **Fig. 26**.[54,55] Embryologically, the ductal plate is comprised of a cylindric tube of cells surrounding a portal vein branch. Biliary ducts form by remodeling and partial involution of these cylindric plates. Ductal malformations arise as ductal plate components are unevenly resorbed. The different types of malformations reflect the time and stage of development at which the embryogenesis and remodeling are disturbed (large ducts versus small ducts, intrahepatic versus extrahepatic). In human beings, a simplified classification scheme divides entities into six groups: (1) congenital hepatic fibrosis, (2) Caroli's syndrome, (3) von Meyenberg complexes, (4) simple hepatic cysts, (5) polycystic liver disease, and (6) choledochal cysts. Group 1 causes portal hypertension secondary to extensive hepatic fibrosis and, subsequently, acquired portosystemic shunting and hepatic encephalopathy. Group 2 reflects ductal plate malformations affecting the largest intrahepatic bile ducts and causes macroscopic cystic lesions that may be complicated by cholangitis, cholelithiasis, and carcinoma within cystic malformations; these may become mineralized. Group 3 involves microscopic intrahepatic malformations that cause few clinical effects. Groups 4 to 6 involve isolated cystic malformations that usually do not communicate with the biliary tree, unless they are associated with Group 1 malformations. In Group 5, hepatobiliary and renal anomalies frequently coexist in various combinations, suggesting the expression of a common underlying genetic abnormality (abnormal polycystin is implicated in several).[56] Despite the classification scheme described above, the fibropolycystic liver disorders usually do not exist as single entities, but rather as members of a family. The diversity of manifestations can predispose to cholangitis, cause portal hypertension, or can evolve into space-occupying lesions (cystic

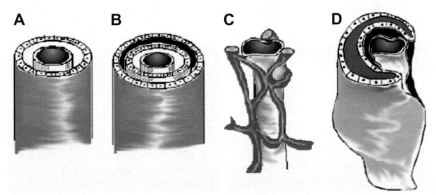

Fig. 26. Diagrammatic interpretation of the embryogenesis of bile ducts explaining ductal plate abnormalities common to fibrocystic malformations. Embryologically the ductal plate is comprised of a cylindric tube of cells surrounding a portal vein branch (*A*). After the plate doubles (*B*), biliary ducts emerge by remodeling and partial involution of segments of the cylindric plates (*C*). Ductal malformations (*D*) arise as ductal plate components are unevenly resorbed. The different types of malformations reflect the time and stage of development at which the embryogenesis and remodeling are disturbed (large ducts versus small ducts, intrahepatic versus extrahepatic). (*Adapted from* Marchal GJ, Desmet VJ, Proesmans WC, et al. Caroli disease: high-frequency US and pathologic findings. Radiology 1986;158:507–11; with permission.)

structures). There are several genetic causes of polycystic disease involving bile ducts in man; thus far, only a single mutation has been identified in cats (autosomal onset dominant polycystic kidney disease).[57–59] Genetic testing (restriction fragment length polymorphisms or single-nucleotide polymorphisms) can now be used to select breeding founders to reduce syndrome prevalence.[58,60] The "juvenile" and "adult" manifestations vary widely and include hepatic fibrosis, portal hypertension, cholangitis, and polycystic hepatic lesions.

Feline polycystic renal disease is well documented and commonly encountered by feline practitioners. While the phenotypic spectrum is diverse, most cats demonstrate renal rather than biliary malformations. Renal tubular malformations can lead to renal failure in early life or may not progress. The hepatic cystic syndrome may involve few isolated cysts in the liver with or without involvement of the pancreas and/or kidneys but the most severe phenotype involves too numerous to count microscopic cystic structures less than 1 mm in diameter, too small to be clearly detected by US examination (**Fig. 21**A). In some cats, many large hepatic cysts cause profound hepatomegaly and require repeated drainage or marsupialization, or complete or partial surgical resection (**Fig. 27**A). These are generally easy to diagnose with US (**Fig. 21**B). Histologic lesions are characterized by dysplastic maldeveloped bile ductules with irregular lumen and flattened epithelium. A fibrolamellar extracellular matrix surrounds and interdigitates between dysplastic structures (**Fig. 27**). There is a paucity of normal hepatic parenchyma in severely affected cats. Extensive connective tissue causes intrahepatic portal hypertension, a firm large liver, and development of acquired shunts and signs of hepatic encephalopathy. Some cats with the extensive polycystic liver phenotype have presented for related clinical signs only after development of hyperthyroidism.

There are several case reports describing biliary dysplastic syndromes in young dogs associated with renal cystic malformations. Lesions in puppies have been reported in Cairn Terriers, West Highland White Terriers, and Golden Retrievers, and two reports of case series from the same hospital describe lesion in dogs of varying ages.[61–65] Case series involved various breeds with ages ranging from 6 months to

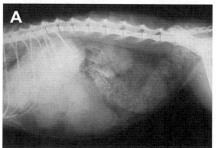 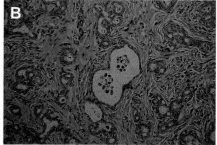

Fig. 27. (*A*) Radiograph of a 9-year-old castrated male Himalayan cat with severe polycystic liver disease. Massive hepatomegaly is associated with too numerous to count biliary cystic malformations. This cat developed portal hypertension and acquired portosystemic shunts. (*B*) Photomicrograph of a liver biopsy from a cat with polycystic liver disease. Note numerous malformed small duct-like structures lined with cuboidal epithelial cells. The large dysplastic duct-like structure in the center has flattened epithelium and contains exfoliated cells. A dense fibrolameller connective tissue matix encircles and surrounds cystic structures and caused portal hypertension and acquired portosystemic shunts (hematoxylin and eosin, original magnification ×400). (Part *A Courtesy* of the Section of Diagnostic Imaging, College of Veterinary Medicine, Cornell University, Ithaca, NY.)

3 years. US imaging in one case series disclosed gross cystic dilatations involving calcified intrahepatic bile ducts, consistent with the subclassification of Caroli's syndrome. Calcifications in malformed ducts likely reflected stagnant bile flow or retrograde infection. In all dogs, unlike cats, high ALP and increased fasting bile acids were consistent. Similar to cats with polycystic hepatobiliary disease, the CBD and GB were normal, liver texture firm, and liver size either normal or slightly increased. Cross section of liver lobes disclosed multiple variably sized cysts. Fibrous connective tissue was increased in zone 1 and often bridged between portal regions, as in cats. Four of six dogs had ascites attributable to portal hypertension associated with intrahepatic fibrosis; while acquired shunts were not grossly identified, they most probably existed. The only treatment for these disorders is to palliate hepatic encephalopathy with protein restricted diets, lactulose, and low-dose metronidazole, to judiciously use diuretics to mobilize ascites and restrict sodium intake. Human beings with similar syndromes are treated with organ transplantation.

Choledochal Cyst

Choledochal cyst is a congenital cystic dilation of the bile duct that has been recognized in cats associated with the distal segment of the CBD. Clinical signs include fever, abdominal pain, and jaundice associated with cyst infection. Because ultrasonographic detection of cystic lesions associated closely with the duodenum and CBD can be difficult, surgical exploration has been required for definitive diagnosis. Extirpation of the cystic structure or marsupialization into the CBD has been successful in the small number of cases seen (Center SA, unpublished data).

Biliary Cystadenoma

Biliary cystadenomas are relatively uncommon, benign tumors found in elderly cats. Well-demarcated and unencapsulated, cystadenomas may occur as focal discrete or multifocal-complex lesions. Because they can invade adjacent hepatic parenchyma, causing compressive atrophy, the most perilous location is within the porta hepatis where they can impose space-occupying effects on essential vasculature and bile ducts. These lesions have been variably termed cystadenomas, bile-duct adenomas, cholangiocellular adenomas, cystic cholangiomas, or hepatobiliary cytadenomas. Cyst contents range from clear, watery fluid to viscous material, and some tumor sections may be solid. Cyst sizes are variable, ranging from 1 mm to 8 cm, with tumor mass ranging from 5 mm to 12.5 cm.[66] Cysts are lined by a simple columnar to cuboidal but attenuated epithelium. On US evaluation, cystic contents are usually anechoic (**Fig. 21**C). Cystadenomas may be serendipitously discovered (no clinical signs, no biochemical abnormalities) during US examinations for other health issues, may be discovered because of investigation of biochemical changes indicative of liver injury or cholestasis, or discovered because of identification of a cranial abdominal mass. Surgical excision is the treatment of choice, as this eliminates mechanical compression of vital structures as the tumor expands. A good prognosis is warranted following complete excision. If complete excision is not possible, partial resection may delay complications from mechanical invasion of normal tissue. Repeated aspiration, catheter drainage, marsupialization, and partial excision have been used for palliative management. Mistaken diagnosis of polycystic liver lesions as biliary cystadenomas is seemingly common (see above).

Extrahepatic Bile Duct Obstruction

Obstruction of the CBD is associated with diverse primary conditions (**Box 1**) and leads to serious hepatobiliary injury within just a few weeks.[67–74] Following complete

---

Box 1
Primary conditions associated with EHBDO

Cholelithiasis

Choledochitis

Neoplasia

    Bile duct adenocarcinoma

    Pancreatic adenocarcinoma

    Lymphosarcoma

    Local tumor invasion

    Biliary cystadenoma

Malformations

    Choledochal cyst

    Polycystic liver disease

Parasitic

    Trematode infestation

Extrinsic compression

    Lymph nodes

    Pancreatic mass

    Entrapment in pancreatic inflammation

    Entrapment in diaphragmatic hernia

Fibrosis

    Blunt trauma

    Peritonitis

    Pancreatitis

Stricture

    Blunt trauma

    Iatrogenic surgical

EHBDO, hepatomegaly and distention of intrahepatic bile ducts promptly follow (**Fig. 28**). Obstructed flow of bile leads to cellular membrane and organelle damage as a result of stagnation of bile acids, lysolecithin, and possibly copper. Biliary epithelial injury evolves from eicosanoid and free radical-mediated damage that initiates a cascade of injurious inflammation. Oval cell hyperplasia (hepatic stem cells) and bile ductule proliferation are early histologic features. Distension and tortuosity of large inter- and intralobular bile ducts, devitalization of biliary epithelium, accumulation of necrotic debris and suppurative inflammation within bile-duct lumen, periportal accumulation of neutrophils, lymphocytes, and plasma cells, periductal edema, and multifocal parenchymal necrosis are classic histologic features after several weeks (**Figs. 29** and **30**). With chronicity, irresolvable distention of major bile ducts develops. Periportal fibrosis is obvious within 2 weeks and evolves into an "onion skin" fibrotic lamination surrounding bile ducts. If obstruction resolves within the first several

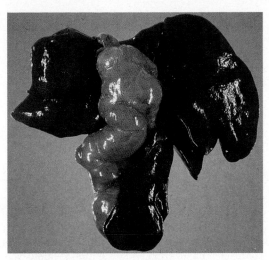

Fig. 28. Gross appearance of a dilated tortuous CBD in a cat with chronic complete extrahepatic CBD obstruction, corresponding to US image demonstrated in **Fig. 14**A.

weeks, periductal fibrosis and bile duct distention may completely resolve. However, persistent obstruction after greater than or equal to 6 weeks predictably evolves biliary cirrhosis, portal hypertension, and acquired portosystemic shunts.

Complete EHBDO may result in formation of white bile, depending on whether or not bilirubin pigments enter the distal "stagnant loop." Increased ductal mucin impressively contributes to continued duct distention. Bacterial colonization of the biliary tree may occur with enteric opportunists hematogenously disseminated from the hepato-biliary-enteric bacterial circulation. Antimicrobial treatment of biliary tree sepsis, without biliary decompression, is ineffective because of inadequate antibiotic penetration and inability to mechanically clear microbial organisms. Some animals are intermittently inappetent while others become polyphagic, reflecting fat maldigestion secondary to the lack of enteric bile acid delivery.

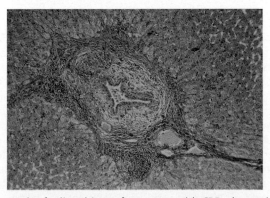

Fig. 29. Photomicrograph of a liver biopsy from a cat with CBD obstruction, demonstrating periductal edema and fibrosis, large duct dilation, ductal luminal inflammatory infiltrate (neutrophils), and periportal inflammatory infiltrates. Connective tissue encircles ducts and bridges between portal triads (Von Gieson's, original magnification ×100).

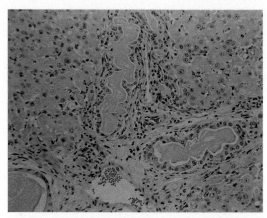

Fig. 30. Photomicrograph of a liver biopsy from a cat with CBD obstruction demonstrating severe bile stasis and tortuosity of large bile ducts. Bile ducts contain large amounts of mucin provoked by epithelial inflammation and distention (hematoxylin and eosin, original magnification ×400).

Clinical signs

Experimental EHBDO has been studied in the dog and cat but represents only a subset of clinical cases because of the acute, severe nature of the experimental model. Clinical scenarios more often have a gradual onset. Acute complete EHBDO leads to lethargy, intermittent fever, and prompt development of jaundice; bilirubin concentration increases within 4 hours. Vomiting may be episodic. Hepatomegaly, acholic feces, and the absence of urine urobilinogen may develop within the first week. Bleeding tendencies may be notable within 3 weeks and seem to be more common in cats. Gastroenteric ulceration at the pyloric-duodenal junction is common and can lead to considerable blood loss.[74] With even miniscule enteric bleeding, bilirubin pigments gain access to the bowel, allowing stools to become brown (sterocobilin formation) and urine to test positive for urobilinogen. Patients with EHBDO have a tendency to become hypotensive and have increased susceptibility to endotoxic shock during surgery and anesthesia.[75–78]

Clinicopathologic features

The major clinicopathologic features of EHBDO are summarized in **Fig. 31**. The hemogram may disclose a neutrophilic leukocytosis and a nonregenerative anemia may develop with chronicity. A strongly regenerative anemia may reflect severe enteric bleeding. As bile stagnates in the biliary tree, serum ALT and AST reflect altered hepatocyte membrane permeability and cell necrosis. Increased serum ALP and GGT activity increases within 8 to 12 hours of obstruction and are substantial within a few days. Parenchymal necrosis and periportal inflammation sustain serum transaminase and cholestatic enzyme activity. In cats, the magnitude of ALP and GGT are less dramatic than in dogs but are nevertheless useful indicators of biliary tree injury. Hypercholesterolemia develops within 2 weeks of complete obstruction, reflecting impaired cholesterol elimination and increased hepatic cholesterol biosynthesis. With chronic obstruction and development of biliary cirrhosis, serum cholesterol declines, reflecting impaired cholesterol synthesis and portosystemic shunting. Coagulopathies associated with vitamin K deficiency may develop within 21 days and are most sensitively detected with a PIVKA (proteins invoked by vitamin

Clinicopaaathologic Features of Extrahepatic Bile Duct Obstruction

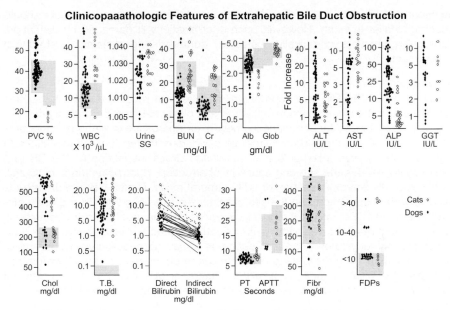

Fig. 31. Clinicopathologic features associated with extrahepatic bile duct obstruction in dogs (*n* = 51) and cats (*n* = 21). (*Courtesy of* College of Veterinary Medicine, Cornell University Medical Center, Ithaca, New York.)

K absence or antagonism) clotting test. Response to vitamin K_1 administration is usually dramatic (**Fig. 32**).

Definitive diagnosis

Confirmation of EHBDO is made with US imaging (see **Figs. 14** and **17**) and exploratory laparotomy. While US imaging may disclose the general location of obstruction, it often cannot determine the underlying cause. In human beings, early diagnosis of EHBDO can be facilitated by feeding a fatty meal before US examination and

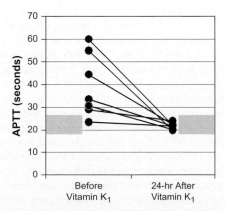

Fig. 32. Graphic depiction of PIVKA clotting time in cats with major bile duct obstruction before and 24 hours after Vitamin K_1 administration (0.5 mg/kg–1.5 mg/kg subcutaneously, three doses at 12-hour intervals). Gray rectangles represent reference range.

monitoring for dimensional changes in duct size.[79-81] An unobstructed duct should become smaller in width. However, once duct elasticity is damaged by distention, duct enlargement is chronically sustained, compromising dynamic postprandial assessments.

Treatment

Confirmation of EHBDO and appropriate management recommendations requires surgical exploration for inspection of the liver and biliary structures and biliary decompression. Liver biopsy by percutaneous needle or laparoscopic methods is inappropriate in EHBDO, as these do not facilitate biliary decompression and may lacerate distended bile ducts, leading to bile peritonitis. Gross inspection of the GB and CBD usually reveals the site and cause of obstruction; duct palpation is essential, as this may disclose the location of an intramural mass. Gentle GB compression is used to verify obstruction and the site of restricted bile flow. Finding a grossly distended tortuous CBD makes the diagnosis apparent. The most difficult obstructions to confirm and resolve involve the hepatic ducts. In some animals, performing a duodenotomy, cholecystotomy, or choledochotomy may be necessary for passage of a flexible catheter into the CBD to verify the site of obstruction and to allow removal of inspissated biliary sludge or choleliths. Treatment of biliary tract sepsis requires mechanical removal of biliary debris and infectious material to allow effective antimicrobial therapy.[1]

Pancreatitis is a common cause of EHBDO in dogs and cats because of periductal fibrosis and duct stricture.[82-85] Controversy exists regarding the need for biliary tree decompression in these patients. In most dogs with EHBDO secondary to pancreatitis, obstruction resolves spontaneously as the acute pancreatitis resolves. In the exceptional case in which EHBDO persists beyond 14 days, temporary or permanent decompression of the biliary tree may be considered.[82-87] Recent study of dogs undergoing extrahepatic biliary surgery reports a 50% mortality in dogs with pancreatitis.[85] Thus, the presence of concurrent pancreatic disease in dogs with EHBDO complicates the decision to pursue surgical options, as surgery may exacerbate the pancreatitis and pose additional risks.

Biliary Decompression

Temporary biliary decompression

Several methods of temporary decompression of the biliary tree in EHBDO have been explored; there is no large database to provide confident recommendations. In human beings this remains a controversial topic. Older retrospective studies that evaluated pre-operative GB decompression reported that it reduced morbidity and mortality when compared with direct surgical treatment.[88,89] It is not clear whether benefit of preoperative decompression reflected treatment or delay in surgery, which allowed for additional supportive care. More recent studies conclude that preoperative biliary drainage in human beings with EHBDO has not improved case outcome, lending to a longstanding controversy. In fact, reviews assessing the impact of preoperative endoscopic or radiologic drainage procedures disclose high complication rates.

Laparoscopic-assisted placement of pigtail catheters into the GB has been investigated experimentally for temporary biliary tree decompression in dogs.[90] There are no case series yet published demonstrating safety or efficacy of this approach. Theoretically, pigtail catheter retention would allow extracorporeal bile drainage for several days. Percutaneous US-guided cholecystocentesis was described in three dogs with acute pancreatitis where it was used to reduce the extent of hyperbilirubinemia and biliary tree distention.[27] One dog had repeated GB aspiration over several days and peritoneal bile leakage necessitated exploratory laparotomy.

Choledochal biliary stenting

Choledochal stenting has been extensively used in human beings to presurgically decompress EHBDO, to stabilize patients before definitive surgery, and for short- or long-term management of obstructive biliary disease because of malignant processes.[91–93] Two small case series of dogs and cats with EHBDO managed with choledochal stenting have been reported.[94,95] Stenting was done after surgical exploration, confirmation of the cause of EHBDO, and demonstration that the CBD could be catheterized through to the major duodenal papilla. An appropriate length of red rubber (Brunswick) feeding tube of appropriate diameter and long enough to span the site of stricture was positioned spanning the region of obstruction (or site of choledochotomy) through the duodenal papilla in dogs. The stent was secured with absorbable suture to the enteric lumen to permit for spontaneous elimination. Spontaneous stent discharge was unpredictable and endoscopic retrieval was needed in one dog. Complications included stent obstruction with bile concretions, duct stricture formation (promoted by stent mechanical trauma), and intralumenal interference with bile drainage that promoted cholangitis. Pancreatitis-associated biliary stricture causing EHBDO in cats ($n = 7$) was managed with choledochal stenting using a 3.5 or 5.0 French red rubber feeding tube or 22-gauge intravenous catheter. Stents were at least 4 cm to 8 cm in length and 2 cm to 4 cm of catheter was extended into the CBD above the compressive lesion, with 2 cm to 4 cm exiting the major duodenal papilla. Stents were anchored to the duodenal submucosa with monofilament absorbable suture; several stents passed in feces postoperatively at 4 to 5 months ($n = 2$), but one cat required endoscopic stent retrieval. Calcium bilirubinate crystallized on stents and two out of seven cats reobstructed within the first postoperative week. Results were less favorable in cats than dogs and there is concern that placement of a stent in the fused feline biliary/pancreatic duct may foster pancreatic inflammation and retrograde infection.[96,97] Experimental choledochal stenting in healthy cats demonstrated biliary tract colonization with duodenal bacteria within 2 weeks of placement.[96] Thus, stenting in cats is associated with considerable complications but the procedure does provide an alternative salvage remedy for distal CBD occlusion in difficult cases.

Clinical use of choledochal stenting requires careful assessment to determine whether this option is appropriate. If the CBD cannot be catheterized across the obstructive lesion, a surgical biliary diversion is more appropriate. When the CBD can be easily catheterized and functional EHBDO confirmed, choledochal stenting remains an option. The CBD and GB must be carefully palpated and debris removed as atraumatically as possible to minimize risk for postoperative stent occlusion. Cholecystectomy should be done if necrotizing cholecystitis is found. If cholecystolithiasis is discovered, diverse treatment options include cholecystectomy and stone removal (possible recurrent obstruction of normal structures or stent may occur), cholecystoenterostomy (out of concern for possible recurrent EHBDO), or cholecystectomy (if primary GB disease or dysmotility exists). However, cholecystectomy must be carefully considered because GB removal limits future cholecystoenterostomy as an option for permanent biliary diversion.

Surgical biliary tree decompression

A large case series of dogs ($n = 60$) requiring biliary tree surgery reported highest postoperative mortality for dogs with pancreatitis (50% versus 28% of all study dogs).[85]

Septic bile peritonitis, increased serum creatinine concentrations, prolonged activated partial thromboplastin time, and refractory postoperative hypotension were significantly associated with failure to survive.[85] Cholecytoenterostomy in cats with EHBDO has dismal success based on several small case series; approximately 50% of operated cats succumb shortly after or during surgical intervention.[98,99] Causes of death included clinical deterioration, enterostomy dehiscence, and cardiopulmonary arrest. As in dogs, refractory hypotension plays a dominant role in acute treatment failure. Reduced vascular responsiveness to vasopressors and decreased myocardial contractility contribute to nonresponsive hypotension.[77,78,100–105] This may reflect systemic endotoxemia or sepsis, increased production of vasodilatory compounds (ie, nitric oxide), vagal stimulation induced by biliary tract manipulations, or inadequate fluid support.[106–111] A decline in glomerular filtration rate and renal tubular injury secondary to refractory hypotension contributes to renal failure as a cause of death. Endotoxin absorption is likely an important factor in the pathophysiology of extrahepatic biliary disease in small animals, as opposed to human beings. In man, mortality is significantly higher in patients with septic complications. Despite advances in preoperative evaluation and postoperative care in human beings, interventions for relief of obstructive jaundice still carry high morbidity and mortality rates associated with sepsis and renal dysfunction.

Systemic and splanchnic endotoxemia derives from increased bacterial translocation of gram-negative organisms into the portal circulation. This reflects a multifactorial syndrome involving disruption of immunologic, biologic, and mechanical barriers. Absence of bile deprives the gut from 90% of secretory IgA, which normally prevents bacterial adherence to intestinal mucosa.[112,113] Overgrowth of E. coli (augmented by the lack of bile acids) and lack of biliary IgA lead to increased attachment of this bacterial strain to the intestinal mucosa.[112] Attachment of enteropathic E. coli disrupts enterocyte tight junctions and paracellular barriers, inducing transmural leakage of bacteria. Up-regulated Kupffer cell (Kupffer cells are the hepatic fixed macrophages) reactivity increases production of inflammatory cytokines and intercellular signaling, amplifying inflammatory responses. Increased splanchnic endotoxin uptake disrupts intestinal microcirculation and promotes enteric hypoxia, further thwarting normal gut integrity and imposing oxidative injury. Dysregulation between enterocyte apoptosis (enhanced) and cell regeneration (reduced) leads to loss of villi tips and ulcerogenic lesions permissive to enteric bacterial translocation. While various interventions have shown select benefits in animal models, a therapeutic cocktail has yet to evolve. Treatments shown to improve select abnormalities include: administration of N-acetylcysteine as a direct enteric thiol donor, α-tocopherol as a membrane stabilizer and antioxidant, glutamine as an enterocyte fuel and for augmenting enterocyte replication, oral bile acids to reduce enteric bacterial overgrowth, and enteric and systemic antibiotics to thwart bowel microbial overgrowth and systemic/portal sepsis. Risk factors associated with biliary tract infection include: advanced age, recent episodes of cholangitis, acute cholecystitis, choledocholithiasis, and obstructive jaundice from any cause. Considerations pertinent to the construction and long-term management of cholecystoenterostomies are discussed in the section "Cholelithiasis."

Cholelithiasis

The advent of routine abdominal US has increased the antemortem diagnosis of cholelithiasis in both dogs and cats. This coordinates with the fact that most choleliths in companion animals are clinically silent. More common in middle-aged to older animals, incidence may be more common in small breed dogs; one study suggested an increased incidence in Miniature Schnauzers and Miniature Poodles.[17] Cholecystoliths are most common but choledocholiths within the CBD, hepatic, and interlobular bile ducts are also recognized. While most choleliths in the CBD initiate from the GB, some choledocholiths seemingly develop within bile ducts as a consequence of bile stasis, inflammation, or infection (see **Figs. 4** and **19**). Choleliths in dogs and cats differ from those in human beings, which are primarily derived from cholesterol crystallization. Most choleliths in dogs and cats contain calcium carbonate and bilirubin pigments and are considered "pigment stones." Many of these do not contain enough mineral for detection on survey radiographs. Pigment gallstones are divided into two categories: "black-pigment" stones composed primarily of bilirubin polymers, and "brown-pigment" stones composed predominantly of calcium bilirubinate. Black-pigment stones reflect prolonged hyperbilirubinemia; in these, bilirubin polymerization occurs after its nonenzymatic deconjugation. Brown-pigment stones are frequently associated with bacterial infections and biliary stasis. In these, bilirubin deconjugation by bacterial β-glucuronidase yields unconjugated bilirubin that promptly precipitates as calcium bilirubinate. Biliary precipitates and micro-calculi promote bacterial colonization by providing a substrate for bacterial retention, and this further augments calcium bilirubinate aggregate formation. Mucin production, enhanced by local inflammation and prostaglandins, entangles calcium bilirubinate and bilirubin polymers into cholelith aggregates, and this process is augmented by GB dysmotility and bile stasis. Obstruction of the cystic duct in dogs has been shown to enhance GB mucin production and cholesterol concentration, as well as formation of pigment sludge.[114–117] Each of these changes favors cholelith precipitation. Mucin-bilirubin complexes form first, and as mucin content increases, sludge particles (1 mm–4 mm in diameter) coalesce and precipitate as gravel and stones. It is widely recognized that GB distension from any cause stimulates local mucin production and that this contributes to cystic duct occlusion by initiating a self-perpetuating cycle involving biliary sludge accumulation and inspissation. Cholecystitis is lithogenic by virtue of its association with prostaglandin-mediated inflammation that drives local mucin production, hemorrhage, bacterial bilirubin deconjugation, and bile stasis. Therefore, it is clear that disease or stasis of bile flow involving the GB and major bile ducts can lead to cholelithiasis as surely as cholelithiasis can injure these structures, leading to bile stasis. Thus, each case must be individually assessed to determine causal factors that deserve interventional therapy.

Clinical signs
Cholelithiasis may be associated with vomiting, anorexia, jaundice, fever, and abdominal pain. However, many animals with choleliths remain asymptomatic. Part of the problem is that pain associated with biliary colic is referred and evanescent. In human beings, intermittent abdominal pain, nausea, and dyspepsia are the most common clinical signs of cholelithiasis.[116] Cholelith movement or impaction within the cystic duct, CBD, especially in the ampulla (fusion of CBD and pancreatic duct, as in the cat), or the sphincter of Oddi (at the duodenal papilla), causes intense but intermittent local and referred pain. Discomfort is not exclusively postprandial and pain is either localized to the right upper abdominal quadrant, to the epigastrium (dermatome of T8/9), radiates to the right scapula or shoulder, or is localized to the retrosternal region. Nausea and vomiting are common, and patients assume a position of relief or walk to relieve their discomfort. Abdominal pain persists for at least 15 to 30 minutes up to several hours. Pain abates if the stone passes into the duodenum or back into a dilated region of the CBD, or an impacted stone in the cystic duct returns to the gallbladder

lumen.[116] Some animals with cholelithiasis have exhibited intermittent vague pain for years on retrospective consideration of their clinical history. These have unfortunately not been investigated by abdominal US. It is possible that biliary sludge or microliths lodged in the distal portion of the CBD in cats initiate idiopathic recurrent pancreatitis, as has been documented in human beings.[116]

Clinicopathologic features

Laboratory features of cholelithiasis most commonly reflect related cholecystitis. Before common use of diagnostic US, most animals diagnosed with cholelithiasis antemortem had EHBDO. In dogs with small duct lithiasis, clinicopathologic features reflect involvement of biliary structures (high ALP and GGT activity). Jaundice is only directly related to cholelithiasis associated with EHBDO or sepsis; thus, a large number of animals with cholelithiasis are not hyperbilirubinemic. While cholelithiasis may occur secondary to infection, stones also may induce infection. Mechanical trauma derived from choleliths may allow opportunistic organisms transiting the hepato-biliary-enteric circulation to assume residence within biliary structures. Thus, a hemogram in an animal with cholelithiasis may be normal or reflect inflammation or infection. A chemistry profile may be normal or disclose high cholestatic enzymes or evidence obstructive jaundice. Diagnostic imaging has been previously described (see above). Ultrasonography can detect stones greater than or equal to 2 mm in diameter in the GB, with more skill and luck needed to recognize stones lodged within the CBD. For animals with small duct cholelithiasis, biopsy and culture of liver tissue are necessary to identify underlying disease processes and associated bacterial infections.

Treatment

Medical treatment of cholelithiasis includes coverage with broad-spectrum antibiotics, considering that enteric opportunists may be involved. Use of a choleretic regimen is reasonable to facilitate clearance of biliary aggregates and bacterial organisms. Treatment with UDCA (15 mg/kg–25 mg/kg by mouth divided into two doses per day given with food) and SAMe (Denosyl, 20 mg/kg–40 mg/kg daily by mouth on an empty stomach) may have advantage for choledocholiths lodged in small intrahepatic bile ducts, as these may reflect chronic inflammatory disease that also may be attenuated with these medications. Whether or not there is benefit from administration of dehydrocholate, to increase bicarbonate rich watery bile, has not been evaluated in animals with spontaneous cholelithiasis. Liver biopsy determines whether immunomodulatory therapy is advisable (eg, chronic nonsuppurative hepatitis or feline CCHS). Alpha tocopherol (vitamin E: 10 U/kg per day) can be safely used for its antioxidant and anti-inflammatory affects without liver biopsy.

Surgical intervention is necessary in animals with choleliths associated with cholecystitis, causing cystic duct obstruction, or occluding the CBD. Successful treatment of cholecystitis and cystic duct occlusion requires cholecystectomy and lavage of the CBD. Care must be given to ensure that the CBD is clear of obstructive residual biliary debris. It may be possible to remove stones lodged in the CBD by choledochotomy; however, the causal factors of cholelith formation must be carefully considered. Retaining a diseased or dysmotile GB imposes risk for recurrent lithiasis or necrotizing cholecystitis. Some patients may benefit from temporary stent placement, as described previously, to allow healing of their surgical site and ensuring bile drainage into the duodenum during recovery. However, limited review of stent performance is available in companion animals (see section on EHBDO). In cases where CBD obstruction is irresolvable, a cholecystoenterostomy should be performed. These animals require long-term monitoring for septic cholangitis because of the potential for retrograde transit of enteric contents into the biliary structures (see **Fig. 25**). Chronic, pulsitile antimicrobial administration may be needed to control retrograde infections of the biliary tree. Biopsy of the biliary structures and liver for histopathologic examination is essential at the time of cholelith removal or biliary-enteric anastomosis, as this determines if an underlying primary inflammatory or neoplastic disease preceded cholelith formation. Tissue (liver, bile duct, GB), bile, and cholelith nidus should be submitted for aerobic and anaerobic bacterial cultures.

Cholecystoduodenostomy and cholecystojejunostomy are the most common cholecystenteric surgical procedures for biliary bypass in small animals. Cystoenteric anastomosis to the proximal duodenum is most physiologic, as it allows bile to enter the duodenum in a position that closely maintains normal physiologic responses in the proximal bowel. The anastomotic stoma must be large enough to allow intestinal reflux to exit the GB (or ducts if choledochoenterostomy) and provide a margin of error for contracture of the stoma during healing (can be up to 50%).[117,118] In small animals, stoma stricture and retrograde cholangitis are less likely when the stoma is greater than or equal to 2.5 cm in diameter at the time of surgery. This seemingly reduces entrapment of intestinal contents in the biliary tree and secondary cholangitis. Mucosal apposition at the stoma site is important to allow optimal stoma size, early smooth re-epithelialization, and to avoid granulation tissue that can impinge on stoma diameter.[118]

FELINE CHOLANGITIS/CHOLANGIOHEPATITIS SYNDROME

The most common necroinflammatory liver disease in the domestic cat involves the portal triad and surrounding hepatic parenchyma (zone 1).[1,119–133] Cholangitis and cholangiohepatitis are more common in the cat than in the dog and should be considered a disease syndrome. First described in the early1980s, feline CCHS has come to be recognized to coexist with inflammatory processes in the duodenum, pancreas, and kidneys (chronic interstitial nephritis).[1,119–123] The anatomic difference between the anatomy of the biliary and pancreatic ducts in cats versus dogs has long been considered the underlying factor influencing this species difference.[1] While it has been speculated that suppurative CCHS initiates an inflammatory process that transforms to a nonsuppurative process, there is no direct evidence for this pathogenesis. A number of conditions have been concurrently identified in cats with CCHS, whether the inflammatory infiltrate is predominantly neutrophilic (suppurative), lymphocytic or lymphoplasmacytic (nonsuppurative), or whether it actively involves bile duct destruction (**Box 2**). A 10-year retrospective study of liver biopsies ($n = 175$) from cats at one university teaching hospital detailed a prevalence of inflammatory liver disease of 26% ($n = 45$) comprised of cats with CCHS.[130] Detailed histopathologic description, clinicopathologic characterization, management, and survival characteristics of 45 cats were segregated into a series of three articles.[130,131,133] These investigators subdivided cats with inflammatory liver disease into three subsets: cats with suppurative inflammation, and cats with nonsuppurative inflammation with and without hepatic parenchymal inflammation or necrosis.[130,131,133] Cats lacking hepatic parenchyma involvement were classified as having lymphocytic portal hepatitis. Cholangiohepatitis was subcategorized as acute or chronic, according to the predominant inflammatory cell type: a large number of neutrophils, fewer lymphocytes, and minimal bile duct hyperplasia and fibrosis were classified as "acute CCHS," while cats with few neutrophils but many lymphocytes and moderate to severe bile duct hyperplasia and fibrosis were classified as "chronic CCHS." Another investigator described chronic progressive

Box 2
Disorders associated with the feline CCHS

Suppurative CCHS	Nonsuppurative CCHS
Primary biliary infection	Primary cholangitis
Systemic bacterial infection	Cholecystitis
Pyelonephritis	Cholelithiasis
Sinusitis	Extrahepatic bile duct obstruction
Splenic abscess	Malformations
Stomatitis	Choledochal cyst
Malformations	Polycystic biliary malformations
Choledochal cyst infection	Chronic pancreatitis
Polycystic biliary malformations	Chronic inflammatory bowel disease
Pancreatitis: acute	Chronic hepatic infection
Duodenitis: acute	Bacterial
Inflammatory bowel disease	Fluke
Cholelithiasis	Lymphoproliferative disease
Extrahepatic bile duct obstruction	Neoplasia
Trematode infection	Gallbladder adenocarcinoma
Toxoplasmosis	Biliary cystadenoma
Neoplasia	Small cell lymphoma
Chemotherapy-induced immunosuppression	Metastatic mast cell tumor
Lymphosarcoma	Chronic interstitial nephritis
Biliary adenocarcinoma → duct occlusion	Hyperthyroidism (augments disease activity)
Infected feeding appliances	—
Immunosuppression for nonsuppurative CCHS	—
Chronic prednisolone	—
Pulse-dosed methotrexate	—
Chlorambucil	—

lymphocytic CCHS in 20 cats and used immunophenotyping antibodies to demonstrate that histologic features fit criteria of an immune-mediated disorder.[132] This work subdivided histologic features into an "active stage" characterized by marked lymphocytic inflammation of portal tracts, particularly surrounding and infiltrating bile ducts, with occasional extension to periportal hepatic parenchyma ("piecemeal necrosis") and accompanied by bile duct proliferation and early portal-to-portal bridging fibrosis. A "chronic stage" was characterized by prominent monolobular fibrosis and a reduction in the intensity of lymphocytic infiltration and extent of bile duct proliferation. While the subdivision of categories could not be immunophenotypically differentiated, this study characterized substantial portal infiltration with T lymphocytes bearing CD3 and major histocompatibility complex Class II markers.[132] Furthermore, it was clearly shown that T cells infiltrated bile ducts and penetrated the limiting plate of zone 1, becoming closely associated with individual hepatocytes. Cytotoxic destruction of targeted cholangiocytes was surmised. Evaluations of liver from clinically healthy cats confirmed that a background population of CD3+ T cells reside within sinusoids and portal areas adjacent to, or within, bile duct epithelium. It was proposed that these T cells may be analogous to enteric interepithelial lymphocytes and are responsible for hepatic immune surveillance. It was hypothesized that these cells may play an important role in initiating the primary response in lymphocytic CCHS. The author of this article and her colleagues have been actively investigating CCHS for more than 25 years in clinical cases and liver biopsies referred to our pathology section, and the following discussion reflects observations derived from 196 cats with this syndrome (**Fig. 33**).

Feline CCHS is inarguably the most common acquired inflammatory liver disease in the domestic cat. Liver lobe involvement is variable and the extent and severity of histologic lesions may not be fully ascertained when only a single liver biopsy is evaluated, especially if only needle biopsies are available. Thus, lymphocytic portal infiltrates may not appear to penetrate the limiting plate or invade bile ducts in one section, while in another section florid duct destruction and hepatitis prevail. The author has observed some sections to detail modest or moderate duct inflammation and hepatitis, while other liver lobes have undergone nearly complete elimination of bile ducts and lack active inflammation (**Fig. 34**). Considering histologic lesions using descriptive morphology is advantageous over assumed "acute" or "chronic" categories. Using immunophenotyping (CD 3, B cell, macrophage markers) and cytokeratin (cytoplasmic intermediate filaments of the cytokeratin type in epithelial cells) stains, the author and colleagues subcategorize feline CCHS into five morphologic groups: suppurative CCHS, nonsuppurative CCHS without destructive duct lesions, nonsuppurative CCHS with destructive duct lesions, zone 1 lymphoproliferative disease, and small cell lymphosarcoma. Extensive immunophenotyping investigations, bacterial cultures, in situ fluorescent hybridization studies (FISH), and T-cell clonality evaluation (T-cell receptor rearrangement) have more fully distinguished disease subsets in this disorder (A. Warren, BSc, BVSc, Sharon A. Center, DVM, S. McDonough, DVM, PhD, K. Simpson, BVM&S, PhD, unpublished data, 2006). Preliminary findings have

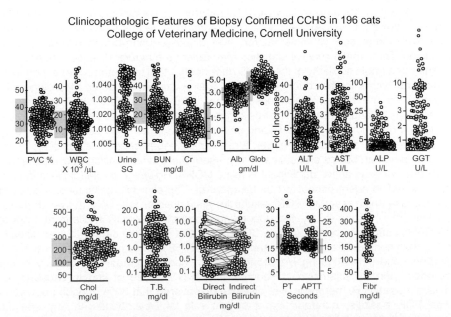

Fig. 33. Clinicopathologic features of 196 cats with the feline CCHS confirmed by liver biopsy. Gray rectangles indicate reference ranges. (*Courtesy of* College of Veterinary Medicine, Cornell University Medical Center, Ithaca, New York.)

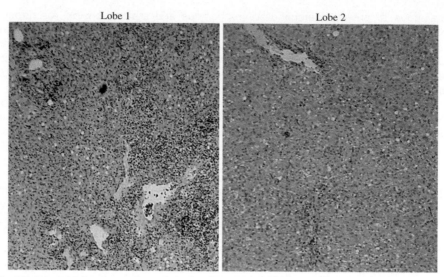

Lobe 1   Lobe 2

Fig. 34. Low-power photomicrograph detailing the difference between two separate liver lobes in a cat with CCHS. In Lobe 1 nonsuppurative inflammation is overt, while in Lobe 2 there is little inflammatory reaction (hematoxylin and eosin, original magnification ×100).

facilitated what appear to be rational therapeutic recommendations. Long-term response and survival with multimodal treatment in this large cohort of cats is being evaluated. Previously published survival statistics in cats with CCHS suggest significantly shorter survival for cats with disease in multiple organ systems; cats with lymphocytic portal hepatitis ($n = 23$) had a mean survival of 37 months and those with CCHS ($n = 15$) a mean survival of 29 months.[133] Treatments (ie, immunomodulation, antioxidant, UDCA) were not consistently provided as study cats were retrospectively diagnosed with inflammatory liver disease during biopsy review for case inclusion. Thus, these survival statistics may reflect the natural disease process.

The remarkable similarity of the CCHS duct destruction to human disorders characterized as "vanishing bile duct syndromes" makes current concepts regarding pathogenesis in the human syndromes relevant. The most recent work for primary sclerosing cholangitis in human beings suggest that biliary epithelial cells may mediate their own destruction by exaggerating innate and adaptive immune responses, initiated by bacterial products in the liver. A role for *Helicobacter* species has been investigated in human beings and cats and at present there is no consistent evidence that *Helicobacter* is an active participant in feline CCHS. However, a role for *Helicobacter* as an initiating agent cannot yet be discounted. The clinical significance of positive polymerase chain reaction (PCR) results for *Helicobacter* spp DNA in liver or bile is unclear.[134,135] In one study, *Helicobacter* was detected by PCR in bile from 4 out of 15 (26%) cats with nonsuppurative CCHS, 8 out of 51 (24%) cats with liver disease other than nonsuppurative CCHS, and 7 out of 12 (58%) cats lacking liver disease.[135] Another study investigating *Helicobacter* sp in human beings with primary biliary cirrhosis, primary sclerosing cholangitis, and liver disease of known cause (alcoholism, hepatitis B, metabolic liver disease) discovered that 30% of each population was PCR positive, contradicting a causal role of *Helicobacter* in any specific disorder.[136] Another feline study using archived paraffin-embedded liver tissue found *Helicobacter* sp in 2 out of 32 (6%) cats with CCHS and 1 out of 17 (6%) control cats (noninflammatory liver disease or healthy cats) by PCR amplification.[134] Positive findings were speciated by sequence confirmation. Using FISH, a single semicurved bacterium (1-2μ long) with *Helicobacter*-like morphology was observed within an intrahepatic bile duct (one cat with suppurative CCHS). DNA of *Helicobacter* spp other than *H. pylori* were confirmed (suppurative CCHS: *H. fennelliae* or *H cinaedi*, *H. bilis* was amplified from a cat with portosystemic vascular anomaly). Silver staining (Steiner stain) was uniformly negative in PCR-positive cats. Discordancy between culture, in-situ localization, and positive-PCR reports are frequent in experimental and clinical studies of *Helicobacter*. Thus, it is possible that PCR detection reflects enterohepatic circulation of intestinal organisms or DNA sojourning the liver rather than true colonization. However, positive reports might also reflect transient tissue colonization and a role for *Helicobacter* in initiation of the nonsuppurative CCHS lesions.

Suppurative Cholangitis/Cholangiohepatitis Syndrome

Suppurative CCHS causes the most overt clinical illness. These cats have a shorter duration of illness before presentation (< 5 days) with young or middle-aged adults predominating (age range 3 months to 16 years). Clinical signs include pyrexia, lethargy, dehydration, inappetence, vomiting, and variable jaundice. Many cats manifest abdominal pain (tender liver on palpation), and some have palpable hepatomegaly (<50%). Clinicopathologic features are similar to the other forms of CCHS, with moderate increases in transaminases (ALT, AST) and more modest increases in ALP and GGT activity. Unexpectedly, cholestatic enzymes may be normal. Most cats are hyperbilirubinemic, some have concurrent renal azotemia, many have a left-shifted leukogram associated with toxic neutrophils. Concurrent hepatic lipidosis may confuse initial assessments. Abdominal US may disclose features consistent with EHBDO, cholecystitis, choledochitis, pancreatitis, or inflammatory bowel disease, and diffuse hepatic parenchymal hyperechogenicity consistent with hepatic lipidosis. A heterogenous hepatic parenchymal pattern may sometimes be recognized reflecting parenchymal inflammation. Thoracic radiography often discloses a large sternal lymph node reflecting abdominal inflammation or sepsis (see **Fig. 5**). Medical and surgical interventions address diagnostic findings. Because of the severity of the patient's clinical presentation, medical treatment is often provided before surgical interventions (biliary decompression surgery for EHBDO, cholecystectomy for cholecystitis, cholecystotomy for cholelithiasis) and liver biopsy acquisition. Aspiration or biopsy imprint cytology of liver and bile usually disclose bacterial organisms. Cytologic assessments are essential as bacteria are usually not identified on routine histologic assessment but rather are suspected, based on the suppurative inflammatory reaction. Gram stain of cytologic specimens demonstrating bacteria is warranted to assist in selection of antimicrobial agents. Histologically, suppurative inflammation involves the bile ducts, is dispersed within the adventitia of the portal triad, and may cross into the hepatic parenchyma. Oval cell hyperplasia and bile duct hyperplasia intermixes with the suppurative inflammatory infiltrates. In some cases single cell necrosis is observed. Treatment involves administration of appropriate antimicrobials, UDCA, SAMe, vitamin E, water-soluble vitamins, enteral alimentation with a specifically feline-formulated maximum calorie diet, and judicious administration of fluids to correct and maintain hydration status and to correct electrolyte abnormalities. Antioxidants are provided during critical illness by administration of n-acetylcysteine (140 mg/kg initial dose, 70 mg/kg thereafter every 8–12 hours, infused IV over 20 minutes); when oral administration is possible, SAMe is given by mouth. Broad-spectrum antimicrobial coverage (against anaerobic and gram-negative enteric opportunists) is essential. Combination of enrofloxacin, metronidazole, and ampicillin/sulbactam is often initially administered. Antimicrobial therapy is thereafter sculpted to sensitivity reports of cultured bacteria from hepatobiliary aspirates or biopsy. Treatment with antimicrobials should be initiated before surgical intervention for EHBDO, cholecystitis, or cholelithiasis, as sepsis greatly compromises postoperative survival. Antimicrobial treatment is continued for 8 to 12 weeks (and sometimes longer) or until liver enzymes normalize. If liver enzymes remain increased, repeat-US assessment is warranted, inspecting for abnormalities of the biliary structures, pancreas, gut, or lymphadenopathy. Repeat aspiration cytology looking for persistent bacterial infection, or liver biopsy to determine whether nonsuppurative CCHS exists, may be necessary. Common coexistent disorders (see **Box 2**) require identification and management.

Nonsuppurative Cholangitis/Cholangiohepatitis Syndrome—Without Destructive Duct Lesions

Affected cats range in age between 2 and 17 years, with most being middle-aged or older. Concurrent infection with feline leukemia virus or feline immunodeficiency virus is uncommon; there is no sex or breed predisposition. Duration of illness ranges between 2 weeks and several years; most have been ill for several months before initial clinical presentation. Clinical signs commonly include intermittent vomiting and diarrhea, and episodic illness that may be associated with self-resolving jaundice. Hepatomegaly is common (> 50%). It is uncommon for nonsuppurative CCHS to cause portal hypertension and abdominal effusion, as cats seem to succumb to the illness before chronic fibrosis and biliary cirrhosis are established. Common coexistent disorders (see **Box 2**) require identification and management. Cats with nonsuppurative CCHS have variable white blood cell counts, but typically do not display a left-shifted leukogram nor toxic neutrophils. Poikilocytes are commonly identified. Hyperglobulinemia is observed in many of these cats, and most have moderate to marked increases in ALT and AST that often initiates the quest for definitive diagnosis. Activity of ALP and GGT are widely variable (see **Fig. 33**). Hyperbilirubinemia is inconsistent and seems cyclic in severity. Some cats are persistently jaundiced secondary to inflammatory obstruction of small- and medium-sized bile ducts and these develop symptomatic coagulopathies responsive to vitamin K administration (0.5 mg/kg–1.5 mg/kg subcutaneously or intramuscularly, three doses at 12-hour intervals is routinely used before biopsy) (see **Fig. 32**). Abdominal US findings overlap with those described for suppurative CCHS. A nonuniform or coarse parenchymal pattern may be identified (see **Fig. 15**); however, the author has observed many cats with marked histologic lesions that have seemingly normal hepatic US findings. Hepatic histologic changes are characterized by portal and periportal nonsuppurative inflammation associated with oval cell hyperplasia, bile duct hypertrophy and hyperplasia, and portal-to-portal bridging (**Figs. 35–38**). Severity of lesions is highly variable within and between liver lobes and between patients (see **Figs. 34** and **35**). Individual hepatocyte necrosis is observed. Cytokeratin staining of biliary epithelium is used to designate classification regarding duct destruction subset (see **Fig. 35**).

Initial treatment with appropriate antimicrobials, UDCA, SAMe, vitamin E, water-soluble vitamins (B vitamin supplementation), enteral alimentation with a specifically feline-formulated maximum calorie diet, and judicious administration of fluids to correct and maintain hydration and to correct electrolyte abnormalities, are essential. As discussed earlier, broad-spectrum antimicrobial coverage (against anaerobic and gram-negative enteric opportunists) is recommended as for suppurative CCHS until the nature of the disease process is clarified by liver biopsy and culture results. Antimicrobial therapy is thereafter tailored to sensitivity reports of bacteria cultured from hepatobiliary aspirates or biopsies. Long-term treatment requires immunomodulation. First-line immunosuppressive therapy is prednisolone, initially administered at 2 mg/kg

Lobe 1   Lobe 2

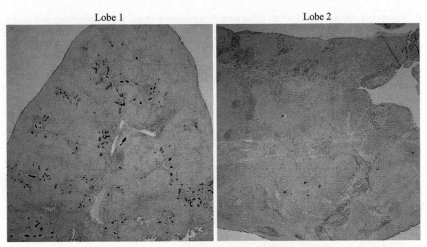

Fig. 35. Low-power photomicrograph detailing the difference between two separate liver lobes in a cat with CCHS (different cat than shown in **Fig. 34**), stained with anticytokeratin (biliary epithelium stains darkly). Findings characterize florid duct inflammation in Lobe 1, where brown stained structures are bile ducts, but nearly complete duct destruction in Lobe 2 (original magnification ×40).

to 4 mg/kg by mouth once a day, with the dose titrated, based on treatment response, to 5 mg to 10 mg per day. Coadministration with metronidazole (7.5 mg/kg by mouth) may assist with immunomodulation and control of associated inflammatory bowel disease. Some clinicians have used Chlorambucil for these cats (2 mg per day, once a day initially, titrated to every other day). Continued administration of SAMe (40 mg/kg–50 mg/kg per day by mouth) and vitamin E (10 U/kg per day) are recommended. The role of silymarin (milk thistle) is not resolved; recent studies in human beings with sclerosing CCHS suggest that silymarin provides an immunomodulatory and anti-inflammatory benefit, but further studies are needed to verify this impression.[137] At present, UDCA is the only medication in human beings that provides an inarguable treatment benefit for "sclerosing cholangitis."[137] Response to treatment in feline nonsuppurative

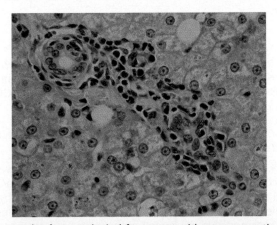

Fig. 36. Photomicrograph of a portal triad from a cat with nonsuppurative cholangitis/cholangiohepatitis. Lymphocytes infiltrate the portal triad and can be observed infiltrating biliary epithelium (hematoxylin and eosin, original magnification ×400).

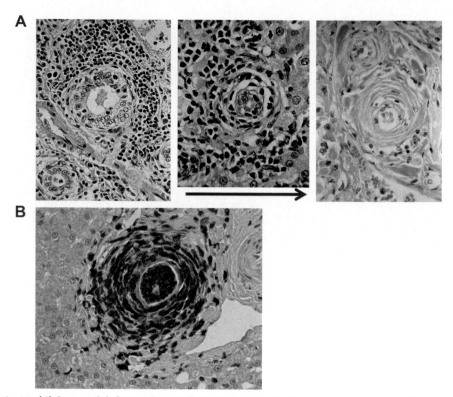

Fig. 37. (*A*) Sequential change in portal triads in cats with the sclerosing or destructive form of CCHS (hematoxylin and eosin, original magnification ×400). (*Left*) Lymphoplasmacytic, cholangiohepatitis, with ducts invaded. (*Middle*) Involuting ducts are consistent with an immune-mediated process. (*Right*) Relative "ductopenia" leaves a trail of "onion ring" sclerosis. (*B*) CD3 lymphocyte staining of the inflammatory infiltrated in nonsuppurative cholangitis/cholangiohepatitis (anti-CD3 lymphocyte immunostaining, original magnification ×200). The CD3 positive lymphocytes appear to target duct epithelium until ducts involute. Thereafter, once ductopenia is achieved, the inflammation subsides, as observed in **Figs. 34** and **35**, previously.

CCHS usually achieves normalization of bilirubin concentrations, but cyclic increases in enzyme activity remain, although the magnitudes of liver enzyme activity are attenuated. Long-term survival (>8 years) has been documented with immunomodulatory treatment (Center SA, unpublished data). The natural biology of CCHS reported in one case series[132–134] suggests that treatment improves survival.

Nonsuppurative Cholangitis/Cholangiohepatitis Syndrome-With Destructive Duct Lesions—Sclerosing Cholangitis

As early as 1983, a destructive duct lesion in cats with CCHS was identified that resembled human sclerosing cholangitis.[121] Cats with this lesion can eventually have widespread small duct destruction that imposes permanent hyperbilirubinemia and acholic stools; the histologic progression to ductopenia is summarized in **Figs. 36** and **37**. Examination of stools collected over a series of 3 days may disclose intermittent acholic feces, consistent with ductopenia (see **Fig. 35**). Cats so affected require weekly vitamin K injections and water-soluble vitamin E (polyethylene glycol

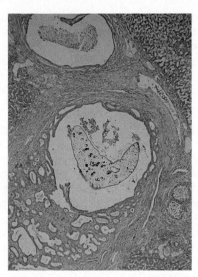

Fig. 38. Photomicrograph of biliary tree damage attributable to chronic fluke infestation. This biopsy demonstrates extensive large duct fibrosis, biliary epithelial hyperplasia and dysplasia, and a fluke within the large bile duct lumen (hematoxylin and eosin, original magnification ×100). (*Courtesy of* P.H. Rowland, VMD, Clifton Park, NY.)

α-tocopherol succinate, 10 U/kg by mouth per day). Care must be given to not over-dose vitamin K_1 as this can cause serious hemolytic anemia. Affected cats should be investigated for severe inflammatory bowel disease and B_{12} adequacy. Hematology and serum biochemistry features are similar to cats with nondestructive CCHS. The author's experience is that immunomodulation with prednisolone does little to moderate enzyme activity or hyperbilirubinemia in this subset. Rather, the author has employed pulse-dosed methotrexate (MTX) at 0.13 mg/kg by mouth every 12 hours up to three doses on a single day (total dose = 0.39 mg per day once every 7–10 days). Alternatively, MTX may be given by intravenous or intramuscular injection with a 50% dose reduction (enhanced bioavailability). Folic acid, 0.25 mg by mouth daily is concurrently administered to prevent MTX-associated hepatotoxicity, as shown in human beings. MTX dosing must be reduced in cats with renal azotemia. Careful inspection for infectious agents before initiating MTX therapy is essential, as this drug imposes profound immunosuppression at the dose used based on the author's clinical experience. It has been observed that cats develop feeding tube abscesses, hepatic abscesses, pyelonephritis, herpes keratitis, and demodecosis subsequent to MTX immunosuppression. Thus, careful monitoring for these complications during therapy is essential. Concurrent treatment with the antioxidant SAMe is recommended as a GSH donor, along with low-dose prednisolone and metronidazole to achieve multimodal immunomodulation. Treatment for concurrent inflammatory bowel disease with a hypoallergenic diet, and weekly supplementation with vitamin B_{12}, is indicated when appropriate.

Lymphoproliferative Disease Masquerading As Lymphocytic Cholangitis/Cholangiohepatitis Syndrome

This category of CCHS includes lesions characterized by dense portal lymphocyte infiltration that penetrate into hepatic sinusoids. However, involved lymphocytes lack convincing microscopic details for classification as a neoplastic population. Immunophenotyping with anti-CD3 antibodies characterize a CD3+-positive population. Lack of clonality (T-cell receptor gene rearrangement) leaves such cases in a lymphoproliferative category. Treatment with chlorambucil has been recommended, using 2 mg given on alternate days, combined with treatments previously characterized for CCHS. Some of these cats have survived for several years with minimal clinical signs.

Small cell lymphoma masquerading as lymphocytic Cholangitis/Cholangiohepatitis Syndrome

This category of CCHS involves cats with dense portal infiltration of CD3+ lymphocytes that penetrate into hepatic sinusoids and generate a single clone T-cell signal (T-cell receptor gene rearrangement). At present, treatment with chemotherapy designed for feline lymphoma is recommended. Judicious administration of nutritional, vitamin, and antioxidant support, as previously described, also is advised. These cats may have coexistent intestinal involvement, although the author has also identified cats with overt liver lymphosarcoma with inflammatory bowel diseases and cats with overt enteric lymphosarcoma and non-neoplastic nonsuppurative CCHS. The author hypothesizes that inflammatory CCHS may evolve to a neoplastic process.

Hepatobiliary Fluke Infection

Infection with liver flukes in endemic regions can cause acute and chronic cholangitis in the cat, and less frequently in dogs. Trematodes of the *Opisthorchiidae* family are involved (**Box 3**).[1,138,139] These require two intermediate hosts, a fresh water snail and a secondary host (eg, fish, reptile, or amphibian) in which metacercariae encyst. The mammalian tertiary host (cat or dog) ingests the fluke by consumption of the secondary host. Young flukes emerge in the intestines, migrate into the CBD, GB, or hepatic ducts, where they mature within 8 to 12 weeks. Embryonated eggs pass from bile into the alimentary canal where they may be detected in feces as early as 12 weeks after infection. Progressive clinical signs in some cats with naturally acquired Platynosomiasis have included weight loss, anorexia, vomiting, mucoid diarrhea, jaundice, hepatomegaly, emaciation, and abdominal distention.[1,138] Severely affected cats die of chronic fluke infestation; however, some exposed animals remain

---

Box 3
Family opisthorchiidae reported in dogs and cats

Genus, species, and geographic distribution

Amphimerus pseudofelineus: North, Central, South America

Clonorchis sinensis: China, Japan, Korea, Taiwan

Metorchis albidus: Northern Europe

Metorchis conjunctus: North America

Metorchis orientalis: South/East Asia

Opisthorchis felineus: Europe, Siberia, Ukraine

Opisthorchis viverrini: South/East Asia

Parametorchis complexus: North America

Pseudoamphistomum truncatum: Europe, India

asymptomatic. First clinical signs develop between 7 and 16 weeks of infection. Some symptomatic cats resolve clinical signs by 24 weeks after infection without treatment. Hematologic changes may include a circulating eosinophilia between 3 and 14 weeks after infestation that may persist. Heavily infected cats develop increased ALT and AST activities; however, normal or only mild increases in ALP activity are seen. Heavily infected cats may become hyperbilirubinemic within 7 to 16 weeks of infection. Histologic changes emerge after 3 weeks and progressively increase in severity in persistent infections. Inflammation and distention of large bile ducts is associated with a mixed neutrophilic and eosinophilic inflammatory infiltrate. By 4 months, severe adenomatous biliary hyperplasia and peribiliary inflammation are established, and by 6 months, progressive fibrosis results in marked fibroplasia surrounding bile ducts (see **Fig. 38**). Relatively, the hepatic parenchyma remains uninvolved, although regional lymphadenopathy may develop. Continued infection evolves to biliary cirrhosis with periductal infiltrates comprised of histiocytes, lymphocytes, and plasma cells, and small numbers of residual neutrophils and eosinophils. Experimental Platynosomiasis in cats established a direct correlation between developmental stage of the parasite in liver and the clinical manifestations of infection. Bile duct distention increases with growth of adult flukes and upon their sexual maturation, bile ducts containing parasites become fibrotic. During this time, serum transaminase activities normalize. Abdominal US may disclose one or more of the following features: (1) biliary obstruction involving the GB, CBD (> 2 mm), or intrahepatic ducts; (2) GB debris with flukes represented as oval hypoechoic structures having echoic centers; (3) a thickened GB wall associated with a double-rim sign (cholecystitis); and (4) hypoechoic hepatic parenchyma with prominent hyperechoic portal regions (ducts), reflecting cholangitis and cholangiohepatitis.

Considering that infected cats may not demonstrate clinical signs, diagnosis of fluke infestation may be difficult. Fecal examination may fail to detect eggs because of their sporadic passage, variable morphology (immature and embryonated forms), the small size of eggs, the insensitivity of routinely used fecal methods for identifying fluke eggs, and the development of bile duct obstruction that precludes passage of eggs into bile and feces. Cholecystocentesis has been used to document fluke eggs in bile but is not recommended as a routine screening method. Rather, treatment with Praziquantel (20 mg/kg subcutaneously every 24 hours for 3–5 days) is recommended when fluke infection is suspected. It is notable that eggs may continue to pass in feces for up to 2 months after successful treatment. Prednisolone is used to reduce eosinophilic inflammation in response to dying flukes at a dose of 15–25 mg/kg PO in two divided doses each day at meal time. Ursodeoxycholic acid is given at a dose of 15–25 mg/kg PO in two divided doses each day at meal time. Broad-spectrum antibiotic coverage is recommended to protect against retrograde infection of the biliary tree with bacteria introduced by migrating flukes, which can be augmented by fluke death in tissues. Antioxidant therapy, as previously suggested for necroinflammatory tissue injury, is also recommended (vitamin E: 10 IU/kg a day by mouth; SAMe: 20 mg/kg–40 mg/kg by mouth daily) until liver enzymes normalize. If necessary, an antiemetic is administered: for example, metoclopramide (0.2 mg/kg–0.5 mg/kg by mouth, subcutaneously every 6–8 hours) or maropitant (Cerenia 1.0 mg/kg per day for no more than 5 consecutive days).

ACKNOWLEDGEMENT

The author thanks Dr. A. Yeager for providing ultrasonography during the last 3 decades at Cornell University.

REFERENCES

1. Center SA. Diseases of the gallbladder and biliary tree. In: Guilford MG, Center SA, Strombeck DA, editors. Strombeck's small animal gastroenterology. 3rd edition. Philadelphia: WB Saunders; 1996. p. 860–88.
2. Etue SM, Penninck DG, Labato MA, et al. Ultrasonography of the normal feline pancreas and associated landmarks: a prospective study of 20 cats. Vet Radiol Ultrasound 2001;42:330–6.
3. Vielgrader HD. Sonographische und klinische Diagnostik bei Gallenblasen-und Gallengangserkrankungen der Katze [dissertation].eterinarmedizinische Universitat Wien, 1998.
4. Kanno N, LeSage G, Glaser S, et al. Functional heterogeneity of the intrahepatic biliary epithelium. Hepatology 2000;31:555–6.
5. Lee TK, Li L, Ballatori N. Hepatic glutathione and glutathione S-conjugate transport mechanism. Yale J Biol Med 1997;70:287–300.
6. Center SA, Warner KL, Erb HN. Liver glutathione concentrations in dogs and cats with naturally occurring liver disease. Am J Vet Res 2002;63: 1187–97.
7. Center SA, Randolph JF, Warner KL, et al. The effects of S-adenosylmethionine on clinical pathology and redox potential in the red blood cell, liver, and bile of clinically normal cats. J Vet Intern Med 2005;19:303–14.
8. Fardel O, Payen L, Courtois A, et al. Regulation of biliary drug efflux pump expression by hormones and xenobiotics. Toxicology 2001;167:37–46.
9. Payen L, Sparfel L, Courtois A, et al. The drug efflux pump MRP-2: regulation of expression in physiopathological situations and by endogenous and exogenous compounds. Cell Biol Toxicol 2002;18:221–33.
10. Yanaura S, Ishikawa S. Choleretic properties of ursodeoxycholic acid and chenodeoxycholic acid in dogs. Jpn J Pharmacol 1978;28:383–9.
11. Feeney DA, Anderson KL, Ziegler LE, et al. Statistical relevance of ultrasonographic criteria in the assessment of diffuse liver disease in dogs and cats. Am J Vet Res 2008;69:212–21.
12. Spaulding KA. Ultrasound corner: gallbladder wall thickness. Vet Radiol Ultrasound 1993;34:270–2.
13. Hittmair KM, Vielgrader HD, Loupal G. Ultrasonographic evaluation of gallbladder wall thickness in cats. Vet Radiol Ultrasound 2001;42:149–55.
14. Shlaer WJ, Leopold GR, Scheible FW. Sonography of the thickened gallbladder wall, a nonspecific finding. AJR Am J Roentgenol 1981;136:337–9.
15. Ramstedt KL, Center SA, Randolph JF, et al. Changes in gallbladder volume in healthy dogs after food was withheld for 12 hours followed by ingestion of a meal or a meal containing erythromycin. Am J Vet Res 2008;69:647–51.
16. Zeman RK, Taylor KJ, Rosenfield AT, et al. Acute experimental biliary obstruction in the dog. Sonographic findings and clinical implications. AJR Am J Roentgenol 1981;136:965–7.
17. Nyland TG, Gillett NA. Sonographic evaluation of experimental bile duct ligation in the dog. Vet Radiol 1982;13:252–60.
18. Nyland TG, Hager DA, Herring DS. Sonography of the liver, gallbladder, and spleen. Semin Vet Med Surg 1989;4:13–31.
19. Aguirre AL, Center SA, Randolph JF, et al. Gallbladder disease in Shetland Sheepdogs: 38 cases (1995–2005). J Am Vet Med Assoc 2007;231:79–88.
20. Pike FS, Berg J, King NW, et al. Gallbladder mucocele in dogs: 30 cases (2000–2002). J Am Vet Med Assoc 2004;224:1615–22.

21. Besso JG, Wrigley RH, Gliatto JM, et al. Ultrasonographic appearance and clinical findings in 14 dogs with gallbladder mucocele. Vet Radiol Ultrasound 2000; 41:261–71.
22. Rothuizen J, van den Brom WE. Quantitative hepatobiliary scintigraphy as a measure of bile flow in dogs with cholestatic disease. Am J Vet Res 1990; 51:253–6.
23. Boothe HW, Boothe DM, Komkov A, et al. Use of hepatobiliary scintigraphy in the diagnosis of extrahepatic biliary obstruction in dogs and cats: 25 cases (1982–1989). J Am Vet Med Assoc 1992;201:134–41.
24. McGahan JP, Phillips HE, Nyland T, et al. Sonographically guided percutaneous cholecystostomy performed in dogs and pigs. Radiology 1983;149:841–3.
25. Voros K, Sterczer A, Manczur F, et al. Percutaneous ultrasound-guided cholecystocentesis in dogs. Acta Vet Hung 2002;50:385–93.
26. Savary-Bataille KCM, Bunch SE, Spaulding KA, et al. Percutaneous ultrasound-guided cholecystocentesis in healthy cats. J Vet Intern Med 2003;17(3): 298–303.
27. Herman BA, Brawer RS, Murtaugh RJ, et al. Therapeutic percutaneous ultrasound-guided cholecystocentesis in three dogs with extrahepatic biliary obstruction and pancreatitis. J Am Vet Med Assoc 2005;227:1782–6.
28. vanSonnenberg E, D'Agostino HB, Goodacre BW, et al. Percutaneous gallbladder puncture and cholecystostomy: results, complications, and caveats for safety. Radiology 1992;183:167–70.
29. Kovatch RM, Hildebrandt PK, Marcus LC. Cystic mucinous hypertrophy of the mucosa of the gallbladder in the dog. Pathol Vet 1965;2:574–84.
30. Kline LW, Karpinski E. Progesterone inhibits gallbladder motility through multiple signaling pathways. Steroids 2005;70:673–9.
31. Tierney S, Nakeeb A, Wong O, et al. Progesterone alters biliary flow dynamics. Ann Surg 1999;229:205–9.
32. Ludwig LL, McLoughlin MA, Graves TK, et al. Surgical treatment of bile peritonitis in 24 dogs and 2 cats: A retrospective study (1987–1994). Vet Surg 1997;26:90–8.
33. Church EM, Matthiesen DT. Surgical treatment of 23 dogs with necrotizing cholecystitis. J Am Anim Hosp Assoc 1988;24:305–10.
34. Holt DE, Mehler SJ, Mayhew PD, et al. Canine gallbladder infarction: 12 cases (1993–2003). Vet Pathol 2004;41:416–8.
35. Friman S, Radberg G, Bosaeus I, et al. Hepatobiliary compensation for the loss of gallbladder function after cholecystectomy-an experimentall study in the cat. Scand J Gastroenterol 1990;25:307–14.
36. Mahour GH, Wakim KG, Soule EH, et al. Effects of cholecystectomy on the biliary ducts in the dog. Arch Surg 1968;97:570–4.
37. Pomare EW, Heaton KW. The effect of cholecystectomy on bile salt metabolism. Gut 1973;14:753–62.
38. Simmons F, Ross APJ, Bouchier IAD. Alterations in hepatic bile composition after cholecystectomy. Gastroenterology 1972;63:466–71.
39. Ropda E, Aldini R, Mazzela G, et al. Enterohepatic circulation of bile acids after cholecystectomy. Gut 1978;19:640–9.
40. Nahrwold DL, Rose RC. Changes in hepatic bile secretion following cholecystectomy. Surgery 1976;80:178–82.
41. Hepner GW, Hofmann AR, Malagelada JR, et al. Increased bacterial degradation of bile acids in cholecystectomized patients. Gastroenterology 1974;66: 556–64.

42. Brewer NF, Jackel S, Dommess P, et al. Fecal bile acid excretion pattern in cholecystectomized patients. Dig Dis Sci 1986;31:953–60.
43. Newell SM, Selcer BA, Mahaffey MB, et al. Gallbladder mucocele causing biliary obstruction in two dogs: Ultrasonographic, scintigraphic, and pathologic findings. J Am Vet Med Assoc 1995;31:467–72.
44. Barie PS, Fischer E, Eachempati SR. Acute acalculous cholecystitis. Curr Opin Crit Care 1999;5:144–58.
45. Sepesy LM, Center SA, Randolph JF, et al. Vacuolar hepatopathy in dogs: 336 cases (1993–2005). J Am Vet Med Assoc 2006;229:246–52.
46. Mawdesley-Thomas LE, Noel PRB. Cystic hyperplasia of the gallbladder in the beagle associated with the administration of progestational compounds. Vet Rec 1967;80(22):658–9.
47. Center SA, Warner KL, McCabe J, et al. Evaluation of the influence of S-adenosylmethionine on systemic and hepatic effects of prednisolone in dogs. Am J Vet Res 2005;66:330–41.
48. Ward A, Brogden RN, Heel RC. Ursodeoxycholic acid: a review of its pharmacological properties and therapeutic efficacy. Drugs 1984;27:95–131.
49. Festi D, Montagnani M, Azzaroli F, et al. Clinical efficacy and effectiveness of ursodeoxycholic acid in cholestatic liver diseases. Curr Clin Pharmacol 2007;2: 155–77.
50. Pusl T, Beuers U. Ursodeoxycholic acid treatment of vanishing bile duct syndromes. World J Gastroenterol 2006;12:3487–95.
51. Jüngst C, Sreejayan N, Zündt B, et al. Ursodeoxycholic acid reduces lipid peroxidation and mucin secretagogue activity in gallbladder bile of patients with cholesterol gallstones. Eur J Clin Invest 2008;38:634–9.
52. Guarino MP, Cong P, Cicala M, et al. Ursodeoxycholic acid improves muscle contractility and inflammation in symptomatic gallbladders with cholesterol gallstones. Gut 2007;56:815–20.
53. Stalker MJ, Hayes MA. Liver and biliary system. In: Maxie MG, editor. Jubb, Kennedy, and Palmer's pathology of domestic animals, vol. 2. 5th edition. Philadelphia: WB Saunders, Elsevier; 2007. p. 298–388.
54. Brancatelli G, Federle MP, Vilgrain V, et al. Fibropolycystic liver disease: CT and MR imaging findings. RadioGraphics 2005;25:659–70.
55. Marchal GJ, Desmet VJ, Proesmans WC, et al. Caroli disease: high-frequency US and pathologic findings. Radiology 1986;158:507–11.
56. Chang MY, Ong AC. Autosomal dominant polycystic kidney disease: recent advances in pathogenesis and treatment. Nephron Physiol 2008;108:1–7.
57. Young AE, Biller DS, Herrgesell EJ, et al. Feline polycystic kidney disease is linked to the PKD1 region. Mamm Genome 2005;16:59–65.
58. Lyons LA, Biller DS, Erdman CA, et al. Feline polycystic kidney disease mutation identified in PKD1. J Am Soc Nephrol 2004;15:2548–55.
59. Eaton KA, Biller DS, DiBartola SP, et al. Autosomal dominant polycystic kidney disease in Persian and Persian-cross cats. Vet Pathol 1997;34:117–26.
60. Helps CR, Tasker S, Barr FJ, et al. Detection of the single nucleotide polymorphism causing feline autosomal-dominant polycystic kidney disease in Persians from the UK using a novel real-time PCR assay. Mol Cell Probes 2007;21:31–4.
61. McAloose D, Casal M, Patterson DF, et al. Polycystic kidney and liver disease in two related West Highland White Terrier litters. Vet Pathol 1998;35:77–81.
62. McKenna SC, Carpenter JL. Polycystic disease of the kidney and liver in the Cairn Terrier. Vet Pathol 1980;17(4):436–42.

63. Last RD, Hill JM, Roach M, et al. Congenital dilatation of the large and segmental intrahepatic bile ducts (Caroli's disease) in two Golden Retriever littermates. J S Afr Vet Assoc 2006;77:210–4.
64. Van den Ingh TS, Rothuizen J. Congenital cystic disease of the liver in seven dogs. J Comp Pathol 1985;95(3):405–14.
65. Görlinger S, Rothuizen J, Bunch S, et al. Congenital dilatation of the bile ducts (Caroli's disease) in young dogs. J Vet Intern Med 2003;17:28–32.
66. Nyland TG, Koblik PD, Tellyer SE. Ultrasonographic evaluation of biliary cystadenomas in cats. Vet Radiol Ultrasound 1999;40:300–6.
67. Stewart HL, Lieber MM. Ligation of the common bile duct in the cat. Arch Pathol 1935;34–46.
68. Cameron GR, Hasan SM. Disturbances of structure and function in the liver as the result of biliary obstruction. J Pathol Bacteriol 1958;75:333–47.
69. Center SA, Castleman E, Roth L, et al. Light microscopic and electron microscopic changes in the livers of cats with extrahepatic bile duct obstruction. Am J Vet Res 1986;47:1278–82.
70. Trams EG, Symeonidis A. Morphologic and functional changes in the liver of rats after ligation or excision of the common bile duct. Am J Pathol 1957;33:13–27.
71. Steiner JW, Carruthers JS. Experimental extrahepatic biliary obstruction. Am J Pathol 1962;40:235–70.
72. Stewart HL, Cantarow A. Decompression of the obstructed biliary system of the cat. Am J Dig Dis Nutr 1935;2:101–8.
73. Van Vleet JF, Alberts JO. Evaluation of liver function tests and liver biopsy in experimental carbon tetrachloride intoxication and extrahepatic bile duct obstruction in the dog. J Am Vet Med Assoc 1968;29:2119–31.
74. Ohlsson EG. The effect of biliary obstruction on the distribution of the hepatic flow and reticuloendothelial system in dogs. Acta Chir Scand 1972;138:159–64.
75. Saito H. Clinical and experimental studies on the hyperdynamic states in obstructive jaundice. J Jap Surg Soc 1981;82:483–97.
76. Sasha SM, Better OS, Chaimovitz C, et al. Hemodynamic studies in dogs with chronic bile duct ligation. Clin Sci Mol Med 1975;50:533–7.
77. Fineberg JPM, Syrop HA, Better OS. Blunted pressor response to angiotensin and sympathomimetic amines in the bile duct ligated dogs. Clin Sci (Lond) 1981;61:535–9.
78. Binah O, Bomzon A, Blendis LM, et al. Obstructive jaundice blunts myocardial contractile response to isoproternol in the dog. A clue to the susceptibility of jaundiced patients to shock. Clin Sci (Lond) 1985;69:647–53.
79. Wilson SA, Gosink BB, van Sonnenberg E. Unchanged size of a dilated common bile duct after a fatty meal. Results and significance. Radiology 1986;160:29–31.
80. Simeone JF, Mueller PR, Ferrucci JT, et al. Sonography of the bile ducts after a fatty meal: an aid in detection of obstruction. Radiology 1982;143:211–5.
81. Simeone JF, Butch RJ, Mueller PR, et al. The bile ducts after a fatty meal. Further sonographic observations. Radiology 1985;154:763–8.
82. Cribb AE, Burgener DC, Reimann KA. Bile duct obstruction secondary to chronic pancreatitis in seven dogs. Can Vet J 1988;29:654–7.
83. Edwards DF, Bauer MS, Walker MA, et al. Pancreatic masses in seven dogs following acute pancreatitis. J Am Anim Hosp Assoc 1990;26:189–98.
84. Fahie MA, Martin RA. Extrahepatic biliary tract obstruction: a retrospective study of 45 cases (1983–1993). J Am Anim Hosp Assoc 1995;31:478–82.

85. Mehler SJ, Mayhew PD, Drobatz KJ, et al. Variables associated with outcome in dogs undergoing extrahepatic biliary surgery: 60 cases (1998–2002). Vet Surg 2004;33:644–9.
86. Martin RA, MacCoy DM, Harvey HJ. Surgical management of extrahepatic biliary tract disease. A report of eleven cases. J Am Anim Hosp Assoc 1986; 22:301–7.
87. Matthiesen DT, Rosin E. Common bile duct obstruction secondary to chronic fibrosing pancreatitis. Treatment by use of cholecystoduodenostomy in the dog. J Am Vet Med Assoc 1986;189:1443–6.
88. Denning DA, Ellison EC, Carey LC. Preoperative percutaneous biliary decompression lowers operative morbidity in patients with obstructive jaundice. Am J Surg 1981;141:61–5.
89. Gobien RP, Stanley JH, Soucek CD, et al. Routine preoperative biliary drainage: effect on management of obstructive jaundice. Radiology 1984; 152:353–6.
90. Murphy SM, Rodríguez JD, McAnulty JF. Minimally invasive cholecystostomy in the dog: evaluation of placement techniques and use in extrahepatic biliary obstruction. Vet Surg 2007;36:675–83.
91. Barthet M, Bernard JP, Duval JL, et al. Biliary stenting in benign biliary stenosis complicating chronic calcifying pancreatitis. Endoscopy 1994;26:569–72.
92. Smits ME, Rauws EA, Van Gulik TM, et al. Long-term results of endoscopic stenting and surgical drainage for biliary stricture due to chronic pancreatitis. Br J Surg 1996;83:764–8.
93. Sewnath ME, Karsten TM, Prins MH, et al. A meta-analysis on the efficacy of preoperative biliary drainage for tumors causing obstructive jaundice. Ann Surg 2002;236:17–27.
94. Mayhew PD, Richardson RW, Mehler SJ, et al. Choledochal tube stenting for decompression of the extrahepatic portion of the biliary tract in dogs: 13 cases (2002–2005). J Am Vet Med Assoc 2006;228:1209–14.
95. Mayhew PD, Weisse CW. Treatment of pancreatitis-associated extrahepatic biliary tract obstruction by choledochal stenting in seven cats. J Small Anim Pract 2008;49:133–8.
96. Zhao P, Tu J, Martens A, Ponette E, et al. Radiologic investigations and pathologic results of experimental chronic pancreatitis in cats. Acad Radiol 1998;5: 850–6.
97. Sung JY, Leung JWC, Shaffer EA, et al. Ascending infection of the biliary tract after surgical sphincterotomy and biliary stenting. J Gastroenterol Hepatol 1992;7:240–5.
98. Buote NJ, Mitchell SL, Penninck D, et al. Cholecystoenterostomy for treatment of extrahepatic biliary tract obstruction in cats: 22 cases (1994–2003). J Am Vet Med Assoc 2006;228(9):1376–82.
99. Mayhew PD, Holt DE, McLear RC, et al. Pathogenesis and outcome of extrahepatic biliary obstruction in cats. J Small Anim Pract 2002;43:247–53.
100. Bomzon A, Monies-Chass I, Kamenetz L, et al. Anesthesia and pressor responsiveness in chronic bile-duct-ligated dogs. Hepatology 1990;11:551–6.
101. Bomzon A, Binah O, Blendis LM. Hypotension in experimental cirrhosis. Is loss of vascular responsiveness to norepinephrine the cause of hypotension in chronic bile-duct-ligated dogs? J Hepatol 1993;17:116–23.
102. Bomzon A, Rosenburg M, Gali D, et al. Systematic hypotension and decreased pressor response in dogs with chronic bile duct ligation. Hepatology 1986;6: 595–600.

103. Finberg JP, Seidman R, Better OS. Cardiovascular responsiveness to vasoactive agents in rats with obstructive jaundice. Clin Exp Pharmacol Physiol 1982;9: 639–43.
104. Jacob G, Nassar N, Hayam G, et al. Cardiac function and responsiveness to beta-adrenoceptor agonists in rats with obstructive jaundice. Am J Physiol 1993;265(2 Pt 1):G314–20.
105. Schafer J, d'Almeida MS, Weisman H, et al. Hepatic blood volume responses and compliance in cats with long term bile duct ligation. Hepatology 1993;18: 969–77.
106. Utkan ZN, Utkan T, Sarioglu Y, et al. Effect of experimental obstructive jaundice on contractile responses of dog isolated blood vessels: role of endothelium and duration of bile duct ligation. Clin Exp Pharmacol Physiol 2000;27:339–44.
107. Wardle EN, Wright NA. Endotoxin and acute renal failure associated with obstructive jaundice. Br Med J 1970;4:472–4.
108. Wilkinson SP, Moodie H, Stamatakis JD, et al. Endotoxaemia and renal failure in cirrhosis and obstructive jaundice. Br Med J 1976;2:1415–8.
109. Bailey ME. Endotoxin, bile salts and renal function in obstructive jaundice. Br J Surg 1976;63:774–8.
110. Pain JA, Cahill CJ, Bailey ME. Perioperative complications in obstructive jaundice: therapeutic considerations. Br J Surg 1985;72:942–5.
111. Deitch EA, Sittig K, Li M, et al. Obstructive jaundice promotes bacterial translocation from the gut. Am J Surg 1990;159:79–84.
112. Assimakopoulos SF, Scopa CD, Vagianos CE. Pathophysiology of increased intestinal permeability in obstructive jaundice. World J Gastroenterol 2007;13: 6458–64.
113. Wells CL, Jechorek RP, Erlandsen SL. Inhibitory effect of bile on bacterial invasion of enterocytes: possible mechanism for increased translocation associated with obstructive jaundice. Crit Care Med 1995;23:301–7.
114. Soloway RD, Powell KM, Senior JR, et al. Interrelationships of bile salts, phospholipids, and cholesterol in bile during manipulation of the enterohepatic circulation in the conscious dog. Gastroenterology 1973;64:1156–62.
115. Bernhoft RA, Pelligrini CA, Broderick WC, et al. Pigment sludge and stone formation in the acutely ligated dog gallbladder. Gastroenterology 1983;85: 1166–71.
116. Portincasa P, Moschetta A, Petruzzelli M, et al. Symptoms and diagnosis of gallbladder stones. Best Pract Res Clin Gastroenterol 2006;20:1017–29.
117. Martin O, Tobias K. Liver and biliary system. In: Slatter D, editor. Textbook of small animal surgery. 3rd edition. Philadelphia: WB Saunders; 2003. p. 708–26.
118. Morrison S, Prostredny J, Roa D. Retrospective study of 28 cases of cholecystoduodenostomy performed using endoscopic gastrointestinal anastomosis stapling equipment. J Am Anim Hosp Assoc 2008;44:10–8.
119. Prasse K, Mahaffey EA, Denovo R, et al. Chronic lymphocytic cholangitis in three cats. Vet Pathol 1982;19:99–108.
120. Hirsch VM, Doige CE. Suppurative cholangitis in cats. J Am Vet Med Assoc 1983;182:1223–6.
121. Edwards DF, McCracken MD, Richardson DC. Sclerosing cholangitis in a cat. J Am Vet Med Assoc 1983;182:710–2.
122. Zawie DA, Garvey MS. Feline hepatic disease. Vet Clin North Am Small Anim Pract 1984;2:1201–30.
123. Lucke VM, Davies JD. Progressive lymphocytic cholangitis in the cat. Small Anim Pract 1984;25:249–60.

124. Center SA. Feline liver disorders and their management. Compend Contin Educ Pract Vet 1986;8:889–901.
125. Shaker EH, Zawie DA, Garvey MS, et al. Suppurative cholangiohepatitis in a cat. J Am Anim Hosp Assoc 1991;27:148–50.
126. Nakayama H, Uchida K, Uetsuka K, et al. Three cases of feline sclerosing lymphocytic cholangitis. Vet Med Sci 1992;54:769–71.
127. Day D. Diseases of the liver. In: Sherding RG, editor. The cat: disease and clinical management. 2nd edition. New York: Churchill Livingstone Inc; 1994. p. 1297–340.
128. Jackson MW, Panciera DL, Hartman F. Administration of vancomycin for treatment of ascending bacterial cholangiohepatitis in a cat. J Am Vet Med Assoc 1994;204:602–5.
129. Center SA, Rowland PR. The cholangitis/cholangiohepatitis complex in the cat. Proc 12th American College of Veterinary Internal Medicine Forum, Orlando, Florida, ACVIM, 1994;766–771.
130. Gagne JM, Weiss DJ, Armstrong PJ. Histopathologic evaluation of feline inflammatory liver disease. Vet Pathol 1996;33:521–6.
131. Weiss DJ, Armstrong PJ, Gagne J. Inflammatory liver disease. Semin Vet Med Surg (Small Anim) 1997;12(1):22–7.
132. Day MJ. Immunohistochemical characterization of the lesions of feline progressive lymphocytic cholangitis/cholangiohepatitis. J Comp Pathol 1998;119: 135–47.
133. Gagne JM, Armstrong PJ, Weiss DJ. Clinical features of inflammatory liver disease in cats: 41 cases (1983–1993). J Am Vet Med Assoc 1999;214:513–6.
134. Greiter-Wilke A, Scanziani E, Soldati S, et al. Association of Helicobacter with cholangiohepatitis in cats. J Vet Intern Med 2006;20:822–7.
135. Boomkens SY, Kusters JG, Hoffmann G, et al. Detection of Helicobacter pylori in bile of cats. FEMS Immunol Med Microbiol 2004;42:307–11.
136. Boomkens SY, de Rave S, Pot RG, et al. The role of Helicobacter spp. in the pathogenesis of primary biliary cirrhosis and primary sclerosing cholangitis. FEMS Immunol Med Microbiol 2005;44:221–5.
137. Maggs JRL, Chapman RW. An update on primary sclerosing cholangitis. Curr Opin Gastroenterol 2008;24:377–83.
138. Taylor D, Perri SF. Experimental infection of cats with the liver fluke Platynososomum concinnum. Am J Vet Res 1977;38:51–4.
139. Bowman DD, Hendrix CM, Lindsay DS, et al. Feline clinical parasitology. 1st edition. Ames (IA): Iowa State University Press/Blackwell Publishing; 2002.

Hepatic Lipidosis in Cats

P. Jane Armstrong, DVM, MS, MBA[a,*], Geraldine Blanchard, DVM, PhD[b]

KEYWORDS

• Fatty liver • Steatosis • Obesity • Fat • Feline • Liver

PREVALENCE

Since the initial description of hepatic lipidosis (HL) in 1977,[1] it has emerged as the most common form of liver disease diagnosed in cats in North America. In a 10-year retrospective study of all feline liver biopsies at the University of Minnesota College of Veterinary Medicine, HL accounted for 50% of all cases.[2] This figure likely under-represents the true prevalence in this hospital population, because the study included only cats undergoing liver biopsy, not fine-needle aspiration. In a 1996 study in which clinical data were collected in primary care small animal practices across the United States, the overall prevalence of the syndrome was 0.06% (E.M. Lund, personal communication, 2009; the study is described by Lund and colleagues.[3] A prevalence of 0.16% was obtained in a population of over 360,000 cats seen at primary care practices in 2008 (E.M. Lund, personal communication, 2009. Data made available by Banfield, The Pet Hospital). There may be some geographic variation in the prevalence of HL. For example, the authors have received reports that HL is relatively common in cats in North America, Great Britain, Japan, and Western Europe and relatively uncommon in Southern European countries and New Zealand. One could speculate that these differences may correspond with the prevalence of obesity in cats in different countries or other regional differences, such as feeding practices.

Although many cats develop lipidosis during periods of anorexia related to an underlying disease (sometimes called "secondary HL"), otherwise healthy cats can also develop the syndrome (so-called "primary HL") due to inadequate intake during periods of forced overly rapid weight loss, unintentional food deprivation, change to a food unacceptable to the cat, sudden change in lifestyle, or stress (eg, boarding). This understanding has emphasized the importance of maintaining food intake in cats that become anorexic for any reason for periods longer than a few days. Although histologic evidence of HL develops in overweight cats within 2 weeks in an experimental model of HL,[4] clinical experience indicates that the clinical syndrome can develop much more rapidly (in approximately 1 week), perhaps related to percent

---

[a] Veterinary Clinical Sciences Department, College of Veterinary Medicine, University of Minnesota, 1352 Boyd Avenue, St. Paul, MN 55108, USA
[b] Animal Nutrition Expertise SARL, Avenue ile de France, Antony, France
* Corresponding author.
E-mail address: armst002@umn.edu (P.J. Armstrong).

Vet Clin Small Anim 39 (2009) 599–616
doi:10.1016/j.cvsm.2009.03.003
0195-5616/09/$ – see front matter © 2009 Elsevier Inc. All rights reserved.

decrease in caloric intake (total fasting vs partial anorexia) and to initial degree of adiposity. The authors have observed that HL develops most rapidly and most consistently when cats with very high body condition scores (BCSs) become anorexic. Epidemiologic data are needed to support this observation.

PATHOGENESIS

During a period of partial or complete anorexia of 1 week or longer, intense peripheral lipolysis occurs through the stimulation of hormone-sensitive lipase.[5–7] The activity of hormone-sensitive lipase is stimulated by numerous hormones (glucagon, thyroid hormones, epinephrine, norepinephrine, glucocorticoids, and growth hormone) and inhibited by insulin. During prolonged anorexia in cats and in cases of HL, several authors have demonstrated impaired glucose tolerance and a decreased insulin response after intravenous (IV) infusion of glucose, suggesting a lack of insulin secretion.[8,9] This has been confirmed in cats with HL by a decreased insulin/glucagon ratio compared with healthy control cats.[5] Lipolysis induces a dramatic increase of the concentration of free fatty acids in the blood.[10] That these fatty acids are taken up by peripheral cells, and finally by the liver, is suggested by the similar composition of the fatty acids in the liver and adipose tissue of cats with HL.[2]

Once in hepatocytes, fatty acids follow one of two main pathways. Fatty acids may enter the mitochondria with the help of L-carnitine and undergo beta oxidation. Oxidation of fatty acids produces acetyl-CoA, which can enter the tricarboxylic acid (Krebs) cycle to provide energy (this requires glucose or pyruvate) and/or form ketone bodies. Acetoacetate and β-hydroxybutyrate are synthesized, exit the liver, and can be used as energy sources by peripheral tissues. Acetone may also be produced, and this oxidation product must be eliminated in urine or expired. In cats with HL, the production of acetone is responsible for the special smell to the breath that can be detected in some cats. An alternative pathway for metabolism, after fatty acids enter the liver, is for them to be esterified into triglycerides. Triglycerides can accumulate in vacuoles within hepatocytes and/or be incorporated into very low-density lipoproteins (VLDL) and secreted into the blood. It has become clear that the latter pathway occurs in two steps, as triglycerides incorporated into secreted VLDL come from lipid vacuoles in hepatocytes.

Several theories on the pathogenesis of HL have been proposed and been the topic of some investigations. L-carnitine is considered a conditionally essential nutrient, as it can be synthesized in the liver. Under conditions of high demand and/or reduced synthesis, dietary supplementation may be required. Since the entry of fatty acids into the mitochondria requires L-carnitine, an L-carnitine deficiency has been proposed to explain the accumulation of fatty acids in the liver. Measurement of L-carnitine concentrations in different tissues from cats affected with HL, however, failed to support this hypothesis.[11–13]

A lack of apolipoprotein B100, as may occur in protein malnutrition, was proposed as a reason for the diminished ability of the liver to secrete VLDL. This hypothesis is contradicted by reports of hypertriglyceridemia in cats with HL[5,14,15] and by the less consistent finding of hypercholesterolemia in affected cats.[16,17] Additionally, Pazak and colleagues 1994,[14] reported increased serum concentrations of VLDL and LDL, associated with a modified composition of some lipoproteins. While VLDL secretion increases, it seems that lipoprotein metabolism is impaired by a series of phenomena. (1) Hypoinsulinemia develops, associated with prolonged anorexia. (2) Relative lack of insulin downregulates the activity of lipoprotein lipase, the enzyme that enables the uptake of triglycerides from circulating lipoproteins to meet the demands of cells in peripheral tissues. The result is that lipoproteins, especially VLDL and LDL, cannot deliver fatty acids to peripheral tissues. (3) The increased concentration of circulating lipoproteins (VLDL and LDL) and a modification of their composition (more triglycerides and less cholesterol in LDL and more cholesterol in high-density lipoprotein 2 [HDL 2] and HDL) suggest a decrease in activity of cholesterol ester transfer protein.[10]

These findings suggest that HL may be the consequence of profound and prolonged anorexia and subsequent dramatic lipolysis. Hepatic secretion of VLDL is actually increased in cats with HL, but even this may not be sufficient to prevent lipid overload of hepatocytes. The triglyceride content in the liver of cats with lipidosis averages 43% compared with 1% in the liver of healthy cats.[2] Obesity likely predisposes cats to HL during periods of reduced food intake because of the quantity of free fatty acids that can be rapidly released from peripheral fat stores as well as some preexisting insulin resistance related to obesity.[18] Baseline hepatic lipid content is likely also higher in obese cats.[19]

HISTORY AND CLINICAL SIGNS

Most cats affected with HL are middle-aged adults (median age, 7 years), although the condition has been reported in a wide age range of cats (0.5–20 years).[20] Most reports fail to show a breed or sex predilection, but one study suggested that female cats are overrepresented.[17] Most cats are overconditioned at presentation or historically. Anorexia is the primary, and sometimes the only, presenting complaint in cats with this syndrome. The period of inappetance or anorexia may be as short as 2 to 7 days[20] but is occasionally of several weeks' duration. Observant owners may report jaundice. Other historical findings are vomiting, weight loss, diarrhea or constipation, and poor haircoat. In the absence of signs associated with an underlying disease, severe hypokalemia or hepatic encephalopathy (HE), HL cats are commonly bright and alert despite profound anorexia and the presence of marked jaundice (**Fig. 1**A–C).

Physical examination commonly reveals dehydration, jaundice (in about 70% of cases), and hepatomegaly. A BCS is often difficult to assign due to the loss of muscle mass even while some fat stores are retained in a formerly obese cat. Characteristically, the falciform fat pad is retained and can be clearly seen on a lateral survey abdominal radiograph. Severe electrolyte depletion, especially hypokalemia, can result in marked muscle weakness. Coagulation abnormalities may result in easy bruising, such as at venipuncture or cystocentesis sites or where an ultrasound probe is applied (**Fig. 2**). Signs of HE (notably ptyalism and depression) occur in a minority of cases (4% of cats in the largest reported case series[20]) (**Fig. 3**). The mental status of such cats may change suddenly, within 24 hours, from alert and responsive to depressed. Measurement of fasting blood ammonia concentration may confirm HE; such patients will benefit from being fed a protein-restricted diet and other treatments for reduction of blood ammonia (see section on treatment).

Any historical signs or physical examination findings related to a concurrent disease can be superimposed on the above signs in cases where anorexia is triggered by another disease (secondary HL). Many different conditions have been described in association with HL. Potentially any disease inducing anorexia, especially in an overweight cat, can cause secondary lipidosis. Concurrent diseases have been recognized in as many as more than 90% of lipidosis cases in some studies and include other hepatic disorders, small intestinal diseases, pancreatitis, neoplasia, kidney disease, and diabetes mellitus.[20]

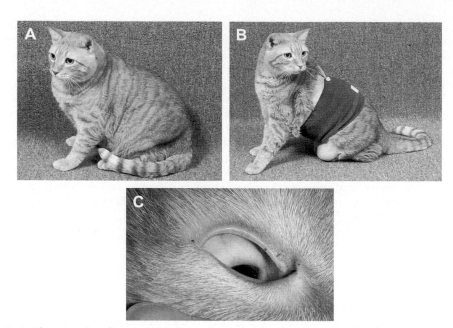

Fig. 1. Photographs of a cat at the time of examination for anorexia related to upper respiratory tract infection (*A*) and 2 weeks later after a gastrostomy tube had been placed for treatment of HL (*B*). Cats with HL are commonly bright and alert despite profound anorexia and the presence of marked jaundice (*C*).

CLINICOPATHOLOGIC FINDINGS

The complete blood cell count is often within normal limits in primary HL. Nonspecific abnormalities that may be encountered are mild to moderate normocytic, normochromic, nonregenerative anemia, lymphopenia, and mild leukocytosis. Poikilocytosis and Heinz bodies are commonly present at admission or may develop during treatment. It

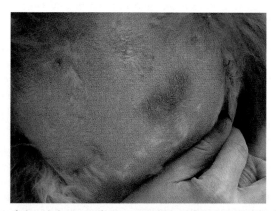

Fig. 2. Photograph of the abdomen of a 2-year-old cat showing the tendency toward easy bruising common in cats with HL. Prothrombin time and activated partial thromboplastin time were within reference ranges; the proteins invoked by vitamin K antagonism or absence (PIVKA) test was not performed. Also, note the marked jaundice.

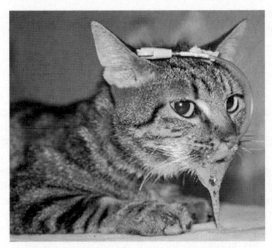

Fig. 3. Spayed female cat with a 3-week history of anorexia following a sudden diet change. She was presented for ptyalism and weakness. Note the amaurosis. She was icteric with hepatomegaly. A nasoesophageal tube was placed to start the nutritional treatment as early as possible.

is important to note that none of the hematologic findings shows any prognostic value.[17]

Clinicopathologic findings in HL are typical of an intrahepatic cholestatic disorder. The most consistent laboratory findings are increases in serum bilirubin and in serum activity of alkaline phosphatase (ALP). Serum activities of alanine aminotransferase (ALT) and aspartate aminotransferase (AST) are less consistently increased than ALP. Increases in serum gamma-glutamyl transpeptidase (GGT) are inconsistently seen. When cats with cholangitis are compared to cats with HL, lipidosis cases tend to have higher total bilirubin concentrations and higher ALT and ALP activities.[5,21,22] Increases in GGT tend to parallel increases in ALP in other forms of liver disease in cats, whereas in HL, GGT activity within the reference range is common.[17] Functional hepatic injury may be recognized by the presence of hypoglycemia, hypoalbuminemia, hyperammonemia, low blood urea nitrogen, and coagulation abnormalities.

Electrolyte alterations are encountered in some cases and are an important cause of morbidity and mortality (see the article by Center elsewhere in this issue). reported hypokalemia in 30% of HL cats, hypomagnesemia in 28%, and hypophosphatemia in 17%.[20] Hypocalcemia is uncommonly encountered and should prompt consideration of acute necrotizing pancreatitis, in which it has been reported to be a negative prognostic indicator.[23] Hypocalcemia should be confirmed by measurement of plasma ionized calcium concentration.

Hypertriglyceridemia is common,[5,10,14] sometimes associated with hypercholesterolemia.[5,14] HL cats may be transiently hyperglycemic, and hyperglycemia is prolonged during a glucose tolerance test.[8] Neither the serum insulin nor glucagon concentration has been found to be correlated with HL.[5] Serum concentrations of thyroxine are lower in cases of HL compared with healthy cats.[5]

Both fasting and postprandial serum bile acid concentrations are increased in HL cats, although these tests are not performed if the cat is jaundiced. Additionally, the profile of bile acids is modified, and some bile acids (cholic and glycocholic acids) are excreted in urine.[17] Serum bile acid concentrations improve once treatment has been started.[20] Urinalysis often shows bilirubinuria and lipiduria (refractile fat globules in urine). Ketonuria and modifications of the urine specific gravity may also be present.[11,17]

IMAGING FINDINGS

Hepatomegaly is a frequent finding in chronic cases; it may not be observed in early cases. On sonographic examination, hyperechoic changes in the hepatic parenchyma are characteristic and may make intrahepatic vessels hard to distinguish.[24] Hyperechogenicity, however, is not pathognomonic and may be seen in other feline hepatic disorders. Indeed, a recent study examined the diagnostic value of changes in sonographic appearance of the liver in cats and dogs and concluded that statistical evaluation of the applied ultrasonographic criteria did not yield clinically acceptable accuracy for discrimination among seven categories of diffuse infiltrative liver diseases (including normal liver) in either species.[25] Additionally, clinically normal obese cats may have a liver that is hyperechoic relative to the fat of the falciform ligament.[19] Lipiduria may impart an unusual sonographic appearance to the urinary bladder. (K.A. Spaulding, DVM, DACVR, personal communication, 2009) (**Fig. 4**).

DIAGNOSIS

The diagnostic goal in cats with HL is two-fold: definitive diagnosis of the presence of lipidosis and simultaneous workup for the presence of an underlying disease process. Careful physical examination and laboratory and imaging evaluation are crucial in cats with signs of lipidosis in order not to overlook concurrent disorders.

The diagnosis of HL is based on compatible history, clinical signs, biochemical and sonographic findings plus cytologic, and/or histologic confirmation. It is important that the diagnosis be substantiated by aspiration cytology or, in some cases, liver biopsy (percutaneous ultrasound guided or obtained by laparoscopy or laparotomy). Reliance on aspiration cytology alone may confirm fatty change in the liver but miss other, potentially more important, diagnoses. In a retrospective study involving 41 cats and 56 dogs, histologic and cytologic diagnoses were categorized as vacuolar

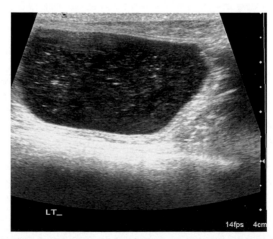

Fig. 4. Ultrasonographic appearance of lipiduria in a cat with HL. Note the sonographic shadowing as a result of lipid globules floating in the urinary bladder. *(Courtesy of* K.A Spaulding, DVM, DACVR, College Station, TX.)

hepatopathy, inflammation, neoplasia, cirrhosis, primary cholestasis, shunt, normal, and other.[26] Vacuolar hepatopathy was the category with the highest percentage of agreement between the histopathologic and cytologic diagnoses, but there was still concordance in only approximately 51% in cats. This study confirmed previous case reports where inflammatory and neoplastic lesions, documented by histopathology and present concurrently with vacuolar change, were not seen on cytologic evaluation.[27] Fine-needle aspiration cytology is a useful diagnostic procedure with many advantages, but care must be taken to avoid diagnosing HL as the cause of illness when an infiltrative hepatic disease may be primarily responsible.

Fine-needle hepatic aspiration cytology typically shows vacuolation of a majority of sampled hepatocytes. When stained with Wright's stain or Diff-Quik, hepatocytes are filled with variably sized, sharply defined, empty-appearing vacuoles (**Fig. 5**). Macrovesicular lipidosis may cause nuclear margination (so-called signet ring appearance) and make hepatocytes difficult to recognize. Both microvesicular and macrovesicular change, or a combination, are consistent with a diagnosis of HL.[28] Severely affected hepatocytes may be easily disrupted, leading to a background of free lipid and other cytoplasmic contents between clusters of intact hepatocytes. It is important to identify hepatocytes, as aspiration of falciform or subcutaneous fat may otherwise erroneously be interpreted as HL.

As discussed in the treatment section, it is often prudent to delay anesthesia in HL cats until they have been fed for a few days. This sequence of events lends itself to initial feeding via a nasoesophageal (NE) tube and performing fine-needle aspiration cytology (sedation generally not required) with ultrasound guidance during the initial evaluation of the cat, followed by a short anesthesia for indwelling feeding tube placement a few days later. It is not necessary, or even prudent, to perform a biopsy on every HL cat. It is important, however, to obtain biopsy confirmation of the diagnosis if any inflammatory cells are seen on cytology or if the cat fails to respond as expected to nutritional support. For example, roughly a 50% reduction in the degree of hyperbilirubinemia is expected within about a week of initiation of therapy.[20] Failure to show this degree of improvement should raise concern that a concurrent hepatobiliary disease exists. Such cases should definitely be reevaluated sonographically and a liver biopsy obtained. Core biopsy procedures carry risk for iatrogenic injury, such as inadvertent sampling of major bile ducts, in cats. Caution should always be exercised in using a spring-loaded biopsy gun in cats if bile duct dilation is present (see another

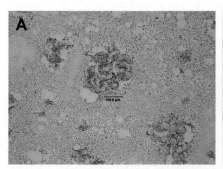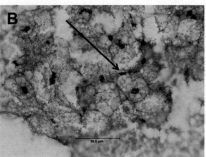

Fig. 5. A hepatic aspirate from an anorectic, icteric cat (Wright's stain). *A* shows clumps of intact hepatocytes in a background of material from disrupted cells (original magnification x10). The cytoplasm of the hepatocytes in *B* is distended with clear vacuoles of varying sizes (original magnification x50). Hepatocytes can be difficult to recognize due to nuclear margination *(arrow)*. *(Courtesy of* Jed Overmann, DVM, DACVP, St. Paul, MN.)

article elsewhere in this issue). For these reasons, when biopsies are indicated, sampling by laparoscopy is preferred by many internists. This approach also minimizes the risk of discordance between core needle and larger tissue samples.[29,30]

The liver parenchyma is typically very friable in cats with HL. In a series of 195 dogs and 51 cats undergoing ultrasound-guided, fine-needle aspiration and/or biopsy of abdominal organs at one institution, only three animals, two of them cats, had major postbiopsy complications, and both cats were diagnosed with HL.[31] Complications did not develop after any fine-needle aspirations. Another retrospective study found that 10.5% of cats undergoing percutaneous ultrasound-guided biopsy of an organ or tissue experienced a hemorrhagic complication requiring intervention.[32] The lowest hematocrit was usually reached within 5 hours postbiopsy, but in some cats, it took as long as 18 hours. Cats had an increase in hemorrhagic complications if the platelet count was less than 80,000/uL.[32] Other tests of coagulation can present a somewhat confusing picture regarding biopsy risk. It was reported that coagulation tests were abnormal in 45% of severe HL cats tested, but few showed clinical bleeding tendencies.[17] In a later report, prolonged clotting time was more reliably detected with a coagulation test sensitive to vitamin K deficiency (PIVKA or proteins invoked by vitamin K antagonism or absence), and there was generally a good response to administering three doses of vitamin K_1. Center[20] and Bigge and colleagues[32] found an activated partial thromboplastin time (aPTT) greater than 1.5 times the upper reference interval value correlated with an increased risk of hemorrhage; this study was not limited to hepatic biopsies. A fibrinogen level below 50% of the lower end of the reference interval may contraindicate taking a biopsy (see another article found elsewhere in this issue). Overall, biopsy-related risks warrant careful selection of cats for biopsy, prebiopsy screening for a coagulation disorder, prebiopsy treatment with vitamin K_1 if indicated, atraumatic biopsy technique, and careful postbiopsy monitoring. Minor postbiopsy hemorrhage may be detected ultrasonographically; these cats should be monitored especially closely for a few hours postbiopsy.

Laparotomy or laparoscopy shows an enlarged liver, with a homogenous dark apricot color, with reddish spots. Histopathology of the liver typically reveals diffuse, mixed microvesicular and microvesicular lipidosis (see another article elsewhere in this issue) (**Fig. 6**). In some cases, the steatosis is macrovesicular, where the accumulation of lipids forms vacuoles that are larger than the hepatocyte nuclei and tend to displace them. Intrahepatic cholestasis, seen as the presence of bile in fine linear deposits between hepatocytes, is commonly found. On ultrastructural examination, the number and form of peroxisomes in the hepatocytes may be impaired.[33]

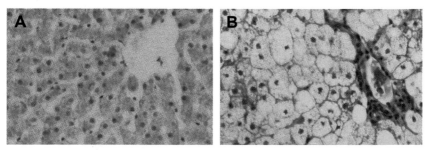

Fig. 6. (*A*) Liver biopsy from a healthy 2-year-old domestic shorthair cat. (*B*). Liver biopsy from a 2-year-old domestic shorthair cat with clinical findings of anorexia (3 week), weakness, lethargy, and jaundice. Note the diffuse hepatic vacuolization associated with HL. (hematoxylin-eosin, original magnification x40).

Peroxisomes are a major oxidation site for long-chain fatty acids. Hepatic histopathology gradually returns to normal following clinical recovery (**Fig. 7**).

Postmortem examination confirms the signs already described and related ones: diffuse hepatic steatosis (**Fig. 8**) and cholestasis, fatty infiltration of the bone marrow, retention of dramatic fat stores even in the face of marked weight loss and stores and loss of muscle mass, and occasionally Wallerian degeneration of the brain compatible with HE.

Treatment

Fluid and electrolyte therapy

Successful recovery of cats with HL requires correction and careful monitoring of fluid and electrolyte abnormalities (especially hypokalemia and hypophosphatemia), but the cornerstone of therapy is enteral nutritional support concentrating on meeting protein and caloric needs. This is best achieved by inserting an NE tube on the day of admission (see **Fig. 3**) followed a few days later by placement of either an esophagostomy or gastrostomy tube. An important component of treatment is recognition and management of any underlying process initially promoting the onset of HL.

On admission, attention must be given to rehydration therapy and correcting electrolyte imbalances primarily resulting from vomiting and lack of intake. Electrolyte abnormalities are an important cause of morbidity and mortality in HL cats. Potassium chloride needs to be judiciously added to the fluids according to a conventional sliding scale based on serum K (no more than 0.5 mEq/kg body weight [BW]/h). Hypokalemia may persist in the face of appropriate supplementation if there is concurrent hypomagnesemia. Magnesium is present in enteral diets in quantities sufficient to normalize serum levels. This is the preferred route of supplementation, but occasionally IV administration is necessary.[34] Fluid and enteral nutritional therapy should be accompanied by regular monitoring of serum electrolytes, especially potassium and phosphate concentrations, as these may drop precipitously in refeeding syndrome. In particular, potassium must be followed carefully (once or twice a day is recommended) for the first 72 hours and provided at a level of at least 0.6% dry matter in the diet. Enteral supplementation with potassium gluconate syrup, gel, or granules (starting at 2 mEq potassium per day per os) can be used when necessary, especially as parenteral fluid therapy is discontinued.[35]

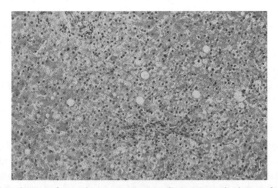

Fig. 7. Follow-up liver biopsy from the cat in **Fig. 6** taken 4 months later after supportive care and enteral feeding when the cat was clinically and biochemically normal. Note the few remaining fatty inclusions (hematoxylin-eosin, original magnification x16).

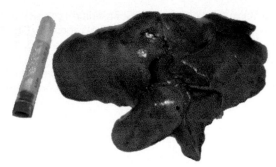

Fig. 8. Liver of a cat with HL. Note the yellow-orange color and hepatomegaly. The volume and weight of the liver are increased by three- to four fold.

Fluid supplementation with dextrose is contraindicated, as cats with HL are intolerant to glucose and such supplementation may exacerbate hyperglycemia.[8] Impaired lactate metabolism is suspected in some cats with HL and is the reason that some authors advise against using lactate-containing fluids. This seems more of a concern in theory than in practice. A balanced, polyionic crystalloid solution (with appropriate supplements) such as Ringer's is ideal, but lactated Ringer's solution is routinely used with success.

ENTERAL FEEDING
Tube Selection

Enteral feeding must be initiated as early as possible in the course of HL and sustained until voluntary intake resumes. The most useful methods for enteral support are feeding via NE, esophagostomy, or percutaneous gastrostomy tube (**Table 1**). Oral forced feeding is of limited benefit in cats that have been anorectic for prolonged periods and can be stressful when performed. It should only be attempted for a short time and abandoned in favor of a tube-feeding technique if unsuccessful in inducing significant voluntary food intake within 1 to 2 days. Concern also exists about inducing learned food aversion when forced feeding is used.

An NE is inexpensive, does not require anesthesia for placement, and is easy to use and remove but requires closer observation of the cat ± use of an Elizabethan collar, as it is more easily removed by the cat than either an esophagostomy or gastrostomy tube (**Fig. 9**A). Feeding through an NE tube necessitates feeding a liquid diet. Placement of either an esophagostomy or percutaneous non-endoscopic gastrostomy tube requires a short anesthesia, but either tube allows the use of a blended solid (canned) food and is sufficiently durable for reliable use in a home environment (**Fig. 9**B, C). Propofol can be safely used in HL cats as an anesthetic agent, such as for placement of a feeding tube.[36] Liquid oral medications may also be administered through any type of feeding tube.

Diet Selection

The first diets used for enteral forced feeding of cats with HL were those designed for human patients, relatively poor in protein and lipid and rich in carbohydrates, especially glucose. The work of Biourge and colleagues[4,37] indicates that dietary protein is the nutrient class that is most efficient at reducing hepatic lipid accumulation in cats in negative energy balance. Small amounts of protein administered to obese cats during fasting significantly reduced accumulation of lipid in the liver, prevented increases in

Table 1 Enteral feeding tube choices		
Tube	Size	Use/Remarks
Nasoesophageal	8 Fr with radiopaque marker (5 Fr for very small cats and brachycephalic breeds)	Available for immediate placement in any anorectic cat even while diagnostic tests are pending. Does not require sedation or anesthesia for placement. Verify correct positioning radiographically. Duration of use usually <2 weeks.
Esophagostomy	14 Fr	Requires short anesthesia for placement. Place after enteral support given for several days. Suitable for longer duration use (weeks to a few months).
Percutaneous gastrostomy	18 Fr	Requires short anesthesia for placement. Place after enteral support given for several days. Suitable for very long duration use (months).

Abbreviation: NE, nasoesophageal.

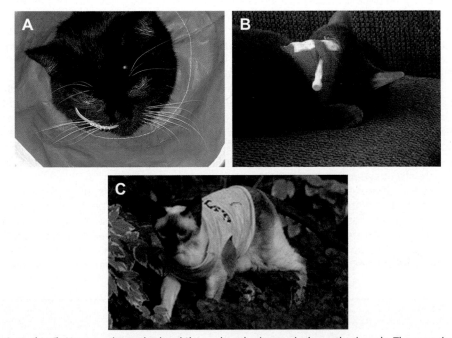

Fig. 9. (*A–C*). Nasoesophageal tubes (*A*) are placed using topical anesthesia only. They require close observation of the cat than either an esophagostomy or gastrostomy tube, as they are more easily removed by the cat. Use of an Elizabethan collar with an NE tube is prudent in most cats; flexible collars (*A*) are comfortable and interfere minimally with normal activities. Esophagostomy (*B*) and gastrostomy (*C*) tubes are well suited to home use by owners. (Fig. 9C *courtesy of* Kristy Walker, Minneapolis, MN.)

ALP activity, eliminated negative nitrogen balance, and appeared to minimize muscle catabolism. These findings emphasize the importance of providing HL cats with adequate protein during recovery. In these studies, carbohydrate supplementation reduced hepatic lipid accumulation, but metabolic abnormalities still developed.

Carbohydrates are usually less well tolerated than lipids as a source of calories in cats. Diarrhea, abdominal cramping, borborygmus, and hyperglycemia may be associated with the use of diets that are too high in carbohydrates, as confirmed by Simpson and Michel[38] and the authors' own experience.

As a result of the above considerations, the diet selected to feed a cat with HL should be rich in protein (30%–40% of the energy), moderate in lipids (about 50% of the energy), and relatively poor in carbohydrate (about 20%, preferably as glucose, which requires no digestion but constitutes a good energy source for enterocytes). (**Table 2**). Liquid diets balanced for cats and meeting these criteria are now commercially available for use through an NE tube (eg, EnteralCare HLP, PetAg, Inc., Hampshire, Illinois, per 100 g: 76.5 g water, 125.9 kcal, 10.7g protein, 6.1 g fat, 5.3 g carbohydrate; and FORTOL C+, Intervet/Schering-Plough Animal Health-Angers Technopole, Beaucouze, France, per 100 g: 80.1 g water, 100 kcal, 8.0 g protein, 5.3 g fat, 5.0 g carbohydrate). Recovery formula commercial canned diets are suitable for feeding through an esophagostomy or a gastrostomy tube.

Refeeding Program

Many cats with lipidosis are initially volume sensitive. The feeding schedule is determined by the patient's ability to tolerate food and the logistics of feeding. Two aspects have to be considered: the amount of food per day and per meal and the interval between consecutive meals. The stomach volume of a cat with HL may be dramatically reduced to as little as 10% of its original volume (**Fig. 10**A–D). To avoid vomiting, it is best to use a continuous rate infusion (CRI) or provide a small amount of food at a time, with an interval of 2.5 to 3 hours between meals.

Nutritional support should aim to deliver sufficient amounts of a nutritionally balanced food to meet the cat's resting energy requirement (RER) at its current weight when the BCS is 3/5 (5/9) or less. In most cats, 50 to 60 kcal/kg BW/d approximates RER. Cats with a BCS greater than 3/5 (or >5/9) generally have the same muscle mass as those with a BCS of 3/5; therefore, RER is calculated based on estimated optimal weight to prevent overfeeding. This is an important consideration as many cats with HL are still obese at presentation.

Feeding approximately 20% of RER on day 1 (in divided feedings) and then increasing the amount by 10% every 24 hours (**Table 3**) may be better tolerated than schedules that reach RER faster. Some cats, especially those that experienced a relatively short period of anorexia, will tolerate reaching full feeding more rapidly (3–5 days). Foods should be warmed to room temperature, but not higher than body temperature, before feeding. Food boluses must be infused slowly (over

Table 2
Diet profile for cats with hepatic lipidosis

Energy Source	Caloric Distribution (%)	Other Nutrients	
Protein	>32	Essential amino acids including arginine and taurine	Minerals
Fat	>40	Essential fatty acids	Trace elements
Carbohydrate	≈20	Preferably glucose	Vitamins

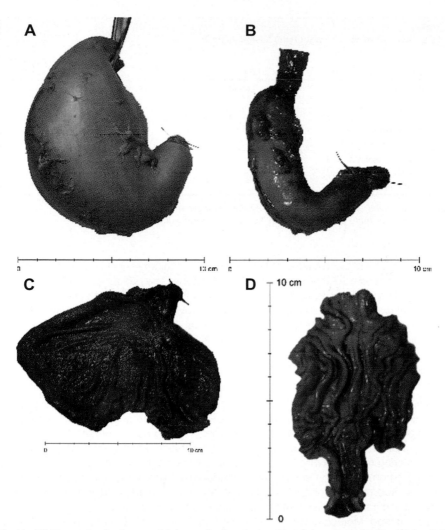

Fig. 10. (*A*) Stomach of a 2-year-old domestic shorthair x Abyssinian cat weighing 2.2 kg (BCS 3/5) that died after being hit by a car. The stomach was examined immediately postmortem, ligated at the cardia, and carefully filled by syringe. The volume of the stomach was 140 mL. Note the light pink color of the serosa and overall appearance of the normal stomach. (*B*) Stomach of a 2-year-old domestic shorthair x Abyssinian cat weighing 2.2 kg (BCS 3/5) that died of HL. The stomach was handled in the same manner as the stomach in *A*. The volume of the stomach was 15 mL. Note the yellowish discoloration due to icterus. (*C*) Same stomach as in *A*, opened along the greater curvature. Note the normal light pink color of the gastric mucosa. (*D*) Same stomach as in *B*, opened along the greater curvature. Note the pale, dull appearance of the mucosa and the persistence of rugal folds despite post-mortem distention with fluid.

approximately 1 minute) to allow gastric expansion. Daily food dosage should be divided into several meals, usually four to five, when feeding is begun and three to four per day as volume tolerance increases. Feeding should be stopped at the first sign of gulping, retching, or salivating, the meal size reduced by 50% for 12 hours and then increased gradually. Each meal must be followed by a water flush to clear

Table 3
Suggested refeeding plan for cats with hepatic lipidosis

Day of Refeeding	D1	D2	D3	D4	D5	D6 to D9	Until Appetite is Recovered
% of MER to cover	10–20	20–30	30–40	40–50	50–60	60–100	100
Kcal ME/kg optimal body weight	5–12	10–18	15–24	20–30	25–36	30–60	50 to 60[a]
Number of meals (at least 3 h between meals)	4–5	4–5	4	4	4	4	4 to 3

Abbreviations: ME, metabolizable energy; MER, maintenance energy requirement.
[a] MER for neutered cats is 50 kcal ME/kg optimal body weight.

the feeding tube of food residue. When the patient is volume sensitive, it is important to know the minimum volume required to flush the tube. The patient's daily fluid requirement must be met, and additional water may be administered through the feeding tube to meet that requirement. The amount of water provided by the liquid diet must be deducted from the total water requirement of the cat. The water bolus may be provided 30 minutes before a meal.

OTHER THERAPEUTIC CONSIDERATIONS
Antiemetic Therapy

Vomiting is a common clinical problem in cats with HL and often persists during the first week of refeeding despite use of a CRI or gradual introduction of increasing meal volumes. The authors have observed that vomiting can sometimes be alleviated by minimizing handling of the patient at the time of feeding and immediately afterward. Administering the meal while the cat is in its hospital cage (or in the cat's usual sitting area in the home environment) is recommended if gulping, apparent nausea, or vomiting occur soon after feeding. It is critical to continue to feed some food even if some vomiting occurs (see earlier section), and use of antiemetics will often facilitate reintroduction of food. Metoclopramide (CRI of 1–2 mg/kg/d or 0.2–0.5 mg/kg q8h subcutaneously (SC) 30 minutes before feeding) is often a first-choice drug because of availability and low cost, and because it has both antiemetic and prokinetic effects. Metoclopramide is a weak antiemetic in cats, however, and better control of emesis may be obtained by use of maropitant (Cerenia, Pfizer; 1 mg/kg IV, SC or orally q24h),[39] dolasetron (Anzemet, Hoecht Marion Russel; 0.5–0.6 mg/kg q24h IV, SC, or orally), or ondansetron (0.22 mg/kg q8–12h IV). An H_2 receptor antagonist (famotidine 0.5–1.0 mg/kg q12–24h IV or orally) is often used to protect the lower esophagus from acid damage and to help alleviate possible gastritis.

Cobalamin Therapy

Evaluation of plasma B_{12} (cobalamin) concentrations in cats with lipidosis revealed that 40% had subnormal values.[38] All cats with concurrent diagnoses of HL and inflammatory bowel disease had subnormal concentrations. Cobalamin deficiency is occasionally severe enough to produce neuromuscular signs, such as neck ventroflexion, anisocoria, papillary dilatation, vestibular signs, postural reaction deficits, and seizures. The route of choice for cobalamin supplementation is parenteral injection (250 µg/injection once weekly for 6 weeks, once every 2 weeks for 6 weeks, and then monthly as assessed by measurement of serum cobalamin concentration).

Treatment of Coagulation Disorders

Vitamin K deficiency is frequently suspected in cats with HL,[20,40] and supplementation may be beneficial in cats with impaired coagulation.[20] Response to vitamin K suggests that prolongation of coagulation tests in cats with HL is more often the result of vitamin K deficiency than decreased factor production because of failure of liver function. Vitamin K deficiency likely arises because of reduced absorption of fat-soluble vitamins due to impaired enterohepatic circulation of bile acids.[20] This makes parenteral, rather than oral, supplementation important. If coagulation abnormalities are present, administer 2 to 3 doses of vitamin K_1 (0.5–1.5 mg/kg SQ or intramuscularly at 12-hour intervals using a 25-g needle). This treatment is particularly important if a biopsy is to be obtained. More severe coagulopathies, disseminated intravascular coagulation, for example, may require treatment with fresh-frozen plasma or blood products ± heparin.

Other Nutrients

Supplementation with other nutrients has been suggested by several authors,[20,41,42–44] but beyond meeting the nutritional requirements, supplement use is still poorly scientifically documented in the cat. To date, no prospective clinical trials have been conducted to evaluate specific nutrients or supplements in cats with spontaneous HL. Prescribing multiple supplements and medications risks decreasing client compliance with feeding instructions.

L-carnitine is the nutrient that has been studied the most. It seems to have an interesting effect in fatty acid oxidation in cats with negative energy balance and in the early treatment of HL.[11,20] L-carnitine may be provided orally at a dose of 250 to 500 mg/d.[20] Some authors advocate routinely providing L-carnitine to HL cats (250 mg orally/d) for the theoretical reason of promoting fatty acid oxidation and retention of lean body mass. This metabolic response to L-carnitine has recently been proven in obese healthy cats undergoing weight loss,[11] but evidence is lacking that it provides any benefit in recovery from HL.

Treatment of Hepatic Encephalopathy

Treatment for HE is primarily achieved by improving hepatic function by enteral nutritional support and modulating the level of protein supplied in the enteral formula selected (see earlier section). In the small percentage of HL cats that show signs of HE at admission or have high blood ammonia concentrations, lactulose (0.3–0.5 mL/kg q8h orally) and neomycin (22 mg/kg q8h PO) are administered initially. Both medications may be given through an NE tube. Lactulose may also be given by retention enema.

Appetite Stimulants

The use of appetite stimulants, such as mirtazapine, cyproheptadine, and clonazepam, is not recommended in cats with HL. Although such drugs may increase appetite transiently, they are unreliable for ensuring adequate caloric intake and encourage a false sense of nutritional success. Additionally, drug metabolism may be impaired in cats with HL, making dosing and side effects unpredictable. Benzodiazepine agonists (diazepam, oxazepam) and $5-HT_2$ agonists (cyproheptadine) can exacerbate preexisting HE, and diazepam, oxazepam, and cyproheptadine have been reported to cause fulminant liver failure in individual cases.[20]

Heinz Body Anemia

Even if not present initially, Heinz bodies may develop during treatment, warranting close monitoring of the hematocrit. Cats showing Heinz body hemolytic anemia may benefit from IV administration of a thiol substrate donor, such as n-acetylcysteine, followed by supplemental s-adenosylmethionine (SAMe) for several weeks.[20] N-acetylcysteine is administered at a rate of 140 mg/kg (20% solution diluted 1:4 or greater with saline) IV through a 0.2-μm nonpyrogenic filter over 20 minutes. Once enteric feeding is underway, SAMe replaces n-acetylcysteine therapy (see another article elsewhere in this issue). Low hepatic glutathione concentrations in the liver of cats with HL compared with healthy control feline liver are consistent with reduction in tissue antioxidant availability.[20]

PROGNOSIS

The two most important factors affecting the outcome for cats with HL are the presence or absence of a serious, irreversible concurrent disease and how early enteral nutritional support is begun. In the absence of diagnosis of a fatal underlying condition, recovery rates of 80% to 88%[10,45] can be expected if enteral feeding is initiated as early as possible in the course of the disease and sustained until voluntary intake resumes. Cats may need tube feeding for several (3–6) weeks, requiring the owner to be an active participant in their cat's recovery.

Positive prognostic factors have been reported by Center and colleagues[17] as younger age (which was also associated with a diagnosis of primary vs secondary HL) and higher median serum potassium concentration and hematocrit. Cats making a successful clinical recovery from HL demonstrate a gradual reduction in laboratory abnormalities over time. Expect the total bilirubin concentration to decline by 50% or more within 7 to 10 days, even though serum liver enzyme activities may remain close to values documented at the time of case admission.[20] Once a cat recovers from HL, recurrence is unlikely.

REFERENCES

1. Barsanti JA, Jones BD, Spano JS, et al. Prolonged anorexia associated with hepatic lipidosis in three cats. Feline Pract 1977;7:52–7.
2. Hall JA, Barstad LA, Connor WE. Lipid composition of hepatic and adipose tissues from normal cats and cats with idiopathic hepatic lipidosis. J Vet Intern Med 1997;11:238–42.
3. Lund EM, Armstrong PJ, Kirk CA, et al. Health status and population characteristics of dogs and cats examined at private veterinary practices in the United States. J Am Vet Med Assoc 1999;214:1336–41.
4. Biourge V, Massat B, Groff JM, et al. Effects of protein, lipid, or carbohydrate supplementation on hepatic lipid accumulation during rapid weight loss in obese cats. Am J Vet Res 1994a;55:1406–15.
5. Brown B, Mauldin GE, Armstrong J, et al. Metabolic and hormonal alterations in cats with hepatic lipidosis. J Vet Intern Med 2000;14(1):20–6.
6. Burrows CF, Chiapella AM, Jesyk P. Idiopathic feline hepatic lipidosis: the syndrome and speculations on the pathogenesis. Florida Vet J 1981;18–20.
7. Center SA, Baldwin BH, Dillingham S, et al. Diagnostic value of serum gamma-glutamyl transferase and alkaline phosphatase activities in hepatobiliary disease in the cat: 1975–1990. J Am Vet Med Assoc 1986;188(5):507–10.

8. Biourge V, Nelson RW, Feldman EC, et al. Effect of weight gain and subsequent weight loss on glucose tolerance and insulin response in healthy cats. J Vet Intern Med 1997;11(2):86–91.

9. Zawie DA, Garvey MS. Feline hepatic disease. Vet Clin North Am Small Anim Pract 1984;14(6):1210–6.

10. Blanchard G, Paragon BM, Sérougne C, et al. Plasma lipids, lipoprotein composition and profile during induction and treatment of hepatic lipidosis in cats and the metabolic effect of one daily meal in healthy cats. J Anim Physiol Anim Nutr (Berl) 2004;88(3–4):73–87.

11. Blanchard G, Paragon BM, Milliat F, et al. Dietary L-carnitine supplementation in obese cats alters carnitine metabolism and decreases ketosis during fasting and induced hepatic lipidosis. J Nutr 2002;132(2):204–10.

12. Jacobs G, Cornelius L, Keene B, et al. Comparison of plasma, liver, and skeletal muscle carnitine concentrations in cats with idiopathic hepatic lipidosis and in healthy cats. Am J Vet Res 1990;51(9):1349–51.

13. Jones BR, Wallace A, Hancock WS, et al. Cutaneous xanthomata associated with diabetes mellitus in a cat. J Small Anim Pract 1985;26:33–41.

14. Pazak HE, Bartges JW, Cornelius LC, et al. Characterization of serum lipoprotein profiles of healthy, adult cats and idiopathic feline hepatic lipidosis patients. J Nutr 1998;128(12 Suppl):2747S–50S.

15. Thornburg LP, Simpson S, Digilio K. Fatty liver syndrome in cats. J Am Anim Hosp Assoc 1982;18:397–400.

16. Biourge V, MacDonald MJ, King L. Feline hepatic lipidosis: pathogenesis and nutritional management. Comp Cont Educ Pract Vet [Small Animal] 1990;12:1244–58.

17. Center SA, Crawford MA, Guida L, et al. Retrospective study of 77 cats with severe hepatic lipidosis: 1975–1990. J Vet Intern Med 1993;7:349–59.

18. Hoenig M, Thomaseth K, Waldron M, et al. Insulin sensitivity, fat distribution, and adipocytokine response to different diets in lean and obese cats before and after weight loss. Am J Physiol Regul Integr Comp Physiol 2007;191:R227–34.

19. Nicoll RG, O'Brien RT, Jackson MW. Qualitative ultrasonography of the liver in obese cats. Vet Radiol Ultrasound 1998;39(1):47–50.

20. Center SA. Feline hepatic lipidosis. Vet Clin North Am Small Anim Pract 2005;35(1):225–69.

21. Gagne JM, Armstrong PJ, Weiss DJ, et al. Clinical features of inflammatory liver disease in cats: 41 cases (1983–1993). J Am Vet Med Assoc 1999;214(4):513–6.

22. Hubbard BS, Vulgamott JC. Feline hepatic lipidosis. Comp Cont Educ Pract Vet [Small Animal] 1992;14:459–564.

23. Kimmel SE, Washabau RW, Drobatz KJ. Incidence and prognostic value of low plasma ionized calcium concentration in cats with acute pancreatitis: 46 cases (1996–1998). J Am Vet Med Assoc 2001;219(8):1105–10.

24. Yeager AE, Mohammed H. Accuracy of ultrasonography in the detection of severe hepatic lipidosis in cats. Am J Vet Res 1992;53(4):597–9.

25. Feeney DA, Anderson KL, Ziegler LE, et al. Statistical relevance of ultrasonographic criteria in the assessment of diffuse liver disease in dogs and cats. Am J Vet Res 2008;69(2):212–21.

26. Wang KY, Panciera DL, Al-Rukibat RK, et al. Accuracy of ultrasound-guided fine-needle aspiration of the liver and cytologic findings in dogs and cats: 97 cases (1990–2000). J Am Vet Med Assoc 2004;224(1):75–8.

27. Willard MD, Weeks BR, Johnson M. Fine-needle aspirate cytology suggesting hepatic lipidosis in four cats with infiltrative hepatic disease. J Feline Med Surg 1999;1(4):215–20.

28. Meyer D. The liver. In: Raskin R, Meyer DJ, editors. Atlas of canine and feline cytology. Philadelphia: W.B. Saunders; 2001. p. 231–52.

29. Cole TL, Center SA, Flood SN, et al. Diagnostic comparison of needle and wedge biopsy specimens of the liver in dogs and cats. J Am Vet Med Assoc 2002; 220(10):1483–90.

30. Dimski DS, Taboada J. Feline idiopathic hepatic lipidosis. Vet Clin North Am Small Anim Pract 1995;25(2):357–72.

31. Léveillé R, Partington BP, Biller DS, et al. Complications after ultrasound-guided biopsy of abdominal structures in dogs and cats: 246 cases (1984–1991). J Am Vet Med Assoc 1993;203(3):413–5.

32. Bigge LA, Brown DJ, Penninck DG. Correlation between coagulation profile findings and bleeding complications after ultrasound-guided biopsies: 434 cases (1993–1996). J Am Anim Hosp Assoc 2001;37(3):228–33.

33. Center SA, Guida L, Zanelli E, et al. Ultrastructural hepatocellular features associated with severe hepatic lipidosis in cats. Am J Vet Res 1993;54(5):724–31.

34. Holan KM. Feline hepatic lipidosis. In: Bonagura JD, editor. Kirk's current veterinary therapy XIV. Philadelphia: Elsevier; 2008. p. 570–5.

35. Laflamme DP. Nutritional management of liver disease. In: Bonagura JD, editor. Kirk's current veterinary therapy XIII. Philadelphia: W.B. Saunders; 2000. p. 693–7.

36. Posner LP, Asakawa M, Erb HN. Use of propofol for anesthesia in cats with primary hepatic lipidosis: 44 cases (1995-2004). J Am Vet Med Assoc 2008; 232(12):1841–3.

37. Biourge V, Groff JM, Fisher C, et al. Nitrogen balance, plasma free amino acid concentrations and urinary orotic acid excretion during long-term fasting in cats. J Nutr 1994b;124:1094–103.

38. Simpson KW, Michel KE. Medical and nutritional management of feline pancreatitis. Presented at the Proceedings of the 18th American College of Veterinary Internal Medicine, Seattle, Washington, 2000.

39. Hickman MA, Cox SR, Mahabir S, et al. Safety, pharmacokinetics and use of the novel NK-1 receptor antagonist maropitant (Cerenia™) for the prevention of emesis and motion sickness in cats. J Vet Pharmacol Ther 2008;31:220–9.

40. Lisciandro SC, Hohenhaus A, Brooks M. Coagulation abnormalities in 22 cats with naturally occurring liver disease. J Vet Intern Med 1998;12(2):71–5.

41. Center SA. Nutritional support for dogs and cats with hepatobiliary disease. J Nutr 1998;128:2733S–46S.

42. Center SA, Warner K, Corbett J, et al. Proteins invoked by vitamin K absence and clotting times in clinically ill cats. J Vet Intern Med 2000;14(3):292–7.

43. Roudebush P, Davenport DJ, Dimski DS. Hepatobiliary disease. In: Hand MS, Thatcher CD, Remillard RL, et al, editors. Small animal clinical nutrition. 4th edition. Topeka (KS): Mark Morris Institute; 2000. p. 811–47.

44. Simpson KW, Fyfe J, Cornetta A, et al. Subnormal concentrations of serum cobalamin (vitamin B12) in cats with gastrointestinal disease. J Vet Intern Med 2001;15: 26–32.

45. Kuehn NF. Nutritional management of feline hepatic lipidosis. In: Reinhart GA, Carey DP, editors. Recent advances in canine and feline nutrition, vol.III. 2000 Iams Nutrition Symposium Proceedings. Wilmington (OH): Orange Frazier Press; 2000. p. 333–8.

Hepatobiliary Neoplasia in Dogs and Cats

Cheryl Balkman, DVM

KEYWORDS

- Liver • Hepatic • Biliary • Hepatobiliary
- Neoplasia • Dog • Cat

The liver is a site of both primary and secondary neoplasia. The prevalence of primary hepatobiliary neoplasia ranges from 0.6% to 2.6% of dogs based on necropsy studies.[1–3] Secondary tumors of the liver occur more frequently, with metastasis to the liver occurring in 30.6% to 36.8% of dogs with primary nonhepatic neoplasia.[3,4] Metastasis to the liver is most common from tumors of the spleen, pancreas, and gastrointestinal tract.

The prevalence of primary hepatobiliary tumors in cats has been reported to be 1.5%[5] and 2.3%[6] of cats undergo necropsies. When hematopoietic neoplasms were excluded in one study, 6.9% of tumors were hepatic in origin.[7] Currently, there are no comprehensive studies regarding the prevalence of metastatic liver disease in cats.

TUMOR TYPES

Primary hepatobiliary tumors can develop from the hepatocyte (hepatocellular adenoma, hepatocellular carcinoma); bile duct epithelium (biliary adenoma, biliary carcinoma); neuroendocrine cells (neuroendocrine carcinoma or carcinoid); or stromal cells (sarcomas). These can be further characterized based on their morphologic appearance: massive involving a large mass in one lobe, nodular with discrete nodules in several lobes, or diffuse where the entire liver or part of it is infiltrated with neoplastic cells.[1] Other neoplastic conditions that often involve the liver include lymphoma, disseminated histiocytic sarcoma, and systemic mastocytosis.

AGE, GENDER, AND BREED PREDILECTION

Hepatobiliary tumors are usually found in older animals between the ages of 9 and 12 years.[1–3,8–12] Carcinoids in dogs are usually diagnosed in slightly younger animals with a mean age of 8 years[1,13]; this may also be true for cats.[14] Some studies have reported

Department of Clinical Sciences, College of Veterinary Medicine, C3-506 Clinical Programs Center, Box 31, Cornell University, Ithaca, NY 14853–6401, USA
E-mail address: ceb11@cornell.edu

Vet Clin Small Anim 39 (2009) 617–625
doi:10.1016/j.cvsm.2009.01.001
0195-5616/09/$ – see front matter © 2009 Elsevier Inc. All rights reserved.

vetsmall.theclinics.com

more male dogs diagnosed with hepatocellular carcinoma[8] and more male cats with carcinoids[14] and bile duct tumors[10]; other studies have shown no differences between genders.[3,11] There are no breed predilections in either dogs or cats.

CLINICAL SIGNS
Dogs

Clinical signs for dogs with hepatobiliary tumors are nonspecific with anorexia, lethargy, vomiting, and weight loss the most common.[1–4,8,12,15] Other clinical signs reported include polyuria, polydipsia, abdominal distention, diarrhea, jaundice, dyspnea, seizures, myelopathy, hematochezia and melena less frequently.[1,15] In one study, 5 of 18 dogs had no clinical signs at the time of diagnosis.[16]

Cats

Anorexia, lethargy, and vomiting are the most common reported clinical signs in cats.[10,11,14] Cats with malignant tumors are more likely to show clinical signs than those with benign tumors.[11]

PHYSICAL EXAMINATION

Hepatomegaly or cranial abdominal mass is the most common physical examination abnormality in both dogs and cats.[2,3,8,12,16] Abdominal pain, ascites, and icterus are less frequent.[10,14]

LABORATORY
Dogs

Hematologic and biochemical changes in dogs are common but not specific for liver tumors. Anemia (20%–53%) and leukocytosis (26%–90%) are reported frequently.[1,8,12,13,16] Forty-six percent of dogs with massive hepatocellular carcinoma had thrombocytosis.[12] Abnormalities in coagulation profiles have been documented in dogs with primary hepatic neoplasia[12,17] and should be evaluated before invasive procedures. Liver enzymes are commonly elevated but are not specific for the diagnosis of neoplasia.[1–3,12,16,18] One report showed an association between liver enzyme elevations and prognosis.[12] Other biochemical abnormalities documented include hypoalbuminemia, hyperglobulinemia, hypoglycemia, and elevated bile acids.[1,2,12,16,19,20]

Cats

As with dogs, cats with hepatobiliary tumors have nonspecific hematologic and biochemical abnormalities. Twenty-eight percent of cats in one study had a leukocytosis.[10] Alanine aminotransferase, aspartate aminotransferase, and total bilirubin were higher in cats with malignant tumors compared with benign tumors in another study[11] but cannot be used to differentiate the two. Cats with neuroendocrine carcinomas of the bile duct or gallbladder are more likely to have liver specific biochemical abnormalities than cats with hepatic neuroendocrine carcinomas.[14] Azotemia was the most common biochemical abnormality in one report but was not characterized as primary renal or other[10] and may be a reflection of the age of the cats at diagnosis (11–14 years).

PARANEOPLASTIC SYNDROMES

Paraneoplastic hypoglycemia has been reported with hepatocellular carcinoma, hepatic leiomyosarcoma, and hemangiosarcoma in dogs.[21,22] Alopecia has been reported in cats with hepatocellular and bile duct carcinomas.[23,24] Thrombocytosis has been documented in 18 of 39 dogs with massive hepatocellular carcinoma and is currently being investigated to determine if this is a paraneoplastic phenomenon.[12]

IMAGING

Abdominal radiographs can be used to detect cranial abdominal masses in dogs and cats; however, ultrasound is the preferred method of imaging.[12,15,16] Ultrasound allows for the characterization of morphologic features of the tumor (massive, nodular, or diffuse) and also can be used to detect intra-abdominal metastasis. Ultrasound-guided fine-needle aspirate of a liver mass is a minimally invasive procedure that can be helpful in obtaining a diagnosis. Limitations of this diagnostic procedure should be acknowledged because agreement between cytology and histopathology has varied among studies from 14% to 86%.[25,26] Ultrasound-guided needle biopsy is a relatively safe procedure in patients with greater than 50,000/µL platelets and normal coagulation parameters.[27] Results of needle biopsies for liver tumors correlated with wedge biopsies in 7 of 10 cases in one study.[28] Three-view thoracic radiographs should be performed to rule out pulmonary metastasis. CT with contrast enhancement and MRI may help in determining the resectability of a tumor (discussed elsewhere in this issue).

TREATMENT AND PROGNOSIS OF SELECTED TUMOR TYPES
Hepatocellular Tumors

Hepatocellular adenomas are benign tumors found in both dogs and cats (**Fig. 1**).[3,11] They are more common than hepatocellular carcinoma in cats[11] and less common in dogs.[3] Hepatocellular carcinoma is the most common primary liver tumor in dogs (**Fig. 2**).[8] They are classified as massive, nodular, or diffuse. In one study, the majority were massive (61%), followed by nodular (29%) and diffuse (10%).[8] Liver lobectomy is the treatment of choice for dogs and cats with a solitary massive hepatocellular tumor. In one report of dogs with massive hepatocellular carcinoma, the perioperative mortality rate was 11.9% (5 of 42) with two dogs dying intraoperatively because of exsanguination; the complication rate was 28.6% (10 of 42 mild to moderate hemorrhage and 2 of 42 vascular compromise to adjacent liver lobe). Dogs with right-sided liver tumors are more likely to have surgical complications caused by the proximity to the caudal vena cava. The median survival time for dogs undergoing surgery was

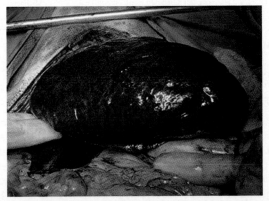

Fig. 1. Hepatocellular adenoma in a dog. (*Courtesy of* James Flanders, Ithaca, NY.)

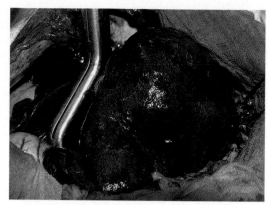

Fig. 2. Hepatocellular carcinoma in a dog. (*Courtesy of* James Flanders, Ithaca, NY.)

greater than 4 years.[12] Tumor recurrence is rare and reported to be 0% to 13% after liver lobectomy.[12,16] Dogs not undergoing surgical resection (N = 6) had a median survival time of 270 days with five of six dogs dying because of progressive disease.[12] The metastatic rate for hepatocellular carcinoma ranges from 4.8% to 61%.[3,8,12] The morphologic type and histopathologic features influence biologic behavior.[1,8] In one report 100% of the diffuse type, 93% of the nodular type, and 37% of the massive type had metastatic disease at necropsy.[8] Early detection may also influence the rate of metastasis because the lowest rate was from a report on dogs that underwent curative intent surgery. The most common sites of metastasis are local lymph nodes, lung, and peritoneum.[3,8] Data on cats with hepatocellular carcinoma are limited; in one report two of eight cats had metastatic disease at necropsy.[9]

Bile Duct Tumors

Bile duct adenomas are benign tumors derived from biliary epithelium. They are rarely documented in dogs.[3] Bile duct adenocarcinomas occur more commonly[1,3] and behave aggressively with metastasis documented in 60% to 88% of necropsy cases. The most common sites of metastasis are local lymph nodes and lungs with other abdominal organs and bone reported less frequently.[1,3] In cats benign bile duct adenomas (also referred to as "biliary adenomas," "biliary cystadenomas," or "cholangiocellular adenomas") are the most common hepatobiliary tumor (**Fig. 3**) followed by bile duct adenocarcinomas (cholangiocarcinomas).[10,11] As in dogs, carcinomas of the biliary system behave aggressively in cats with metastasis detected in 80% in one report[9]; in another report all 10 cats with bile duct carcinomas died or were euthanized during hospitalization.[11] Bile duct tumors that are solitary or confined to one liver lobe with no evidence of lymph node or distant metastasis should be surgically excised. Effective chemotherapy agents have not been identified.

Neuroendocrine Tumors (carcinoids)

In dogs hepatic neuroendocrine tumors are uncommon and typically have a diffuse morphology[13,29] making surgical excision rarely an option. Effective therapy remains to be determined. A few case reports have documented neuroendocrine tumors of the gallbladder in dogs.[30–32] All dogs seemed to have localized disease and had cholecystectomies performed. Long-term follow-up is lacking but one dog lived 8 months before recurrent gastrointestinal signs developed and another lived 10 months without evidence of recurrent disease before being lost to follow-up.[31,32] Neuroendocrine

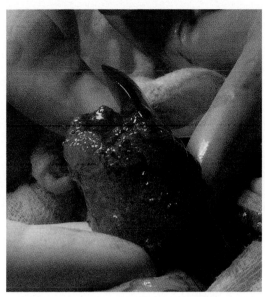

Fig. 3. Multifocal biliary cystadenoma in a cat. (*Courtesy of* James Flanders, Ithaca, NY.)

tumors in cats can be intrahepatic or extrahepatic involving the bile duct and rarely involve the gallbladder.[14] One cat with a composite tumor (elements of both epithelial and neuroendocrine carcinoma) lived for over a year before dying of another unrelated tumor, and two cats with extrahepatic tumors lived for over a year before being lost to follow-up.[14] The remaining 14 cats were euthanized during or soon after surgery. Four cats underwent necropsies; all had metastatic disease. Sites of metastasis included lymph nodes, lungs, and intestine, and all had carcinomatosis.

Sarcomas

Hepatic sarcomas make up less than 13% of primary hepatic tumors in the dog.[1,3] Hemangiosarcoma, leiomyosarcoma, fibrosarcoma, osteosarcoma, malignant mesenchymoma, and chondrosarcoma have been reported.[1,3,33–37] Primary sarcomas of the liver tend to behave aggressively having either a diffuse morphology or metastatic disease at diagnosis (**Fig. 4**).

Primary sarcomas of the liver are also rare in cats. Case reports and case series have documented hemangiosarcoma, leiomyosarcoma, rhabdomyosarcoma, and osteosarcoma.[9–11,38–40] Most cats with hemangiosarcoma had metastatic disease at diagnosis.[9,38] A cat with a primary extraskeletal hepatic osteosarcoma was treated with surgery and carboplatin and was alive 42 months after diagnosis with no clinical evidence of disease.[40]

Lymphoma

Lymphoma is a common neoplasia in both dogs and cats.[41] In dogs the liver can be involved in variable forms including multicentric, alimentary,[41,43–45] or hepatosplenic lymphoma.[46,47] A study in cats documented that abdominal lymphoma is currently the most common anatomic location[48] and the liver occasionally is the only organ involved.[48–50] Low-grade lymphocytic lymphoma affects the intestinal tract of older, feline leukemia virus negative cats and has a better prognosis than high-grade lymphoma.[50–52] In two reports the liver was involved in 20% to 24% of cats with

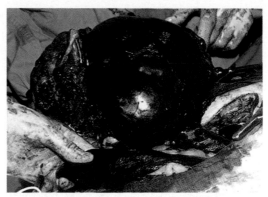

Fig. 4. Primary hepatic anaplastic sarcoma in a dog. (*Courtesy of* James Flanders, Ithaca, NY.)

lymphocytic lymphoma,[49,50] although the number of cats that had liver biopsies was small so the true extent of liver involvement is unknown. Median survival times are reported to be 2 years or more with prednisone and chlorambucil chemotherapy.[50,52] Studies are ongoing to determine if some of the inflammatory liver diseases in cats are small cell lymphocytic lymphoma (Sharon Center, personal communication, 2008). Another type of lymphoma that often affects the liver of cats is lymphoma of large granular lymphocytes, which is thought to originate in the small intestine. Hepatomegaly was documented in 80% of cats in one study and 12 of 13 had histologic confirmation of lymphoma in the liver.[42] Alanine aminotransferase and total bilirubin were increased in 7 of 12 and 7 of 13 cats respectively.[52]

The best treatment to date for high-grade lymphomas in dogs and cats is a combination protocol that contains doxorubicin, vincristine, cyclophosphamide, and prednisone.[41] Careful evaluation of liver function is necessary before starting chemotherapy because many drugs undergo hepatic metabolism and altered hepatic clearance may lead to unpredictable and potentially increased toxicity.[53]

Histiocytic Sarcoma

Disseminated histiocytic sarcoma of dogs frequently involves the liver and other organs.[54,55] CCNU has shown some efficacy with 46% of dogs responding with a median remission duration of 85 days and median survival time of 172 days.[55]

Mast Cell Tumors

Mast cell tumors can metastasize to the liver of dogs in advanced disease and rarely have been implicated as the primary site.[55–57] The overall prognosis of dogs with disseminated mast cell tumor is grave. The median survival times reported in one study was 43 days despite therapy with various chemotherapy agents.[58] Chemotherapeutic drugs most active against mast cell tumors include vinblastine and lomustine.[59,60] Recently, tyrosine kinase inhibitors have shown some promise.[61]

Primary visceral mast cell tumors are more common in cats than dogs. The spleen is usually the primary site with metastasis to the liver and bone marrow common.[62] Survival time with splenectomy alone can be a year or more. Recently, lomustine (CCNU) has been shown to be active against feline mast cell tumors.[63]

SUMMARY

Hepatobiliary tumors are uncommon in dogs and cats. They generally occur in older animals with nonspecific clinical signs usually relating to the gastrointestinal tract. Liver enzyme concentrations are commonly elevated. Early detection for massive-type lesions may allow for surgical resection and prolonged survival especially for hepatocellular carcinomas. Chemotherapy, in general, is not effective for primary liver tumors.

REFERENCES

1. Patnaik AK, Hurvitz AI, Lieberman PH. Canine hepatic neoplasms: a clinicopathologic study. Vet Pathol 1980;17:553–64.
2. Strombeck DR. Clinicopathologic features of primary and metastatic neoplastic disease of the liver in dogs. J Am Vet Med Assoc 1978;173(3):267–9.
3. Trigo FJ, Thompson H, Breeze RG, et al. The pathology of liver tumors in the dog. J Comp Pathol 1982;92:21–39.
4. McConnell MF, Lumsden JH. Biochemical evaluation of metastatic liver disease in the dog. J Am Anim Hosp Assoc 1983;19:173–8.
5. Engle GC, Brodey RS. A retrospective study of 395 feline neoplasms. J Am Anim Hosp Assoc 1969;5:21–31.
6. Schmidt RE, Langham RF. A survey of feline neoplasms. J Am Vet Med Assoc 1967;151:1325–8.
7. Patnaik AK, Liu SK, Hurvitz AI, et al. Nonhematopoietic neoplasms in cats. J Natl Cancer Inst 1975;54:855–60.
8. Patnaik AK, Hurvitz AI, Lieberman PH, et al. Canine hepatocellular carcinoma. Vet Pathol 1981;18:427–38.
9. Patnaik AK. A morphological and immunocytochemical study of hepatic neoplasms in cats. Vet Pathol 1992;29:405–15.
10. Post G, Patnaik AK. Nonhematopoietic hepatic neoplasms in cats: 21 cases (1983–1988). J Am Vet Med Assoc 1992;201:1080–2.
11. Lawrence HJ, Erb HN, Harvey HJ. Nonlymphomatous hepatobiliary masses in cats: 41 cases (1972 to 1991). Vet Surg 1994;23:365–8.
12. Liptak JM, Dernell WS, Monnet E, et al. Massive hepatocellular carcinoma in dogs: 48 cases (1992–2002). J Am Vet Med Assoc 2004;225:1225–30.
13. Patnaik AK, Newman SJ, Scase T, et al. Canine hepatic neuroendocrine carcinoma: an immunohistochemical and electron microscopic study. Vet Pathol 2005;42:140–6.
14. Patnaik AK, Lieberman PH, Erlandson RA, et al. Hepatobiliary neuroendocrine carcinoma in cats: a clinicopathologic, immunohistochemical, and ultrastructural study of 17 cases. Vet Pathol 2005;42:331–7.
15. Evans SM. The radiographic appearance of primary liver neoplasia in dogs. Vet Rad 1987;28:192–6.
16. Kosovsky JE, Manfra-Marretta S, Matthiesen DT, et al. Results of partial hepatectomy in 18 dogs with hepatocellular carcinoma. J Am Anim Hosp Assoc 1989;25:203–6.
17. Badylak SF, Dodds J, Van Vleet JF. Plasma coagulation factor abnormalities in dogs with naturally occurring hepatic disease. Am J Vet Res 1983;44:2336–40.
18. Center SA, Slater MR, Manwarren T, et al. Diagnostic efficacy of serum alkaline phosphatase and gamma-glutamyltransferase in dogs with histologically confirmed hepatobiliary disease: 270 cases (1980–1990). J Am Vet Med Assoc 1992;201:1258–64.

19. Center SA, Baldwin BH, Erb HN, et al. Bile acid concentrations in the diagnosis of hepatobiliary disease in the dog. J Am Vet Med Assoc 1985;187:935–40.
20. Center SA, ManWarren T, Slater MR, et al. Evaluation of twelve-hour preprandial and two hour postprandial serum bile acids concentrations for diagnosis of hepatobiliary disease in dogs. J Am Vet Med Assoc 1991;199:217–26.
21. Leifer CE, Peterson ME, Matus RE, et al. Hypoglycemia associated with nonislet cell tumor in 13 dogs. J Am Vet Med Assoc 1985;186:53–5.
22. Zini E, Glaus TM, Minuto F, et al. Paraneoplastic hypoglycemia due to an insulin-like growth factor type-II secreting hepatocellular carcinoma in a dog. J Vet Intern Med 2007;21:193–5.
23. Marconato L, Albanese F, Viacava P, et al. Paraneoplastic alopecia associated with hepatocellular carcinoma in a cat. Vet Dermatol 2007;18:267–71.
24. Pascal-Tenorio A, Olivry T, Gross TL, et al. Paraneoplastic alopecia associated with internal malignancies in the cat. Vet Dermatol 1997;8:47–52.
25. Wang KY, Panciera DL, Al-Rukibat RK, et al. Accuracy of ultrasound-guided fine-needle aspiration of the liver and cytologic findings in dogs and cats: 97 cases (1990–2000). J Am Vet Med Assoc 2004;224:75–8.
26. Roth L. Comparison of liver cytology and biopsy diagnoses in dogs and cats: 56 cases. Vet Clin Pathol 2001;30:35–8.
27. Bigge LA, Brown DJ, Penninck DG. Correlation between coagulation profile findings and bleeding complications after ultrasound-guided biopsies: 434 cases (1993–1996). J Am Anim Hosp Assoc 2001;37:228–33.
28. Cole TL, Center SA, Flood SN, et al. Diagnostic comparison of needle and wedge biopsy specimens of the liver in dogs and cats. J Am Vet Med Assoc 2002;220:1483–90.
29. Patnaik AK, Lieberman PH, Hurvitz AI, et al. Canine hepatic carcinoids. Vet Path 1981;18:445–53.
30. Lippo NJ, Williams JE, Brawer RS, et al. Acute hemobilia and hemocholecyst in 2 dogs with gall bladder carcinoid. J Vet Intern Med 2008;22:1249–52.
31. Morrell CN, Volk MV, Mankowski JL. A carcinoid tumor in the gall bladder of a dog. Vet Path 2002;39:756–8.
32. Willard MD, Dunstan RW, Faulkner J. Neuroendocrine carcinoma of the gall bladder in a dog. J Am Vet Med Assoc 1988;192:926–8.
33. Patnaik AK, Liu S, Johnson GF. Extraskeletal osteosarcoma of the liver in a dog. J Small Anim Pract 1976;17:365–70.
34. Kapatkin AS, Mullen HS, Matthiesen DT, et al. Leiomyosarcoma in dogs: 44 cases (1883–1988). J Am Vet Med Assoc 1992;201:1077–9.
35. Jeraj K, Yano B, Osborne CA, et al. Primary hepatic osteosarcoma in a dog. J Am Vet Med Assoc 1981;179:1000–3.
36. McDonald RK, Helman RG. Hepatic mesenchymoma in a dog. J Am Vet Med Assoc 1986;188:1052–3.
37. Chikata S, Nakamura S, Katayama R, et al. Primary chondrosarcoma in the liver of a dog. Vet Path 2006;43:1033–6.
38. Culp WTN, Drobatz KJ, Glassman MM, et al. Feline visceral hemangiosarcoma. J Vet Intern Med 2008;22:148–52.
39. Minkus G, Hillemanns M. Botryoid-type embryonal rhabdomyosarcoma of liver in a young cat. Vet Pathol 1997;34:618–21.
40. Dhaliwal RS, Johnson TO, Kitchell BE. Primary extraskeletal hepatic osteosarcoma in a cat. J Am Vet Med Assoc 2003;222:340–2.
41. Vail DM, Young KM. Hematopoietic tumors. In: Withrow & MacEwen's small animal clinical oncology. 4th edition. St. Louis (MO): Saunders; 2007.

42. Roccabianca P, Vernau W, Caniatti M, et al. Feline large granular lymphocyte (LGL) lymphoma with secondary leukemia: primary intestinal origin with predominance of a CD3/CD8αα phenotype. Vet Pathol 2006;43:15–28.
43. French RA, Seitz SE, Valli VEO. Primary epitheliotropic alimentary T-cell lymphoma with hepatic involvement in a dog. Vet Pathol 1996;33:349–52.
44. Coyle KA, Steinberg H. Characterization of lymphocytes in canine gastrointestinal lymphoma. Vet Pathol 2004;41:141–6.
45. Frank JD, Reimer SB, Kass PH, et al. Clinical outcomes of 30 cases (1997–2004) of canine gastrointestinal lymphoma. J Am Anim Hosp Assoc 2007;43:313–21.
46. Cienava EA, Barnhart KF, Brown R, et al. Morphologic, immunohistochemical, and molecular characterization of hepatosplenic T-cell lymphoma in a dog. Vet Clin Path 2004;33:105–10.
47. Fry MM, Vernau W, Pesavento PA, et al. Hepatosplenic lymphoma in a dog. Vet Pathol 2003;40:556–62.
48. Louwerens M, London CA, Pedersen NC, et al. Feline lymphoma in the post feline leukemia virus era. J Vet Intern Med 2005;19:329–35.
49. Gabor LJ, Malik R, Canfield PJ. Clinical and anatomical features of lymphosarcoma in 118 cats. Aust Vet J 1998;76:725–32.
50. Kiselow MA, Rassnick KM, McDonough SP, et al. Outcome of cats with low-grade lymphocytic lymphoma: 41 cases (1995–2005). J Am Vet Med Assoc 2008;232:405–10.
51. Carreras JK, Goldschmidt M, Lamb M, et al. Feline epitheliotropic intestinal malignant lymphoma: 10 cases (1997–2000). J Vet Intern Med 2003;17:326–31.
52. Fondacaro JV, Richter KP, Carpenter JL, et al. Feline gastrointestinal lymphoma: 67 cases (1988–1996). Eur J Comp Gastroenterol 1999;4:5–11.
53. Collins J, Supko J. Pharmacokinetics. In: Chabner DL, Longo BA, editors. Cancer chemotherapy and biotherapy. 4th edition. Philadelphia: Lippincott, Williams, and Wilkins; 2006.
54. Affolter VK, Moore PF. Localized and disseminated histiocytic sarcoma of dendritic cell origin in dogs. Vet Pathol 2002;39:74–83.
55. Skorupski KA, Clifford CA, Paoloni MC, et al. CCNU for the treatment of dogs with histiocytic sarcoma. J Vet Intern Med 2007;21:121–6.
56. O'Keefe DA, Couto CG, Burke-Schwartz C, et al. Systemic mastocytosis in 16 dogs. J Vet Intern Med 1987;1:75–80.
57. Takahashi T, Kadosawa T, Nagase M, et al. Visceral mast cell tumors in dogs: 10 cases (1982–1997). J Am Vet Med Assoc 2000;216:222–6.
58. Marconato L, Bettini G, Giacoboni C, et al. Clinicopathological features and outcome for dogs with mast cell tumors and bone marrow involvement. J Vet Intern Med 2008;22:1001–7.
59. Thamm DH, Mauldin EA, Vail DM. Prednisone and vinblastine chemotherapy for canine mast cell tumor: 41 cases (1992–1997). J Vet Intern Med 1999;13:491–7.
60. Rassnick KM, Moore AS, Williams LE, et al. Treatment of canine mast cell tumors with CCNU (Lomustine). J Vet Intern Med 1999;13:601–5.
61. Isotani M, Ishida N, Tominaga M, et al. Effect of tyrosine kinase inhibition by Imatinib Mesylate on mast cell tumors in dogs. J Vet Intern Med 2008;22:985–8.
62. Liska WD, MacEwen EG, Zaki FA, et al. Feline systemic mastocytosis: a review and results of splenectomy in seven cases. J Am Anim Hosp Assoc 1979;15:589–97.
63. Rassnick KM, Williams LE, Kristal O, et al. Lomustine for treatment of mast cell tumors in cats: 38 cases (1999–2005). J Am Vet Med Assoc 2008;232:1200–5.

Hepatic Chemoembolization: A Novel Regional Therapy

KEYWORDS

- Liver • Hepatocellular carcinoma • Cancer
- Chemoembolization • Regional tumor therapy
- Embolization • Interventional radiology

Nonresectable and metastatic liver tumors are difficult challenges in veterinary patients. As such, these animals have traditionally been treated conservatively and symptomatically. The relatively limited efficacy of routine (intravenous) chemotherapy for macroscopic disease, and the cost and potential deleterious side effects associated with radiation therapy have led investigators to evaluate increasingly novel therapeutic modalities. Similar difficulties in human oncology have inspired various creative, image-guided, regional tumor therapies in the continuously developing subspecialty of interventional radiology termed "interventional oncology." Regional tumor therapies, as suggested by the name, have been designed to increase local tumor control without increasing systemic toxicities and side effects. These techniques are not indicated for all oncology patients, just those patients in whom surgery and radiation are not indicated, and where systemic therapies have failed to control the local disease. Regional techniques, such as percutaneous tumor ablation (including radiofrequency ablation, microwave ablation, laser thermal ablation, cryoablation, and percutaneous ethanol injection), and transcatheter arterial chemoembolization have been demonstrated to improve response rates and local control, and enhance tumor necrosis when compared with traditional therapies.[1] Percutaneous tumor ablation techniques used in the liver of humans tend to be most effective in patients with a few (<3), small (<4 cm diameter) lesions. Because these circumstances are less commonly encountered in the author's clinical experience in veterinary medicine, patients are more commonly candidates for chemoembolization for the palliative treatment of nonresectable and metastatic liver neoplasia.

In general, "embolotherapy" involves the use of fluoroscopy and other advanced imaging modalities to access specific vascular structures selectively to deliver embolic materials to control hemorrhage, occlude vascular malformations, or reduce tumor growth. These techniques are commonly used in human medicine for

Veterinary Hospital of the University of Pennsylvania, Philadelphia, PA 19104, USA
E-mail address: weissec@vet.upenn.edu

Vet Clin Small Anim 39 (2009) 627–630
doi:10.1016/j.cvsm.2009.01.003
0195-5616/09/$ – see front matter © 2009 Elsevier Inc. All rights reserved.
vetsmall.theclinics.com

embolization of arteriovenous malformations, intractable epistaxis or gastrointestinal bleeding, and uterine artery embolization for symptomatic uterine fibroids in women.

Chemoembolization involves selective intra-arterial chemotherapy delivery in conjunction with subsequent particle embolization. This technique has been demonstrated to result in a 10- to 50-fold increase in intratumoral drug concentrations when compared with systemic intravenous chemotherapy administration.[2] The subsequent particle embolization results in tumor cell necrosis and paralyzes tumor cell excretion of chemotherapy resulting in minimized systemic toxicity. This procedure is most commonly used in the treatment of diffuse hepatocellular carcinoma in humans but has also been used to treat other tumors of the liver and elsewhere in the body. Most hepatic tumors rely on hepatic arterial blood supply (up to 95%) for growth in contrast to the normal liver parenchyma, which receives most of its blood supply by the portal vein (approximately 80%).[3] Hepatic artery embolization should theoretically cause more ischemia to the liver tumor while the remaining normal hepatic parenchyma obtains sufficient oxygenation from the portal venous system. In addition, the chemotherapy is often mixed with Lipiodol, (Melville Laboratories, Savage, New Jersey), a carrier agent that is an oily substance that supplies radiographic contrast to the chemotherapy and acts as a tumor localizer. Because hepatic tumors lack Kupffer cells, which are important for metabolizing oily substances in normal hepatic parenchyma, the Lipiodol and accompanying chemotherapy are concentrated in the liver tumor rather than the surrounding healthy hepatic parenchyma (**Fig. 1**).[4] More recently, drug-eluting beads that bind to various chemotherapeutics have been evaluated to enhance the concentration and extend the duration of tumor-chemotherapy exposure.

Although often performed under conscious sedation in humans, the veterinary patients in the author's interventional radiology service are placed under general anesthesia and the entire chemoembolization procedure is performed in an angiography suite. Arterial access is usually achieved by cut-down to the femoral artery and the procedure is performed under fluoroscopic guidance using a combination of appropriately sized sheaths, catheters, and guidewires. Microcatheters and microwires are passed coaxially through the larger catheters to superselect very small vessels when necessary.

An intimate knowledge of vascular anatomy is required to ensure the tip of the catheter is beyond any branch points that may supply normal tissue. Once appropriate catheter placement has been confirmed angiographically, a slurry of chemotherapy (standard systemic dose) and Lipiodol, and appropriately sized particulate material

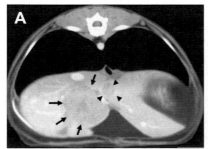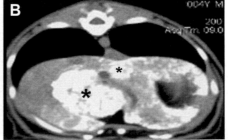

Fig. 1. Prechemoembolization and postchemoembolization CT scans of a cat with hepatocellular carcinoma. (*A*) Prechemoembolization axial CT demonstrating primary tumor (*arrows*) and metastatic lesion (*arrowheads*) within the liver. (*B*) Postchemoembolization axial CT demonstrating enhanced uptake of oily chemotherapy mixture (*asterisks*) caused by enhanced vascularity of tumor versus normal liver parenchyma.

(typically polyvinyl alcohol particles), are injected under fluoroscopic guidance until complete stasis of blood flow is achieved. Repeat selective and nonselective angiograms are performed to document complete embolization (**Fig. 2**). The vascular sheaths are removed and hemostasis is typically achieved by ligation of the femoral artery or direct manual compression for 20 minutes.

Reported complications in the human literature include hemorrhage at the vascular access site; nontarget embolization complications (skin necrosis, damage to normal parenchyma); hepatic infarction and abscessation; and postembolization syndrome, a collection of clinical signs characterized by malaise, fever, and pain.[5] It is premature to speculate if similar complications will occur in the veterinary population; however, the author has not yet identified other, unreported complications in patients. The goal of these therapies is generally palliative (reduced tumor growth); however, some tumors can shrink (**Fig. 3**) and chemoembolization may play a role in neoadjuvant therapy for larger solitary liver tumors.

Regional tumor therapies, such as chemoembolization, offer a new option for treatment of nonresectable and diffuse metastatic tumors. In human patients, chemoembolization of diffuse hepatocellular carcinoma has been shown to improve survival rates.[1] Median survival times of 3 to 6 months are expected, with systemic chemotherapy response rates of only approximately 20%.[1] Chemoembolization has improved median survival times to 1 to 2 years with positive biologic response (as determined by decreasing alpha fetoprotein levels) in 70% to 85% of subjects and morphologic response in 36%.[1]

In veterinary medicine, patients with relapsed tumors or progressive disease comprise a population for which few therapeutic options exist. Interventional radiology

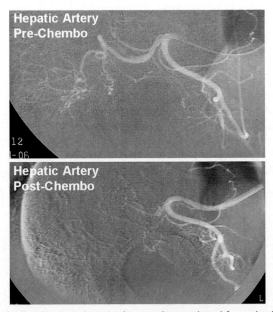

Fig. 2. Prechemoembolization arteriogram by a catheter placed from the femoral artery into the common hepatic artery demonstrating branching and arborization of hepatic artery branches and gastrodudodenal artery (*top*). Postchemoembolization arteriogram demonstrating complete embolization of hepatic artery branches with patent gastroduodenal artery (*bottom*).

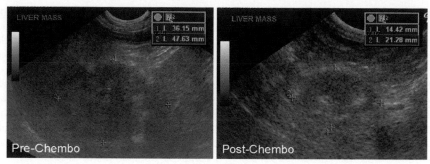

Fig. 3. Prechemoembolization and postchemoembolization abdominal ultrasonography images in a dog with recurrent hepatocellular carcinoma at the porta hepatis. (*Left panel*) Notice defined hepatic tumor with approximate 3.6 × 4.7 cm measurements. (*Right panel*) Six weeks following single chemoembolization treatment demonstrating similar appearance of tumor but with 1.4 × 2.1 cm measurements (partial remission). This dog had subsequent surgery to remove this mass as much as possible.

techniques offer the potential to prolong survival times and quality of life in these patients with minimal systemic toxicity risks. In the author's interventional radiology service, these techniques have been performed and reported on for diffuse hepatocellular carcinoma, metastatic bone tumors, and uterine fibroids among others.[6]

REFERENCES

1. Soulen MC. Multimodality image-guided therapy for liver tumors. Presented at the SIR Annual Meeting. Salt Lake City, UT, March 27–April 4, 2003.
2. Dyet J, Ettles D, Nicholson A, et al, editors. Textbook of endovascular procedures. 1st edition. Philadelphia: Churchill Livingstone; 2000. p. 357–67.
3. Breedis C, Young G. Blood supply of neoplasms of the liver. Am J Pathol 1954;30: 969–72.
4. Sichlau MJ. Regional therapy for hepatic malignancies. Applied Radiology 1999; 28(Suppl):3–10.
5. Hemingway AP, Allison DJ. Complications of embolization: analysis of 410 procedures. Radiology 1988;166(3):669–72.
6. Weisse C, Clifford CA, Holt D, et al. Percutaneous arterial embolization and chemoembolization for treatment of benign and malignant tumors in three dogs and a goat. JAVMA 2002;221(10):1430–6.

Therapeutic Use of Cytoprotective Agents in Canine and Feline Hepatobiliary Disease

Cynthia R.L. Webster, DVM[a], Johanna Cooper, DVM[b],*

KEYWORDS

- S-adenosylmethionine • N-acetylcysteine • Ursodeoxycholate
- Silymarin • Vitamin E • Glutathione

Hepatocytes by virtue of their pivotal role in metabolism and their anatomic juxtaposition between the intestinal lumen and the systemic circulation are uniquely susceptible to injury. As the principal site of metabolism and detoxification of endogenous metabolites, drugs, and xenobiotics, hepatocytes are routinely exposed to potentially toxic reactive intermediates. Because hepatocytes receive the majority of their blood supply from a venous rather than an oxygen-rich arterial circulation, they are susceptible to ischemic injury. In addition, as this blood supply drains, the gastrointestinal tract hepatocytes are exposed to anything toxic that is absorbed by enterocytes, including bacterial by-products and components such as lipopolysaccharide. The liver is also home to a large population of macrophages, the Kupffer cells, which stand poised and ready for activation with subsequent release of inflammatory and toxic cytokines. These cytokines, particularly tumor necrosis factor alpha (TNF-α), can augment and perpetuate liver injury.[1] Additionally, the liver contains a population of vitamin A–storing stellate cells that can transform during liver injury (under the influence of another cytokine, transforming growth factor beta [TGF-β]) into extracellular matrix–producing myofibroblasts that lead to hepatic fibrosis.[1,2]

Given this hostile environment, hepatocytes have developed several ways to protect themselves from harm. These protections include enzymatic (catalase, superoxide dismutase [SOD], and glutathione [GSH] peroxidase and transferase) and nonenzymatic (GSH, vitamin E, ascorbate) defense mechanisms.[2,3] Hepatocytes also respond to toxic insults by initiating intracellular prosurvival signaling pathways. These pathways are controlled by hormones (eg, glucagon) and growth factors (eg,

[a] Department of Clinical Sciences, Tufts Cummings School of Veterinary Medicine, 200 Westborough Road, North Grafton, MA 01589, USA
[b] Tufts VETS, Walpole, MA, USA
* Corresponding author.
E-mail address: jcoope02@gmail.com (J. Cooper).

Vet Clin Small Anim 39 (2009) 631–652
doi:10.1016/j.cvsm.2009.02.002
0195-5616/09/$ – see front matter © 2009 Elsevier Inc. All rights reserved.

hepatocyte growth factor), and work through the modulation of survival kinases.[4] Many medicinal, nutraceutical, and botanic extracts have cytoprotective properties in the liver.[3-12] These agents enhance natural defense mechanisms to inhibit inflammation and fibrosis, prevent apoptosis, or protect against oxidant injury by maintenance of an appropriate redox balance.

MECHANISMS OF HEPATOCYTE CELL DEATH

Injured hepatocytes die by either apoptosis or necrosis, and both forms of cell death accompany naturally occurring hepatobiliary disease in human and veterinary patients.[13,14] Necrosis is a random, nonenergy-dependent event that occurs secondary to overwhelming cellular damage, particularly to mitochondria. Severe mitochondrial damage that results in ATP depletion leads to widespread membrane disruption, loss of plasma membrane integrity, osmotic imbalances, cell swelling, and, ultimately, cell rupture. The subsequent release of cellular contents generates an intense inflammatory response.[13,14]

Apoptosis is a genetically controlled pathway of cell death that requires maintenance of mitochondrial ATP generation. Membrane integrity is preserved, and the resultant apoptotic bodies are cleared by phagocytic cells without stimulating an inflammatory response. Apoptosis relies on the sequential activation of cellular proteases called caspases. Caspases are classified as initiator (caspases 8, 9, and 10) or effector caspases (caspase 3). Initiator caspase activation occurs by either an extrinsic death receptor or an intrinsic mitochondrial-mediated pathway. In the death receptor pathway, binding of death receptor ligands such as TNF-α or Fas to their respective death receptor causes receptor oligomerization and activation. This activation results in the recruitment and binding of adapter molecules which, in turn, recruit the initiator caspases 8, 10, or both to the death receptor. This recruitment results in cleavage and activation of caspase 8 or 10. In type II cells such as hepatocytes, caspase 8 and 10 cleave a cytosolic protein, called Bid, to generate tBid.[14] tBid leads to mitochondrial translocation or activation of the pro-apoptotic proteins Bax and Bak. Once activated, Bax and Bak lead to permeabilization of the outer mitochondrial membrane. Mitochondrial outer membrane permeabilization (MOMP) is accompanied by the formation of a pore and the release of inner mitochondrial matrix protein, cytochrome C, into the cytosol. Cytochrome C stimulates the assembly of the apoptosome, a complex of Apaf-1 (apoptotic protease activating factor 1), procaspase 9, and ATP. Caspase 9 is activated within the apoptosome and goes on to cleave and activate effector caspase 3. Once activated, caspase 3 performs the demolition phase of apoptosis and is responsible for initiating the destruction of cellular components and, ultimately, for the morphologic changes that characterize apoptosis, such as nuclear condensation and DNA fragmentation. In the intrinsic mitochondrial pathway, the trigger for apoptosis is cellular stress such as exposure to ultraviolet radiation, growth factor withdrawal, microtubular disruption, or DNA damage. These signals lead to direct Bax/Bak activation and subsequent MOMP leading to cytochrome C release.[13,14]

OXIDATIVE STRESS

Oxidative stress is defined as an imbalance between oxidant and antioxidant systems (such as an excess of reactive oxygen species [ROS] or a deficiency in antioxidants) in the cell which leads to tissue damage.[2] Oxidative stress has a major role in most forms of hepatobiliary injury.

Normally, the level of ROS in the cell is maintained by a balance between production via aerobic metabolism and elimination via antioxidant systems. In health, most ROS are generated via oxidative phosphorylation in the mitochondria. In hepatobiliary disease, activated inflammatory cells (neutrophils, Kupffer cells), cytochrome P450 enzymes (particularly uncoupled CYP2E1 isoforms), and damaged mitochondria all contribute to ROS production.[2] ROS cause cell damage via a variety of mechanisms, including the oxidation of lipids, proteins, and DNA, and the generation of toxic species (peroxides, alcohols, aldehydes, and ketones). Oxidative stress may also activate pro-apoptotic protein kinases (eg, c Jun N-terminal kinase [JNK]), proinflammatory transcription factors (nuclear factor kappa beta [NF-κβ]), and modulators of apoptosis (caspases, death receptors).[2]

Enzymatic Antioxidant Pathways

The liver possesses a complex, interactive, antioxidant network that can be divided into enzymatic and nonenzymatic pathways. Enzymatic antioxidant pathways include SOD, catalase, and GSH peroxidases. SOD, found in the cytosol and the mitochondria, catalyzes the dismutation of superoxide anion to hydrogen peroxide.[3] Catalase, located predominantly in peroxisomes, catalyzes the conversion of hydrogen peroxide to water. GSH peroxidases, a family of cytosolic and mitochondrial enzymes, convert lipid and hydrogen peroxides to water and stable alcohols by oxidizing reduced GSH to its disulfide form (GSSG) **(Fig. 1)**.[3,15]

Nonenzymatic Antioxidant Pathways

Nonenzymatic defenses include GSH, vitamin E, and ascorbate. GSH is a ubiquitously expressed tripeptide of cysteine, glycine, and glutamine. It is the most abundant nonprotein thiol in cells.[3,15,16] The rate limiting steps in the biosynthesis of GSH are

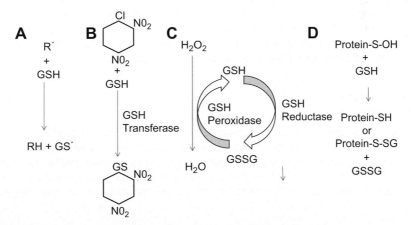

Fig. 1. Major antioxidant mechanisms in the liver involving glutathione (GSH). (*A*) GSH can nonenzymatically act directly on free radicals such superoxide radical, hydroxyl radical, nitric oxide, and carbon radical and aid in their removal. (*B*) Cytosolic and mitochondrial GSH transferases can catalyze the nucleophilic attack by reduced GSH on nonpolar compounds that contain an electrophilic carbon, nitrogen, or sulfur atom. (*C*) In conjunction with GSH peroxidase, GSH can remove hydro- and organic peroxides from the cell. The resultant oxidized glutathione disulfide (GSSG) is reduced back to GSH by GSH reductase. (*D*) GSH can help to maintain protein sulfhydryl groups by nonenzymatically reducing protein sulfenic acids groups or forming protein-GSH mixed disulfides.

the availability of cysteine and the activity of the first enzyme in the biosynthetic pathway, γ-glutamylcysteine synthetase (GCS) (**Fig. 2**). Cysteine is derived from the diet and the breakdown of protein. The liver also has the unique ability to enzymatically convert methionine to cysteine via the transsulfuration pathway (**Fig. 3**). The short half-life of GSH (2–3 hours) and the requirement for dietary cysteine make hepatic GSH levels highly dependent on nutritional conditions. Starvation for 48 hours results in 50% to 75% reductions in hepatic GSH levels in normal rats, which normalize within a few hours of refeeding.[15] Hepatocyte GSH is synthesized in the cytosol and transported into intracellular organelles, particularly the mitochondria.[15,16] GSH transport across the mitochondrial membrane is vital in maintaining mitochondrial defense against oxidant injury. Mitochondrial GSH depletion is an early event in many forms of toxic liver injury and sensitizes hepatocytes to cell death.[17]

GSH serves several vital defense mechanisms in the liver. It exists principally in two forms—a thiol reduced form (GSH) and a disulfide oxidized form (GSSG).[15,16] Normally, the ratio of GSH to GSSG is about 95:1 and is maintained by GSH redox cycling (see **Fig. 1**). The GSH redox cycle involves the oxidation of GSH (GSSG) catalyzed by GSH peroxidase and the recovery of GSH by reduction of GSSG catalyzed by GSH reductase. During this redox recycling, GSH can remove hydrogen and organic peroxides from the cell. Conjugation and removal of endogenous and exogenous toxins from the cell through a family of glutathione S-transferase via the mercapturic acid pathway is another important cytoprotective pathway for GSH. Reduced GSH can also nonenzymatically react with free radicals, including superoxide radicals, hydroxyl radicals, and nitric oxide. In addition, GSH can aid in the reduction of other antioxidants such as tocopherol and ascorbate. GSH also maintains protein sulfhydryl groups. GSH can reduce protein sulfenic acids and bind to sulfhydryl groups to form protein-GSH mixed disulfides (see **Fig. 1**).[15,16]

Vitamin E (α-tocopherol) is an essential nutrient derived from food and nutritional supplements. Vitamin E is considered the predominant lipid-soluble antioxidant protecting membrane phospholipids from lipid peroxidation. Ascorbate (vitamin C) is a water-soluble reducing agent that protects against ROS such as hydrogen peroxide. When vitamin E works as an antioxidant, it is oxidized to a potentially harmful radical, which needs to be reduced back to α-tocopherol by vitamin C.[18]

CYTOPROTECTIVE AGENTS
S-Adenosylmethionine

S-adenosylmethionine (SAMe) is generated from L-methionine and ATP in a two-step reaction catalyzed by methionine adenosyltransferase (MAT) (see **Fig. 3**).[7,12] MAT activity is decreased in many types of liver disease, resulting in decreased hepatocellular levels of SAMe.[7,12,19–21] Reactive oxygen and nitrogen species inactivate MAT secondary to oxidation or nitrosylation of a cysteine residue on the enzyme.[22]

$$\text{Cysteine + Glutamate} \xrightarrow[\substack{\gamma\text{-glutamylcysteine} \\ \text{synthetase}}]{\text{ATP}} \gamma\text{-Glutamylcystiene + Glycine} \xrightarrow[\substack{GSH \\ \text{synthetase}}]{\text{ATP}} \text{GSH}$$

Fig. 2. Biosynthesis of glutathione. Glutathione (GSH) is synthesized from three amino acid precursors: cysteine, glutamate, and glycine. The rate limiting step in its formation is the availability of cysteine which, in the liver, is largely dependent on dietary sources of cysteine and methionine.

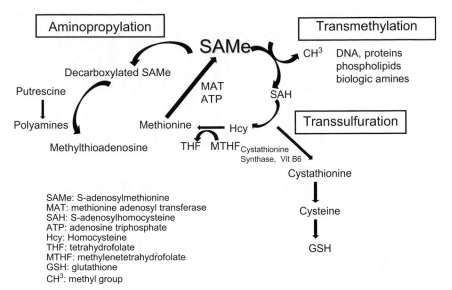

Fig. 3. Hepatic SAMe metabolism. SAMe is generated from methionine in a reaction catalyzed by MAT. The methyl group of SAMe is donated in transmethylation reactions, and the propylamino group is donated for polyamine synthesis (aminopropylation) with MTA being a by-product of this reaction. SAH is a by-product of transmethylation reactions and is hydrolyzed to form homocysteine and adenosine through a reversible reaction catalyzed by SAH hydrolase. Homocysteine can be remethylated to form methionine or can undergo the transulfuration pathway to form cysteine.

Inactivation can be reversed by increasing GSH or overcome by exogenous administration of SAMe.

Within the liver, SAMe is metabolized via three pathways—transmethylation, transulfuration, and aminopropylation (see **Fig. 3**).[7] Most of the SAMe generated is used in transmethylation reactions (85%). In these reactions, SAMe donates its methyl group to a variety of compounds, including nucleic acids, proteins, phospholipids, and biologic amines in reactions catalyzed by methyltransferases. The by-product of these transmethylation reactions, S-adenosylhomocysteine (SAH), is subsequently hydrolyzed to homocysteine and adenosine by SAH hydrolase. Homocysteine is then either remethylated to methionine or undergoes transulfuration. Remethylation requires two enzymes, methionine synthase and betaine methyltransferase, folate, and vitamin B_{12}. In the transulfuration pathway, homocysteine is converted by a series of enzymatic steps in the presence of vitamin B_6 to cysteine. Cysteine can then be used to form GSH (see **Fig. 2**).

The aminopropylation pathway results in the decarboxylation of SAMe, with transfer of its aminopropyl group first to putrescine and then to spermidine to form polyamines.[7] Methyladenosine (MTA) is an important intermediate in this pathway. Exogenous SAMe can also spontaneously convert to MTA, which is stable and can freely pass through cell membranes.

The cytoprotective benefits of SAMe in hepatobiliary disease include (1) augmentation of hepatocyte GSH levels, (2) improvement in membrane fluidity, (3) modification of cytokine expression, (4) alterations in DNA/histone methylation, and (5) modulation of apoptosis (**Table 1**).[7,20,21]

Table 1
Cytoprotective agents

Cytoprotective Agent	Mechanisms of Action	Dose	Side Effects/Drug Interactions	Indication
S-adenosylmethionine	Antioxidant: increases GSH Stabilization of membrane function Modulation of cytokine expression Anti-apoptotic in normal cells	20 mg/kg/d PO Food decreases bioavailability	No side effects	Necro-inflammatory hepatopathies Metabolic hepatopathies (FHL) Cholestatic hepatopathies APAP toxicity
N-acetylcysteine	Antioxidant: increases GSH Anti-inflammatory Improves hepatic microcirculation Improves tissue oxygen delivery	140 mg/kg IV once, then 70 mg/kg IV q 6 h (APAP and ALF) 100 mg/kg/24 h CRI (ALF)	Vomiting with oral preparations	APAP toxicity ALF
Ursodeoxycholic acid	Replaces hepatotoxic bile acids Choleretic Anti-apoptotic Immunomodulatory Stabilizes mitochondria	10–15 mg/kg/d PO Food enhances absorption Increase dose (BID) with severe cholestasis	Rarely vomiting May increase bioavailability of vitamin E and cyclosporine	Cholestatic hepatopathies Necro-inflammatory hepatopathies Metabolic hepatopathies Immune-mediated hepatopathies
Silymarin	ROS scavenger Anti-inflammatory Antifibrotic Increases hepatic protein synthesis Choleretic	Silymarin: 20–50 mg/kg/d divided q 6–8 PO Siliphos: 3–6 mg/kg/d PO	No side effects Inhibits the activity of drug metabolizing enzymes	Amanita mushroom toxicity Hepatotoxicity Cholestatic hepatopathies Necro-inflammatory hepatopathies
Vitamin E	Antioxidant Anti-inflammatory	10–15 IU/kg/d PO of α-tocopherol acetate	None May inhibit the absorption of other fat-soluble vitamins when administered at high doses	Cholestatic hepatopathies Necro-inflammatory hepatopathies

Abbreviations: ALF, acute liver failure; APAP, acetaminophen; FHL, feline hepatic lipidosis; GSH, glutathione.

Because SAMe increases the intracellular availability of cysteine, it increases hepatic GSH levels and has antioxidant activity.[12,19–21] Several studies have demonstrated that SAMe can alleviate signs of oxidative and nitrosative stress.[12,19] Particularly striking is the ability of SAMe to reverse signs of mitochondrial damage.[7] Alterations in membrane fluidity, especially in the mitochondrial membrane, accompany hepatobiliary disease. SAMe restores normal membrane fluidity via methylation of mitochondrial membrane phospholipids, thereby re-establishing normal mitochondrial GSH transport.[7,17]

SAMe modulates cytokine expression.[7,12] SAMe inhibits lipopolysaccharide-stimulated release of TNF-α from macrophages. This anti-inflammatory activity is due to inhibition of histone methylation of the TNF-α promoter by SAMe or its by-product, MTA.[22] SAMe also increases the production of anti-inflammatory cytokines such as IL-10.[7]

SAMe regulates hepatocyte apoptosis.[7] It protects normal hepatocytes against okadaic acid and bile acid induced apoptosis.[7,23] MTA recapitulates these actions.[7] In liver cancer cell lines, SAMe is pro-apoptotic.[7,24] One study has linked this disparity to differential activation of the pro-apoptotic kinase, JNK.[24]

SAMe also has growth regulatory effects on hepatocytes. Mice with genetic depletion of MAT develop hepatic hyperplasia, have abnormal hepatic regeneration after partial hepatectomy, and eventually develop hepatocellular carcinoma.[20] SAMe levels are low in proliferating and regenerating hepatocytes and high in quiescent hepatocytes. SAMe inhibits proliferation in hepatoma cells and protects against the development of neoplastic foci in hepatotoxic models of hepatocarcinogenesis. The growth inhibitory effects of SAMe are due in part to inhibition of the mitogenic response to hepatocyte growth factor.[7,20] SAMe is antiproliferative and pro-apoptotic in neoplastic hepatocytes, whereas it is mitogenic and anti-apoptotic in normal hepatocytes.

Literature review
The effects of SAMe administration in hepatobiliary disease have been evaluated in animal models and human clinical trials.[7,12,19,20,25–28] SAMe improves survival in animal models of alcohol, acetaminophen, galactosamine, and thioacetarsamide induced hepatotoxicity and in ischemia-reperfusion induced liver injury. SAMe treatment also decreases fibrosis in rats treated with carbon tetrachloride. SAMe has also shown efficacy in ameliorating hepatic steatosis. Mice with a genetic depletion in MAT develop hepatic steatosis, implying a link between normal SAMe levels and lipid metabolism. In a genetic model of hepatic lipidosis using ob/ob (leptin deficient) mice, SAMe administration reduced triglyceride accumulation as well as apoptosis during treatment with the hepatotoxin pyrazole.[25] In human patients with established steatosis and in patients with chronic hepatitis given prednisone who normally develop steatosis, SAMe administration attenuated or prevented fat accumulation, respectively.

Several human clinical trials with SAMe have been conducted in Europe. A meta-analysis of six placebo-controlled clinical trials evaluating parenteral SAMe administration in acute intrahepatic cholestasis confirmed that it decreased serum bilirubin levels and ameliorated histologic evidence of hepatocellular necrosis.[26] A follow-up study with oral SAMe confirmed continued beneficial effects on biochemical parameters and clinical signs.[27] In human patients with alcoholic liver cirrhosis, long-term oral supplementation with SAMe (2-year period at 1200 g/d) increased survival and decreased the need for liver transplantation in a subgroup of patients with less advanced disease.[28]

Oral SAMe administration has been evaluated in healthy cats and dogs. Normal dogs and cats given 20 mg/kg and 30 to 50 mg/kg orally, respectively, had significantly increased plasma SAMe concentration, increased hepatic GSH levels, and no overt signs of toxicity.[29,30] Additionally, in cats, a decreased concentration of red blood cell thiobarbituate-reacting substances (oxidative membrane products known as TBARs) and increased resilience to osmotic challenge suggested that chronic SAMe treatment may have antioxidant and membrane-stabilizing effects in erythrocytes.[29] Oral SAMe administration ameliorated acetaminophen-induced red blood cell and hepatic damage in cats (85 mg/kg for 3 days followed by 40 mg/kg) and dogs (40 mg/kg followed by 20 mg/kg), respectively.[31,32] In a study of prednisolone-treated dogs, oral SAMe (20 mg/kg) did not prevent the development of hepatic vacuolar changes or the induction of serum hepatic enzyme activity but increased hepatic GSH levels.[30] Neither prednisolone nor SAMe plasma concentrations were altered by coadministration.[30]

Dose and pharmacokinetics
In the United States veterinary market there are two commercially available stable salts: a 1,4-butanediosulfonate salt (Denosyl-SD4, Nutramax Laboratories, Edgewood, Maryland) and a tosylate salt (Zentonil, Vetoquinol, Buena, New Jersey). Tablets are blister packed because the salts are hydroscopic and enteric coated to prevent inactivation in stomach acid. The tablets must not be split or crushed. Food interferes with absorption, requiring that SAMe be given on an empty stomach. The recommended oral dose is 20 mg/kg/d. SAMe has a high hepatic first-pass effect and a low bioavailability (approximately 3%). Measurable plasma and tissue concentrations are obtained, even within the cerebrospinal fluid in the cat and dog.[33] Maximal plasma concentrations are variable but generally are achieved between 1 and 4 hours in dogs and 2 and 8 hours in cats.[29,30] SAMe is rapidly metabolized intracellularly, with the portion not metabolized undergoing renal or fecal excretion.[3]

Side effects and drug interactions
SAMe is well tolerated. Reported side effects include immediate post pill nausea, food refusal, and anxiety.[3] In a few cats, post-dosing emesis has necessitated discontinuation of treatment.[3]

Use in canine and feline hepatobiliary disease
The therapeutic potential of SAMe in companion animals with hepatobiliary disease is largely unknown because no clinical studies have been published. Dogs and cats with naturally occurring liver disease have reductions in hepatic GSH levels. In one study, low hepatic GSH levels were present in 42% and 33% of dogs with necroinflammatory or vacuolar hepatopathies, respectively[34]; however, some dogs and cats with liver disease also had increased GSH levels. In a separate study, dogs with copper toxicosis, extrahepatic cholestasis, and chronic hepatitis had low hepatic GSH levels, and many had concurrent decreases in hepatic mRNA levels for SOD and catalase.[35] Low hepatic GSH levels were present in 80% and 75% of cats with necroinflammatory liver disease and hepatic lipidosis, respectively.[34] Considering the pivotal role of oxidant stress in liver injury, therapies aimed at restoring normal redox balance by normalizing GSH levels would be expected to be of benefit.

Based on animal models, human clinical trials, and what is known about hepatobiliary disease in companion animals, SAMe administration would likely be beneficial in a variety of disorders in dogs and cats. These disorders would include acute intrahepatic or extrahepatic cholestatic disorders (eg, cholecystitis, gallbladder mucocele, choledochitis), necroinflammatory diseases (eg, canine chronic hepatitis, feline cholangitis), metabolic diseases (eg, canine vacuolar hepatopathy, feline hepatic lipidosis), and toxic (eg, acetaminophen) or ischemic hepatopathies.

N-Acetylcysteine

N-acetylcysteine (NAC) is a stable formulation of the amino acid L-cysteine that can be given parenterally to replenish intracellular cysteine and GSH levels. It is a well-recognized antidote for acetaminophen-induced red blood cell and hepatocyte toxicity. NAC also has a myriad of other cytoprotective effects, including an effect on vascular tone that may improve oxygen delivery in acute liver failure (ALF), an ability to enhance hepatic mitochondrial energy metabolism, and anti-inflammatory actions (blocks polymorphonuclear cell (PMN)–endothelial cell adhesion, PMN activation, and cytokine release (TNF-α)).[36]

Literature review

NAC has been evaluated in animal models of hepatotoxicity, ALF, ischemia-reperfusion injury, bile duct obstruction, and cirrhosis. NAC is beneficial in the treatment of several hepatotoxins, acetaminophen being the best studied.[36] Additionally, NAC has been evaluated in cyclosporine A, arsenic, azathioprine, and lipopolysaccharide-mediated liver injury.[37–40] The cytoprotective effect of NAC in these hepatotoxic models is mediated by its ability to increase hepatic GSH levels.

In ALF, administration of NAC improves vasomotor tone in peripheral, cerebral, and sinusoidal vascular beds. Its effects include increased mean arterial pressure, improved oxygen extraction in capillary beds, and decreased cerebral perfusion pressure.[41,42] In ischemia-reperfusion injury, improvements in the hepatic microcirculation and decreased hepatic damage have been seen with NAC pretreatment in rabbit and rodent models, although no benefits were seen in a recent canine study.[43–46] In bile duct ligated rats and dogs, NAC improves portal and hepatic microcirculatory blood flow.[47,48] The effects of NAC on the microcirculation are believed to be related primarily to its antioxidant effects, because ROS are a major stimulus for inflammatory cell recruitment to endothelial cell surfaces.

NAC is currently undergoing human clinical trials in the treatment of non-acetaminophen associated ALF.[49,50] In a retrospective study in children with ALF, a 72-hour infusion of NAC significantly improved survival when compared with placebo.[49] In preliminary reports of a randomized blinded clinical trial in pediatric patients with ALF, NAC infusion was associated with a shorter length of hospital stay, a higher incidence of native liver recovery without transplantation, and a better survival after transplantation.[50] Currently, a similar clinical trial is ongoing in adult patients with ALF.

Dose and pharmacokinetics

In veterinary medicine, NAC is considered to be the antidote of choice for acetaminophen toxicity in small animals. NAC restores intracellular GSH levels that aid in the detoxification of the reactive intermediate generated by CP-450 metabolism of acetaminophen. There are several published studies on the use of NAC in acetaminophen toxicity in the dog and cat.[51–54] NAC is most effective if given within 8 to 16 hours of ingestion; however, in human patients, treatment up to 53 hours after drug ingestion has yielded a positive clinical response. An initial dose of 140 mg/kg is followed by doses of 70 mg/kg intravenously every 6 hours for seven treatments. In human ALF, a constant rate infusion dose of 100 mg/kg/24 h is being evaluated therapeutically. NAC should be administered through a nonpyrogenic filter (0.25 μm) using a 10% solution diluted 1:2 or more with saline. The high incidence of gastric irritation and vomiting limits the oral use of NAC, which is rarely indicated given the availability of oral SAMe for GSH replenishment.

Side effects and drug interactions
Side effects of an intravenous bolus in humans include gastrointestinal upset, allergic reactions, and hemodynamic changes (increased or decreased blood pressure). Allergic reactions are rare but may manifest as rash, pruritus, angioedema, or bronchospasm. Parenteral NAC administration appears to be well tolerated in veterinary patients, with no adverse events reported in the literature. The oral median lethal dose (LD_{50}) in dogs is greater than 1000 mg/kg.

Use in canine and feline hepatobiliary disease
Indications for NAC use in veterinary medicine include acetaminophen toxicity, Heinz body anemia, suspected toxin-related liver injury, and ALF (regardless of underlying etiology). Of particular interest is the use of NAC in ALF caused by suspected toxicosis (eg, carprofen and trimethoprim toxicity in dogs, diazepam and methimazole toxicity in cats) and in cats with severe hepatic lipidosis (given their propensity for Heinz body anemia and oxidant injury). Given that liver transplantation is not an option in veterinary medicine and that NAC in human ALF improves native liver survival, the use of NAC should be considered in any veterinary patient fitting the criteria for ALF.

Ursodeoxycholic Acid
Yutan, a Chinese compound derived from the dried bile of the Chinese black bear, has been used for centuries for its hepatobiliary healing powers. In 1936, ursodeoxycholic acid (UDCA) was identified as the major bile acid responsible for Yutan's hepatoprotective effects.[4] Currently, synthetic forms of UDCA are approved for the treatment of hepatobiliary disease in human patients (Actigal, Novartis, Basel, Switzerlandand URSO, Axcan, Mont-Saint-Hilaire, Canada).

Bile acids are organic anions synthesized exclusively in the liver from cholesterol. The rate-limiting step is the addition of a hydroxyl group in the seventh position of the cholesterol steroid nucleus. Because cholesterol already contains a 3α-OH group, the simplest bile acids are the 3α, 7α di-OH bile acids such as chenodeoxycholate. Additional hydroxylation at the 12α position creates the tri-OH bile acids in the cholate group. The primary bile acids, cholate and chenodeoxycholate, are conjugated in the liver to either glycine or taurine in the dog or exclusively to taurine in cats.[3] The major circulating bile acid in both species is taurocholate. Some bile acids are hepatotoxic. The elements of toxicity are not completely understood but correlate to some degree with hydrophobicity. In general, the more hydroxylated the bile acid, the less hydrophobic and the less toxic. The more hydrophobic bile acids damage hepatocytes primarily by disrupting mitochondrial membranes and activating apoptotic death receptors.[4,55]

UDCA is a cytoprotective hydrophilic dihydroxylated bile acid even though it is almost structurally identical to the much more hepatotoxic bile acid, chenodeoxycholate. The unique cytoprotective action of UDCA is still not fully understood but several mechanisms have emerged, including replacement of more toxic bile acids in the bile acid pool, stimulation of choleresis, anti-apoptotic effects, stabilization of mitochondrial function, and immunomodulatory actions.[4,55] The cytoprotective effects of UDCA are not limited to hepatobiliary cells but have been demonstrated in cardiac myocytes, neuronal cells, and gastrointestinal epithelial cells.[56–58]

Because serum and hepatic retention of bile acids accompanies most hepatobiliary disorders, and because some bile acids are potentially hepatotoxic, they likely contribute to the pathologic progression of cholestatic hepatopathies. One mechanism of UDCA cytoprotection is replacement of more hydrophobic hepatotoxic bile acids in the bile acid pool[3,4,55]; however, this view is overly simplistic, because a correlation between UDCA enrichment of the bile acid pool and its therapeutic effect has been hard to demonstrate. In addition, this effect would be of limited value in dogs and cats because the major circulating bile acid is the relatively nontoxic taurocholate.

UDCA stimulates choleresis, which increases the elimination of endogenous toxins normally excreted in the bile, such as copper, leukotrienes, and bilirubin. Choleresis is the result of an increase in the expression of membrane transporters necessary to generate bile flow and direct stimulation of a bicarbonate-rich bile flow in the bile ducts.[4,55] The secretory capacity of a hepatocyte is dictated by the number and activity of transporter proteins located on its membrane. UDCA increases the canalicular membrane expression of several transporters, including the bile salt excretory pump, BSEP, and the organic anion pump, MRP2. UDCA stimulates the insertion of transporter molecules that are sitting in intracellular endosomal compartments into the membrane.[4] UDCA also increases cholangiocyte excretion of bicarbonate-rich fluid.[4,55] By increasing intracellular Ca^{+2} in cholangiocytes, UDCA activates both Ca^{+2}–dependent Cl^- channels and Cl^-/HCO_3^- exchange.[4]

A major cytoprotective action of UDCA lies in its ability to inhibit apoptosis. UDCA modulates the apoptotic threshold by preserving mitochondrial integrity.[4,57] In cultured hepatocytes, UDCA protects against the loss of mitochondrial membrane potential, the onset of the MOMP, and the loss of cytochrome C, and can decrease the production of ROS that accompanies apoptosis due to various stimuli. UDCA can increase mitochondrial GSH levels by stabilizing mitochondrial membrane transporters or by increasing the activity of MAT. Furthermore, UDCA can induce the expression of the anti-apoptotic mitochondrial protein, Bcl-2, and decrease Bax levels. Additionally, UDCA can promote survival by controlling transcription factors and kinases involved in apoptosis. In primary hepatocytes, UDCA inhibits TGF-β–induced apoptosis by preventing activation of an E2F-1/p53 transcription factor–induced apoptotic pathway. In hepatocytes, neurons, and cardiac myocytes, UDCA cytoprotection requires activation of the lipid prosurvival kinase, phosphoinositide-3-kinase, and its downstream mediator, Akt. UDCA can also act as a molecular chaperone and modulates apoptosis associated with endoplasmic reticulum stress.[59]

UDCA has immunodulatory properties. UDCA down-regulates aberrant major histocompatibility complex expression on hepatobiliary cells induced by cholestasis.[4] This aberrant expression renders the cells more vulnerable to immune targeting by activated lymphocytes, leading to cell damage.[4,55] UDCA also suppresses interleukin-2 and 4 production. Studies show that UDCA can directly activate the glucocorticoid receptor by interacting with a region of the receptor distinct from the cortisol binding site. UDCA binding to the glucocorticoid receptor induces nuclear translocation of the glucocorticoid receptor and suppresses activation of NF-κβ.[60,61] Inhibition of the UDCA–glucocorticoid receptor interaction prevents UDCA's cytoprotective effect in cultured hepatocytes.[60]

Literature review
UDCA use has been evaluated extensively in animal models of hepatotoxicity. In bile duct ligated rats, UDCA prevents GSH depletion (by up-regulating GCS) and prevents changes in mitochondrial membrane potential and lipid content that accompany chronic cholestasis.[4,55,57] In vivo feeding of toxic bile acids to rats causes apoptosis, whereas simultaneous treatment with UDCA inhibits this effect and prevents the movement of Bax to the mitochondria. In an endoplasmic reticulum stress model of

apoptosis in obese diabetic mice, oral UDCA therapy inhibited the up-regulation of endoplasmic reticulum stress markers in the liver and adipose tissue of mice. UDCA can also inhibit hepatocyte triglyceride accumulation in a rat model of hepatosteatosis.[62]

UDCA is cytoprotective in myocytes and neuronal cells. Administration of UDCA in rats just before inducing myocardial infarction results in a reduction in the number of apoptotic myocytes and the area of infarction in a comparison with controls.[56] UDCA also prevents neuronal cell apoptosis in experimental models of Alzheimer's and Huntington's disease in mice.[57]

In humans, UDCA is used to treat a variety of cholestatic hepatopathies, including primary biliary cirrhosis (PBC), primary sclerosing cholangitis (PSC), pediatric cholestatic disorders, cystic fibrosis, and intrahepatic cholestasis associated with pregnancy and prolonged total parenteral nutrition.[63–68] PBC is an immune-mediated, chronic inflammatory hepatobiliary disease that usually results in biliary cirrhosis and eventual liver failure. UDCA is the only approved treatment for PBC even though its effect on long-term survival remains uncertain.[63–65] Although meta-analyses have failed to show benefit in terms of survival or transplantation rates, many individual studies have shown significant improvements in biochemical parameters, clinical signs, and histologic scores, and, in isolated cases, survival benefits.[63–65] Considering the complexities of PBC (eg, its variability in disease progression and the long natural history of the disease) and issues with study design (eg, studies of insufficient duration, small patient numbers, inconsistently defined end points, and suboptimal UDCA dosing), meta-analyses may fail to recognize beneficial effects of UDCA. In PSC, UDCA improves serum liver chemistries and bilirubin but has no effect on disease progression or transplant-free survival.[66] Similar to the studies on PBC, even the largest of these studies was probably too small and the follow-up period too short to allow evaluation of survival. UDCA has proven benefit in children who have genetic abnormalities causing severe cholestasis, for managing bile flow aberrations in cystic fibrosis, and as adjunctive therapy in immunomodulatory protocols in humans who have immune-mediated liver disease.[55,67] UDCA reduces cholestasis, improves serum aminotransferase levels, and decreases pruritus in women with intrahepatic cholestasis related to pregnancy.[68] There is some evidence for an additive effect of concurrent SAMe and UDCA administration in this disease.[68]

Little information is available in the literature in regards to UDCA use in small animals. In a single case report, a dog with chronic hepatitis was given 15 mg/kg/d of UDCA, which resulted in enrichment of UDCA in the serum associated with biochemical (decreases in alanine aminotransferase, alkaline phosphatase, cholesterol, and bilirubin) and clinical improvement (increased appetite and energy level).[69] In four normal cats, 15 mg/kg/d of UDCA for 8 weeks resulted in no adverse clinicopathologic effects.[70]

Dose and pharmacokinetics

The pharmacokinetics of UDCA have been examined in dogs, humans, and rodents. UDCA is absorbed passively, primarily in the small intestine. Absorption is enhanced in the presence of food. Greater than 60% of the oral dose undergoes hepatic uptake where it is conjugated with taurine or glycine and then undergoes enterohepatic circulation. UDCA that escapes enterohepatic circulation is metabolized to lithocholate in the colon and eliminated in the feces or urine. A dose of 15 mg/kg/d has been extrapolated from human medicine. Bioavailability decreases with advanced cholestasis due to decreased absorption, decreased hepatic extraction, and increased renal elimination; therefore, twice daily administration may be necessary in severe cholestatic disease.

Side effects and drug interactions

UDCA is well tolerated. Little or no toxicity has been seen in human patients. The only side effect appears to be diarrhea. Similarly, in small animals, rare side effects include vomiting and diarrhea. Extensive toxicologic studies performed in healthy dogs for Food and Drug Administration approval did not reveal any serious side effects. No adverse effects were noted in normal cats at doses ranging from 10 to 15 mg/kg/d for treatment periods ranging from 2 to 3 months.[70] UDCA treatment may increase the bioavailability of cyclosporine and vitamin E. Concurrent use of aluminum-containing antacids may decrease the absorption of UDCA.[3]

Use in canine and feline hepatobiliary disease

UDCA should be considered as ancillary therapy in a variety of acute and chronic hepatopathies in the dog and cat. In acute hepatobiliary disease, it would be useful as a choleretic agent to treat intra- and extrahepatic cholestasis in the absence of complete bile duct obstruction. Its use could also be considered in animals assessed as having a large amount of hyperechoic sludge in their gall bladders on ultrasound. Additionally, UDCA could be used in asymptomatic or mildly symptomatic patients with gall bladder mucoceles, in the absence of bile duct obstruction, that are poor surgical candidates due to concurrent disease.[71]

Owing to its anti-apoptotic and immunomodulatory actions, UDCA would likely be beneficial in chronic necroinflammatory hepatobiliary disease regardless of etiology. Because bile acid concentrations are particularly high in the bile ducts, UDCA may be particularly beneficial in cats with cholangitis. In dogs, ancillary UDCA treatment would likely be of benefit in cases of chronic hepatitis (breed related [including primary copper storage hepatopathies], infectious, or immune mediated). In some chronic hepatopathies, particularly where corticosteroids are contraindicated, UDCA may be indicated as part of the immunosuppressive regimen. The therapeutic effects of UDCA may be enhanced by concurrent SAMe administration; it is unclear whether this effect may be synergistic or additive.[68] There is some evidence both in vitro and in vivo that the actions of SAMe and UDCA may be additive.[68,72]

Silymarin

The major active ingredient of benefit in milk thistle is silymarin. Silymarin is actually a group of several closely related flavinoids but consists primarily of four isomers: silybin, isosilybin, silydianin, and silychristin. Silybin is the major active component of silymarin.[6,9,10,12]

Silymarin has several beneficial actions useful in the treatment of hepatobiliary disease, including antioxidant, anti-inflammatory, and antifibrotic properties.[6,10,12] Additionally, silymarin has an ability to modulate hepatocyte transport and increase hepatic protein synthesis.[6] Silymarin acts as an antioxidant by reducing free radical production and lipid peroxidation.[6] Silymarin also scavenges ROS and protects against GSH depletion.[6,12] Anti-inflammatory properties include suppression of NF-$\kappa\beta$ activation, inhibition of TNF-α induced cytotoxicity, and increased expression of IL-10.[6,12,73] Silymarin has an inhibitory effect on the 5-lipoxygenase pathway resulting in inhibition of leukotriene synthesis.[6] It has also been shown to protect hepatocytes against T cell–induced injury and inhibits hepatitis C viral replication.[73] Silymarin also exhibits antifibrotic actions, including inhibition of TGF-β secretion and stellate cell activation.[10]

Silymarin modulates hepatocyte transport.[6,10,12] It promotes choleresis by increasing insertion of transporters into the apical membrane of hepatocytes. Additionally, it inhibits hepatocyte uptake of phalloidin, the toxic agent resulting in ALF secondary to *Amanita* mushroom ingestion. Silymarin increases protein synthesis through stimulation of ribosomal RNA polymerase in hepatocytes.[9] Silymarin also accelerates hepatocellular regeneration as a result of increased gene transcription/ translation and enhanced DNA biosynthesis.

Literature review

Substantial in vitro and in vivo evidence suggests that silymarin can protect the liver from a wide variety of toxins, including acetaminophen, ethanol, carbon tetrachloride, aflatoxin, and *Amanita phalloides* toxins, as well as from ischemic, viral, and radiation-induced injury.[6,11,74–77] Antifibrotic properties have been demonstrated in bile duct ligated rats and alcohol fed baboons, in which stellate cell proliferation and collagen production were inhibited.[78,79] Silymarin can also augment the synthesis of DNA, RNA, and protein following partial hepatectomy in rats.[80]

In humans, silymarin use has been evaluated in a variety of liver conditions, including alcoholic liver disease, liver cirrhosis, acute and chronic viral hepatitis, *A phalloides* poisoning, and toxic and drug-induced liver diseases.[6,9,10] Evidence from these studies to support silymarin use in human hepatobiliary disease is conflicting. Some studies have shown improvements in serum transaminases and bilirubin, clinical signs and indicators of oxidative damage, whereas others have failed to show any benefit. The benefits of silymarin therapy in these studies are difficult to interpret and compare due to different methodologies, small sample sizes, inclusion of patients with heterogeneous hepatic pathology, ill-defined end points, variable treatment durations, and the use of nonstandardized products and dosages that are not well justified. Nevertheless, because of the overwhelming evidence for its cytoprotective effects in in vitro and in vivo models, a meeting (sponsored jointly by the National Institute of Diabetes and Digestive and Kidney Disease, the National Center for Complementary and Alternative Medicine, and the National Institute on Alcohol Abuse and Alcoholism) was held in 2004 with two objectives in mind[81]: (1) to develop a standardized reliable silymarin product that could be used in clinical trials, and (2) to plan and initiate clinical trials of this product in liver disease, with a particular focus on nonalcoholic steatohepatitis (NASH) and hepatitis C. Several phase I and II clinical trials as a direct result of this meeting are nearing completion.

In the veterinary literature, silymarin has been evaluated for its protective action against carbon tetrachloride and phalloidin toxicity. A single study found silymarin to be protective against carbon tetrachloride toxicity in dogs.[77] Silybin was found to be completely protective against *A phalloides* intoxication in Beagles at a dose of 50 to 150 mg/kg when given 5 to 24 hours after ingesting an LD_{50} dose of *A phalloides*.[82] Data from an uncontrolled study suggest that the use of silymarin up to 48 hours after ingestion is effective in preventing severe hepatotoxicity.[9] Silymarin prevents binding of the phalloidin toxin to hepatocytes and interrupts the enterohepatic circulation of the toxin.

Dose and pharmacokinetics

Silymarin's bioavailability is low due to erratic absorption from the gastrointestinal tract. It has a short plasma half-life but is preferentially accumulated in the liver.[81] It is excreted in bile as a glucoronide and sulfoglucoronide conjugate and undergoes some enterohepatic circulation. Bile concentrations are 100 times those seen in serum.[3]

The dose required to achieve a therapeutic range in small animal patients is unknown. In human medicine, variable dosing regimens have been used, with doses of 50 to 150 mg/kg given in cases of *A phalloides* intoxication and 7 to 15 mg/kg/d in cases of hepatitis. Extrapolation of the dose from human studies suggests that 20 to 50 mg/kg/d of silymarin divided into three to four doses per day may be of therapeutic value.[81] Therapeutic formulations should contain 70% to 80% silymarin. Unfortunately, despite labeling claims, there are significant variations between commercially available products and no assurance of extract purity.[81]

More recently, a new product (initially called IdB1016) has become available called Siliphos.[6] Siliphos, a formulation of silibin complexed with phosphatidylcholine, is three to five times more bioavailable than silymarin[83,84]; values in rodent studies have shown concentrates in bile 10 times greater with the phosphatidylcholine complexed compound.[85] These results suggest that this compound can be dosed at 3 to 6 mg/kg/d.[83,84] Commercially it is available as a combined product with vitamin E and zinc (Marin, Nutramax, Edgewood, Maryland) or SAMe (Denamarin, Nutramax, Edgewood, Maryland). A recent study demonstrated that this product increased silybin blood levels in dogs, with a peak maximum at 3 hours and restoration of baseline values by 24 hours.[83] A preliminary pharmacokinetic study of Siliphos in normal cats at a dose of 10 mg/kg orally found a bioavailability of 6% to 7%.[86] A separate study demonstrated that this dose increased neutrophil GSH content and neutrophil function as measured by maximal phagocytic and oxidative burst activity.[87]

Side effects and drug interactions

Silymarin is reported to have an extremely low toxicity and has been used extensively in human clinical patients with few reported side effects. Similarly, no serious adverse effects have been reported in animal studies. Mild side effects such as gastrointestinal upset, pruritus, and headache have been rarely reported in humans. The silybin-phosphatidylcholine complex has been evaluated in both acute and chronic use safety studies in dogs. An acute toxicity study in dogs using levels greater than 80 times the amount in Marin revealed no adverse effects. In a chronic toxicity study in monkeys who received a similar dose for 26 weeks, no side effects were seen. Silymarin has also been evaluated in normal cats and found to have no clinical outward signs of toxicity in a preliminary pharmacokinetic study when given at a dose of 10 mg/kg.[86]

Silymarin inhibits the activities of glucoronide transferases, some cytochrome P450 enzymes, and P-glycoprotein. Inhibition of cytochrome P450 enzymes in vitro only occurred at concentrations greatly exceeding physiologically reachable ones.[6] Nevertheless, given the possibility of silymarin use interfering with the metabolism of other drugs, drug interactions should be considered in polymedicated patients.[3,6]

Use in canine and feline hepatobiliary disease

Silymarin may have benefit in cases of hepatotoxicity, hepatobiliary disease associated with cholestasis, and chronic hepatopathies. Silymarin use is indicated in the treatment of *Amanita* mushroom toxicity, although high doses are needed to inhibit uptake of the phalloidin toxin, and intravenous formulations (ie, silybin dihemisuccinate) are not currently available for clinical use in the United States.

In acute and chronic cholestasis, silymarin may promote choleresis and prevent proinflammatory and profibrotic complications associated with the retention of endogenous toxins normally excreted in bile. Given its anti-inflammatory, antioxidant, antifibrotic, and anti-apoptotic effects, silymarin administration should be considered in dogs and cats with chronic necroinflammatory hepatobiliary disease.

Vitamin E

Vitamin E is an essential nutrient derived from food and nutritional supplements. The vitamin E family consists of eight highly lipophilic antioxidant compounds widely distributed in plants. Alpha-tocopherol is the most bioavailable and active form of vitamin E.[1–3,5,12]

Vitamin E has a major role in the protection of membrane phospholipids from oxidative damage. It defends against peroxidative membrane damage by terminating free radical–induced chain reactions.[3] Upon termination of peroxidation reactions, the oxidized tocopheroxy radical produced is then transformed to the reduced state through interactions with other cellular antioxidants, particularly vitamin C.

Vitamin E has additional nonantioxidant functions, including an antiproliferative effect on vascular smooth muscle and an inhibitory influence on platelet aggregation and adhesion.[3] Vitamin E analogues also modulate signal transduction by altering the activity of lipoxygenases, cyclooxygenases, and protein kinase C, and alter gene expression by inhibiting the activation of NF-κβ.[3] Vitamin E additionally suppresses activation of inflammatory cells and protects against Kupffer and stellate cell activation.[1,2]

Literature review

Vitamin E administration has been evaluated in in vitro and animal models of hepatotoxicity. Vitamin E ameliorated oxidant-induced damage in rat hepatocytes exposed to hydrophobic bile acids in vitro, improved liver histology in ethanol-induced liver disease, prevented the development of hepatic steatosis, and reduced mortality associated with carbon tetrachloride toxicity.[12,88,89] In human patients with hepatobiliary disease, results of clinical trials with vitamin E supplementation have been mixed. A few studies have demonstrated biochemical improvement in patients with NASH treated with vitamin E, with some showing improvement in histologic parameters of inflammation and fibrosis.[90,91] In one small clinical trial, a combination of vitamin E and UDCA improved laboratory values and hepatic steatosis scores in patients with NASH better than UDCA therapy alone.[92] The results in alcoholic liver disease and viral hepatitis have been less impressive, although one small pilot study of vitamin E combined with antiviral therapy resulted in a 2.4 times greater chance of a complete response when compared with antiviral therapy alone.[93]

The effects of vitamin E supplementation in veterinary patients with hepatobiliary disease have not been reported except for a small pilot study of 20 dogs with chronic hepatitis fed a vitamin E–supplemented diet for 3 months. In these dogs, increases in serum and hepatic vitamin E concentrations were accompanied by an increased hepatic GSH:GSSG ratio, suggestive of an improved hepatic redox status, but no changes in clinical or histologic scores were noted.[94]

Dose and pharmacokinetics

The recommended oral formulation of vitamin E is the acetate form of α-tocopherol.[5] It is commercially available as d-α–tocopherol, a synthetic form of vitamin E, comprised of the eight possible stereoisomers in equal amounts. A dose of 10 to 15 IU/kg/d is recommended for dogs and cats that have necroinflammatory or cholestatic liver disorders. Higher doses may be indicated in animals with severe cholestatic disorders that compromise fat absorption. An emulsified formulation is available (Vedco, Agri-Labs, St. Joseph, Missouri; Durvet, Blue Springs, Missouri; Schering-Plough,

Kenilworth, New Jersey) for parenteral administration and should be considered in animals with severe cholestasis. In a recent study in a rodent model, emulsified vitamin E ameliorated acute hepatobiliary injury induced by administration of hydrophobic bile acids.[88] This formula may prove to be useful in the management of acute cholestatic hepatopathies such as idiopathic hepatic lipidosis in cats.

Side effects
Vitamin E is generally considered to be of low toxicity. In humans, high doses (>5000 IU/d) can antagonize the absorption of other fat-soluble vitamins, resulting in impaired bone mineralization, reduction in hepatic vitamin A stores, and coagulopathy secondary to vitamin K insufficiency.[5]

Use in veterinary medicine
Vitamin E supplementation should be considered in the management of hepatobiliary disorders likely to involve oxidative membrane injury, such as cholestatic hepatopathies (hepatic lipidosis in cats), specific hepatotoxins, necroinflammatory hepatobiliary disease, ischemia-reperfusion injury, and transition metal toxicity (copper and iron).

SUMMARY

Although studies in in vitro systems and animal models provide compelling data supporting the hepatoprotective benefits of the cytoprotective agents discussed in this article, clinical studies in naturally occurring hepatobiliary disease have not been as convincing. In many cases, especially in veterinary medicine, this problem is due to the lack of well-designed, randomized, controlled trials evaluating the efficacy of these agents. In vitro studies and animal models suggest that these agents augment and enhance natural hepatic defense mechanisms to inhibit inflammation and fibrosis, prevent apoptosis, and protect against oxidant injury; however, these agents do not address the primary cause of liver injury, and their utility in hepatobiliary disease is of an ancillary nature. The importance of obtaining a definitive diagnosis via liver histopathology, cultures of liver and bile, and the use of special histopathologic stains cannot be overemphasized. A favorable prognosis is most likely when a definitive diagnosis is obtained early in the course of the disease with treatment directed at the underlying cause. Once a definitive diagnosis is obtained and the ongoing pathology is understood, the clinician will be able to select the most appropriate cytoprotective agent. Ideally, in the future, we will endeavor to pursue clinical trials of these cytoprotective agents in our patients to provide a more justified rationale for their use.

REFERENCES

1. Vitaglione P, Morisco F, Caporaso N, et al. Dietary antioxidant compounds and liver health. Crit Rev Food Sci Nutr 2004;44:575–86.
2. Medina J, Moreno-Otero R. Pathophysiological basis for antioxidant therapy in chronic liver disease. Drugs 2005;65:2445–61.
3. Center S. Metabolic, antioxidant, nutraceutical, probiotic, and herbal therapies relating to the management of hepatobiliary disorders. Vet Clin North Am Small Anim Pract 2004;34:67–172.
4. Beuers U. Drug insight: mechanisms and sites of action of ursodeoxycholic acid in cholestasis. Nat Clin Pract Gastroenterol Hepatol 2006;3:318–28.
5. Flatland B. Botanicals, vitamins, and minerals and the liver: therapeutic applications and potential toxicities. Comp Contin Educ 2003;25:514–24.

6. Pradhan SC, Girish C. Hepatoprotective herbal drug, silymarin, from experimental pharmacology to clinical medicine. Indian J Med Res 2006;124:491–504.

7. Mato JM, Lu SC. Role of S-adenosyl-L-methionine in liver health and injury. Hepatology 2007;45:1306–12.

8. Fogden E, Neuberger J. Alternative medicines and the liver. Liver Int 2003;23:213–20.

9. Levy C, Seeff LD, Lindor KD. Use of herbal supplements for chronic liver disease. Clin Gastroenterol Hepatol 2004;2:947–56.

10. Verma S, Thuluvath PJ. Complementary and alternative medicine in hepatology: review of the evidence of efficacy. Clin Gastroenterol Hepatol 2007;5:408–16.

11. Dhiman RK, Chawla YK. Herbal medicines for liver diseases. Dig Dis Sci 2005;50:1807–12.

12. Hanje AJ, Fortune B, Song M, et al. The use of selected nutrition supplements and complementary and alternative medicine in liver disease. Nutr Clin Pract 2006;21:255–72.

13. Malhi H, Gores GJ. Cellular and molecular mechanisms of liver injury. Gastroenterologist 2008;134:1641–54.

14. Akazawa Y, Gores GJ. Death receptor mediated liver injury. Semin Liver Dis 2007;27:327–38.

15. Lu S. Regulation of hepatic glutathione synthesis: current concepts and controversies. FASEB J 1999;13:1169–83.

16. Meister A, Anderson ME. Glutathione. Annu Rev Biochem 1983;52:711–60.

17. Garcia-Ruiz C, Fernandez-Checa JC. Mitochondrial glutathione: hepatocellular survival-death switch. J Gastroenterol Hepatol 2006;21(Suppl 3):S3–6.

18. Bowry VW, Ingold KU, Stocker R. Vitamin E in human low-density lipoprotein: when and how this antioxidant becomes a pro-oxidant. Biochem J 1992;288:341–4.

19. Lieber CS. S-adenosyl-L-methionine: its role in the treatment of liver disorders. Am J Clin Nutr 2002;76:1183S–7S.

20. Martinez-Chantar ML, Garcia-Trevijano ER, Latasa MU, et al. Importance of a deficiency in S-adenosyl-L-methionine synthesis in the pathogenesis of liver injury. Am J Clin Nutr 2002;76:1177S–82S.

21. Avila MA, Garcia-Trevijano ER, Martinez-Chantar ML, et al. S-adenosylmethionine revisited: its essential role in the regulation of liver function. Alcohol 2002;27:163–7.

22. Ara AI, Xia M, Ramani K, et al. S-adenosylmethionine inhibits lipopolysaccharide-induced gene expression via modulation of histone methylation. Hepatology 2008;47:1655–66.

23. Webster CR, Boria P, Usechak P, et al. S-adenosylmethionine and cAMP confer differential cytoprotection against bile acid–induced apoptosis in canine renal tubular cells and primary rat hepatocytes. Vet Ther 2002;3:474–84.

24. Ansorena E, Berasain C, López Zabalza MJ, et al. Differential regulation of the JNK/AP-1 pathway by S-adenosylmethionine and methylthioadenosine in primary rat hepatocytes versus HuH7 hepatoma cells. Am J Physiol Gastrointest Liver Physiol 2006;290:G1186–93.

25. Dey A, Caro AA, Cederbaum AI. S-adenosylmethionine protects ob/ob mice from CYP2E1-mediated liver injury. Am J Physiol Gastrointest Liver Physiol 2007;293:G91–G103.

26. Frezza M, Terpin M. The use of S-adenosylmethionine in the treatment of cholestatic disorders: a meta-analysis of clinical trials. Drug Invest 1992;4:101–8.

27. Manzillo G, Piccinio F, Surrenti C, et al. Multicentre double blind placebo controlled study of intravenous and oral S-adenosyl-l-methionine in cholestatic patients with liver disease. Drug Invest 1992;4:90–100.
28. Mato JM, Camara J, Fernandez de Paz J, et al. S-adenosylmethionine in alcoholic liver cirrhosis: a randomized, placebo-controlled, double blind, multicenter clinical trial. J Hepatol 1999;30:1081–9.
29. Center SA, Randolph JF, Warner KL, et al. The effects of S-adenosylmethionine on clinical pathology and redox potential in the red blood cell, liver and bile of clinically normal cats. J Vet Intern Med 2005;19:303–14.
30. Center SA, Warner KL, McCabe J, et al. Evaluation of the influence of S-adenosylmethionine on systemic and hepatic effects of prednisolone in dogs. Am J Vet Res 2005;66:330–41.
31. Webb CB, Twedt DC, Fettman MJ, et al. S-adenosylmethionine (SAMe) in a feline acetaminophen model of oxidative injury. J Feline Med Surg 2003;38:246–54.
32. Wallace KP, Center SA, Hickford FH, et al. S-adenosyl-L-methionine (SAMe) for the treatment of acetaminophen toxicity in a dog. J Am Anim Hosp Assoc 2002;38:246–54.
33. Giulidori P, Stramentinoli G. A radioenzymatic method of S-adenosyl-L-methionine determination in biological fluids. Anal Biochem 1984;137:217–20.
34. Center SA, Warner K, Hollis E. Liver glutathione concentrations in dogs and cats with naturally occurring liver disease. Am J Vet Res 2002;63:1187–97.
35. Spee B, Arends B, van den Ingh TSGAM, et al. Copper metabolism and oxidative stress in chronic inflammatory and cholestatic liver diseases in dogs. J Vet Intern Med 2006;20:1085–92.
36. Zafarullah M, Li WQ, Sylvester J, et al. Molecular mechanisms of N-acetylcysteine actions. Cell Mol Life Sci 2003;60:6–20.
37. Kaya H, Sogut S, Duru M, et al. The protective effect of N-acetylcysteine against cyclosporine A induced hepatotoxicity in rats. J Appl Toxicol 2008;28:15–20.
38. Santra A, Chowdhury A, Ghatak S, et al. Arsenic induced apoptosis in mouse liver is mitochondrial dependent and is abrogated by N-acetylcysteine. Toxicol Appl Pharmacol 2007;220:146–55.
39. Wang H, Xu DX, Lu JW, et al. N-acetylcysteine attenuates lipopolysaccharide induced apoptotic liver damage in D-galactosamine sensitized mice. Acta Pharmacol Sin 2007;28:1803–9.
40. Menor C, Fernandez-Moreno MD, Fueyo JA, et al. Azathioprine acts upon rat hepatocyte mitochondria and stress activated protein kinases leading to necrosis: protective role of N-acetyl-L-cysteine. J Pharmacol Exp Ther 2004; 311:668–76.
41. Ytrebo LM, Korvald C, Nedredal GI, et al. N-acetylcysteine increases cerebral perfusion pressure in pigs with fulminant hepatic failure. Crit Care Med 2001; 29:1989–95.
42. Harrison PM, Wendon JA, Gimson AE, et al. Improvement by acetylcysteine of hemodynamics and oxygen transport in fulminant hepatic failure. N Engl J Med 1991;324:1852–7.
43. Jin X, Wang L, Wu HS, et al. N-acetylcysteine inhibits activation of toll-like receptor 2 and 4 gene expression in the liver and lung after partial hepatic ischemia-reperfusion injury in mice. Hepatobiliary Pancreat Dis Int 2007;6: 284–9.
44. Smyrnoitis V, Arkadopoulos N, Kostopanagiotou G, et al. Attenuation of ischemic injury by N-acetylcysteine preconditioning of the liver. J Surg Res 2005;129:31–7.

45. Fusai G, Glantzounis GK, Hafez T, et al. N-acetylcysteine ameliorates the late phase of liver ischaemia/reperfusion injury in the rabbit with hepatic steatosis. Clin Sci (Lond) 2005;109:465–73.
46. Baumann J, Ghosh S, Szakmany T, et al. Short-term effects of N-acetylcysteine and ischemic preconditioning in a canine model of hepatic ischemia-reperfusion injury. Eur Surg Res 2008;41:226–30.
47. Yang YY, Lee KC, Huang YT, et al. Effect of N-acetylcysteine administration in hepatic microcirculation of rats with biliary obstruction. J Hepatol 2008;49:25–33.
48. Kigawa H, Nakano K, Kumada, et al. Improvement of portal flow and hepatic microcirculatory tissue flow with N-acetylcysteine in dogs with obstructive jaundice produced by bile duct ligation. Eur J Surg 2000;166:77–84.
49. Kortsalioudaki C, Taylor RM, Cheeseman P, et al. Safety and efficacy of N-acetylcysteine in children with non-acetaminophen induced acute liver failure. Liver Transpl 2008;14:25–30.
50. Lee WM, Lorenzo R, Fontana R, et al. Intravenous N-acetylcysteine improves spontaneous survival in early stage non-acetaminophen acute liver failure. Hepatology 2007;46:268A.
51. Hjelle JJ, Grauer GF. Acetaminophen-induced toxicosis in dogs and cats. J Am Vet Med Assoc 1986;188:742–6.
52. Buck WB, Gonzalez JM. Ibuprofen, aspirin and acetaminophen toxicosis and treatment in dogs and cats. Vet Hum Toxicol 1998;40:156–62.
53. Aronson LR, Drobatz K. Acetaminophen toxicosis in 17 cats. J Vet Emerg Crit Care 1996;6:65–9.
54. Ilkiw JE, Ratcliffe RC. Paracetamol toxicity in a cat. Aust Vet J 1987;64:245–7.
55. Paumgartner G. Medical treatment of cholestatic liver diseases: from pathobiology to pharmacological targets. World J Gastroenterol 2006;12:4445–51.
56. Rivard AL, Steer CJ, Kren BT, et al. Administration of tauroursodeoxycholic acid (TUDCA) reduces apoptosis following myocardial infarction in rat. Am J Chin Med 2007;35:279–95.
57. Ramalho RM, Viana RJ, Low WC, et al. Bile acids and apoptosis modulation: an emerging role in experimental Alzheimer's disease. Trends Mol Med 2008;14:54–62.
58. Bernardes-Silva CF, Damiao AO, Sipahi AM, et al. Ursodeoxycholic acid ameliorates experimental ileitis counteracting intestinal barrier dysfunction and oxidative stress. Dig Dis Sci 2004;49:1569–74.
59. Ozcan U, Yilmaz E, Ozcan L, et al. Chemical chaperones reduce ER stress and restore glucose homeostasis in a mouse model of type 2 diabetes. Science 2006;313:1137–40.
60. Sola S, Amaral JD, Castro RE, et al. Nuclear translocation of UDCA by the glucocorticoid receptor is required to reduce TGF-beta1-induced apoptosis in rat hepatocytes. Hepatology 2005;42:925–34.
61. Weitzel C, Stark D, Kullman F, et al. Ursodeoxycholic acid induced activation of the glucocorticoid receptor in primary rat hepatocytes. Eur J Gastroenterol Hepatol 2005;17:169–277.
62. Okan A, Astarcioglu H, Tankurt E, et al. Effect of ursodeoxycholic acid on hepatic steatosis in rats. Dig Dis Sci 2002;47:2389–97.
63. Paumgartner G. Ursodeoxycholic acid for primary biliary cirrhosis: treat early to slow progression. J Hepatol 2003;39:112–4.
64. Gong Y, Huang Z, Christensen E, et al. Ursodeoxycholic acid for patients with primary biliary cirrhosis: an updated systematic review and meta-analysis of randomized clinical trials using Bayesian approach as sensitivity analyses. Am J Gastroenterol 2007;108:1799–807.

65. Shi J, Wu C, Lin Y, et al. Long-term effects of mid-dose ursodeoxycholic acid in primary biliary cirrhosis: a meta-analysis of randomized controlled trials. Am J Gastroenterol 2006;101:1529–38.
66. Lindor KD. Ursodiol for primary sclerosing cholangitis: Mayo Primary Sclerosing Cholangitis-Ursodeoxycholic Acid Study Group. N Engl J Med 1997; 336:691–5.
67. Desmond CP, Wilson J, Bailey M, et al. The benign course of liver disease in adults with cystic fibrosis and the effect of ursodeoxycholic acid. Liver Int 2007;27:1402–8.
68. Binder T, Salaj P, Zima T, et al. Randomized prospective comparative study of ursodeoxycholic acid and S-adenosyl-L-methionine in the treatment of intrahepatic cholestasis in pregnancy. J Perinat Med 2006;34:383–91.
69. Meyer DJ, Thompson MB, Senior DF. Use of ursodeoxycholic acids in a dog with chronic hepatitis: effects on serum hepatic tests and endogenous bile acid compositions. J Vet Intern Med 1997;11:195–7.
70. Nicholson BT, Center SA, Randolph JF. Effects of oral ursodeoxycholic acid in healthy cats on clinicopathological parameters, serum bile acids and light microscopic and ultrastructural features of the liver. Res Vet Sci 1996;61:258–62.
71. Walter R, Dunn ME, d'Anjou M-A. Nonsurgical resolution of gallbladder mucocele in 2 dogs. J Am Vet Med Assoc 2008;232:1688–93.
72. Milkiewicz P, Mills CO, Roma MG, et al. Tauroursodeoxycholate and S-adenosyl-L-methionine exert an additive ameliorating effect on taurolithocholate-induced cholestasis: a study in isolated rat hepatocyte couplets. Hepatology 1999;29: 471–6.
73. Polyak SJ, Morishima C, Shuhart MC, et al. Inhibition of T-cell inflammatory cytokines, hepatocyte NF-kappaB signaling, and HCV infection by standardized Silymarin. Gastroenterology 2007;132:1925–36.
74. Campos R, Garrido A, Guerra R, et al. Silybin dehemisuccinate protects against glutathione depletion and lipid peroxidation induced by acetaminophen on rat liver. Planta Med 1989;5:417–9.
75. Wang M, Grange LL, Tao J. Hepatoprotective properties of *Silybum marianum* herbal preparation on ethanol induced liver damage. Fitoterapia 1996;67: 167–71.
76. Muriel P, Mourelle M. Prevention by silymarin of membrane alterations in acute CCl4 liver damage. J Appl Toxicol 1990;10:275–9.
77. Paulova J, Dvorak M, Kolouch F, et al. Evaluation of the hepatoprotective and therapeutic effects of silymarin in liver damage experimentally produced with carbon tetrachloride in dogs. Vet Med (Praha) 1990;35:629–35.
78. Boigk G, Stroedter L, Herbst H, et al. Silymarin retards collagen accumulation in early and advanced biliary fibrosis secondary to complete bile duct obliteration in rats. Hepatology 1997;26:643–9.
79. Lieber CS, Leo MA, Cao Q, et al. Silymarin retards the progression of alcohol-induced hepatic fibrosis in baboons. J Clin Gastroenterol 2003;37:336–9.
80. Sonnenbitchler J, Goldberg M, Hane L, et al. Stimulatory effect of silybin on the DNA synthesis in partially hepatectomized rat livers: nonresponse in hepatomo and other malignant cell lines. Biochem Pharmacol 1986;20:888–93.
81. Silymarin as therapy of liver disease. Presented at a workshop sponsored by the National institute of Diabetes and Digestive and Kidney Diseases (NIDDK), National Center for Complementary and Alternative Medicine (NCCAM), and National Institute on Alcohol Abuse and Alcoholism (NIAAA). Bethesda (MD). Available at: http://

www2.niddk.nih.gov/NR/rdonlyres/0AECDEC8-10B4-47A1-A7BA0939D1050E53/
0/DDICC_March_22_2004_workshop_summary.pdf. Accessed March 22, 2004.

82. Vogel G, Tuchweber B, Trost W, et al. Protection by silibinin against *Amanita phalloides* intoxication in beagles. Toxicol Appl Pharmacol 1984;73:355–62.

83. Filburn CR, Kettenacker R, Griffin DW. Bioavailability of a silybin-phosphatidylcholine complex in dogs. J Vet Pharmacol Ther 2007;30:132–8.

84. Kidd P, Head K. A review of the bioavailability and clinical efficacy of milk thistle phytosome: a silybin-phosphatidylcholine complex (Siliphos). Altern Med Rev 2005;10:193–203.

85. Morazzoni P, Montalbetti A, Malandrino S. Comparative pharmacokinetics of silipide and silymarin in rats. Eur J Drug Metab Pharmacokinet 1993;18:289–97.

86. Webb CB, Samber BJ, Gustafson D, et al. Bioavailability following oral administration of a silibinin-phosphatidylcholine complex in cats. J Vet Intern Med 2008;22:812A.

87. Webb CB, McCord KW, Twedt DC. Oxidative stress and neutrophil function following oral supplementation of a silibinin-phosphatidylcholine complex in cats. J Vet Intern Med 2008;22:808A.

88. Soden JS, Devereaux MW, Haas JE, et al. Subcutaneous vitamin E ameliorates liver injury in an in vivo model of steatocholestasis. Hepatology 2007;46:485–95.

89. Parola M, Leonarduzzi G, Biasi F, et al. Vitamin E dietary supplementation protects against carbon tetrachloride-induced chronic liver damage and cirrhosis. Hepatology 1995;22:1474–81.

90. Harrison SA, Torgerson S, Hayashi P, et al. Vitamin E and vitamin C treatment improves fibrosis in patients with nonalcoholic steatohepatitis. Am J Gastroenterol 2003;98:2485–90.

91. Vajro P, Mandato C, Franzese A, et al. Vitamin E treatment in pediatric obesity-related liver disease: a randomized study. J Pediatr Gastroenterol Nutr 2004;38:48–55.

92. Dufour JF, Oneta CM, Gonvers JJ, et al. Randomized placebo-controlled trial of ursodeoxycholic acid with vitamin E in nonalcoholic steatohepatitis. Clin Gastroenterol Hepatol 2006;4:1537–43.

93. Look MP, Gerard A, Rao GS, et al. Interferon/antioxidant combination therapy for chronic hepatitis C: a controlled pilot trial. Antiviral Res 1999;43:113–22.

94. Twedt DC, Webb CB, Tetrick MA. The effect of dietary vitamin E on the clinical laboratory and oxidant status of dogs with chronic hepatitis. J Vet Intern Med 2003;17:418A.

Index

Note: Page numbers of article titles are in **boldface** type.

A

Abdominal ultrasound, in portosystemic vascular anomalies evaluation, 527

Abscess(es), hepatic, in dogs and cats, WSAVA classification of, 413

N-Acetylcysteine, for hepatobiliary disease in dogs and cats, 645–646

Acute hepatocellular necrosis and inflammation, infectious causes of, in dogs and cats, WSAVA classification of, 408–410

Adenoma(s)
    cholangiocellular, in dogs and cats, WSAVA classification of, 414
    hepatocellular, in dogs and cats, WSAVA classification of, 414

S-Adenosylmethionine, for hepatobiliary disease in dogs and cats, 640–645

Adenovirus, acute hepatocellular necrosis and inflammation in dogs and cats due to, WSAVA classification of, 408

Age, as factor in hepatobiliary neoplasia in dogs and cats, 623

Agenesis, gallbladder, 567

Alopecia, hepatobiliary neoplasia and, in dogs and cats, 624–625

Ammonia metabolism, in hepatic encephalopathy, 429–431

Amyloidosis, in dogs and cats, morphologic classification of, of WSAVA, 405–406

Anemia, Heinz body, hepatic lipidosis management in cats and, 620

Angiography
    CT, in portosystemic vascular anomalies evaluation, 527–528
    MR, in portosystemic vascular anomalies evaluation, 528

Antiemetic(s), in hepatic lipidosis management in cats, 618

Apoptosis, in dogs and cats, WSAVA classification of, 406–408

Appetite stimulants, in hepatic lipidosis management in cats, 619

Arteriovenous malformations, hepatic, treatment of, surgical, 535

Ascites, liver disease and, 426–427

Atresia, biliary, 567

B

Bacterial diseases, acute hepatocellular necrosis and inflammation in dogs and cats due to, WSAVA classification of, 408

Bedlington terrier, copper accumulation secondary to cholestasis in, 496

Benign ciliary cysts, 574

Bile, pathologic changes in, 554–555

Bile acid deconjugation, 554–555

Bile duct(s), disorders of, 574–587
    benign ciliary cysts, 574
    biliary cystadenoma, 577
    biliary decompression, 582–584
    choledochal cyst, 577
    cholelithiasis, 584–587

Vet Clin Small Anim 39 (2009) 653–666
doi:10.1016/S0195-5616(09)00051-5
0195-5616/09/$ – see front matter © 2009 Elsevier Inc. All rights reserved.

vetsmall.theclinics.com